Iodine Intake: Essential Element for Health and Wellness

Iodine Intake: Essential Element for Health and Wellness

Editor: Chester Cooke

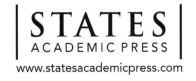

STATES
ACADEMIC PRESS

www.statesacademicpress.com

States Academic Press,
109 South 5th Street,
Brooklyn, NY 11249, USA

Visit us on the World Wide Web at:
www.statesacademicpress.com

ISBN 978-1-63989-784-1 (Hardback)

Cataloging-in-Publication Data

Iodine intake : essential element for health and wellness / edited by Chester Cooke.
   p. cm.
Includes bibliographical references and index.
ISBN 978-1-63989-784-1
1. Iodine in the body. 2. Iodine--Physiological effect. 3. Iodine--Therapeutic use.
4. Iodine--Health aspects. 5. Iodine--Toxicology. 6. Body composition. 7. Health.
I. Cooke, Chester.
QP535.I1 I53 2023
612.392 4--dc23

Contents

Preface...VII

Chapter 1   **Vegans, Vegetarians and Omnivores: How Does Dietary Choice Influence Iodine Intake?**...1
Elizabeth R. Eveleigh, Lisa J. Coneyworth, Amanda Avery and Simon J. M. Welham

Chapter 2   **Iodine Intake in Norwegian Women and Men: The Population-Based Tromsø Study 2015–2016**...21
Ahmed A Madar, Espen Heen, Laila A Hopstock, Monica H Carlsen and Haakon E Meyer

Chapter 3   **Low-Salt Intake Suggestions in Hypertensive Patients do not Jeopardize Urinary Iodine Excretion**...34
Natale Musso, Lucia Conte, Beatrice Carloni, Claudia Campana, Maria C. Chiusano and Massimo Giusti

Chapter 4   **Iodine Status Assessment in South African Adults According to Spot Urinary Iodine Concentrations, Prediction Equations and Measured 24-h Iodine Excretion**...........................42
Karen E. Charlton, Lisa J. Ware, Jeannine Baumgartner, Marike Cockeran, Aletta E. Schutte, Nirmala Naidoo and Paul Kowal

Chapter 5   **Iodine and Pregnancy — A Qualitative Study Focusing on Dietary Guidance and Information**...56
Maria Bouga, Michael E. J. Lean and Emilie Combet

Chapter 6   **Iodine Status in Schoolchildren and Pregnant Women of Lazio, a Central Region of Italy**...75
Enke Baldini, Camilla Virili, Eleonora D'Armiento, Marco Centanni and Salvatore Ulisse

Chapter 7   **Interference on Iodine Uptake and Human Thyroid Function by Perchlorate-Contaminated Water and Food**..82
Giuseppe Lisco, Anna De Tullio, Vito Angelo Giagulli, Giovanni De Pergola and Vincenzo Triggiani

Chapter 8   **Stable Iodine Nutrition During Two Decades of Continuous Universal Salt Iodisation in Sri Lanka**...99
Renuka Jayatissa, Jonathan Gorstein, Onyebuchi E. Okosieme, John H. Lazarus and Lakdasa D. Premawardhana

Chapter 9   **Nutraceuticals in Thyroidology: A Review of in Vitro and in Vivo Animal Studies**..108
Salvatore Benvenga, Silvia Martina Ferrari, Giusy Elia, Francesca Ragusa, Armando Patrizio, Sabrina Rosaria Paparo, Stefania Camastra, Daniela Bonofiglio, Alessandro Antonelli and Poupak Fallahi

Chapter 10   **Dietary Relationship with 24 h Urinary Iodine Concentrations of Young Adults in the Mountain West Region of the United States**.................................130
Demetre E. Gostas, D. Enette Larson-Meyer, Hillary A. Yoder,
Ainsley E. Huffman and Evan C. Johnson

Chapter 11   **The Joint Role of Thyroid Function and Iodine Status on Risk of Preterm Birth and Small for Gestational Age: A Population-Based Nested Case-Control Study of Finnish Women**.................................147
Alexandra C. Purdue-Smithe, Tuija Männistö, Griffith A. Bell, Sunni L. Mumford,
Aiyi Liu, Kurunthachalam Kannan, Un-Jung Kim, Eila Suvanto, Heljä-Marja Surcel,
Mika Gissler and James L. Mills

Chapter 12   **Nutraceutical Supplements in the Thyroid Setting: Health Benefits beyond Basic Nutrition**.................................158
Salvatore Benvenga, Ulla Feldt-Rasmussen, Daniela Bonofiglio and Ernest Asamoah

Chapter 13   **Endemic Goiter and Iodine Prophylaxis in Calabria, a Region of Southern Italy: Past and Present**.................................177
Cinzia Giordano, Ines Barone, Stefania Marsico, Rosalinda Bruno,
Daniela Bonofiglio, Stefania Catalano and Sebastiano Andò

Chapter 14   **Sodium, Potassium and Iodine Intake, in a National Adult Population Sample of the Republic of Moldova**.................................186
Lanfranco D'Elia, Galina Obreja, Angela Ciobanu, Joao Breda, Jo Jewell
and Francesco P. Cappuccio

Chapter 15   **Association between Iodine Nutrition Status and Thyroid Disease-Related Hormone in Korean Adults: Korean National Health and Nutrition Examination Survey VI (2013–2015)**.................................199
Sohye Kim, Yong Seok Kwon, Ju Young Kim, Kyung Hee Hong and
Yoo Kyoung Park

Chapter 16   **Protective Effects of Myo-Inositol and Selenium on Cadmium-Induced Thyroid Toxicity in Mice**.................................214
Salvatore Benvenga, Herbert R. Marini, Antonio Micali, Jose Freni, Giovanni Pallio,
Natasha Irrera, Francesco Squadrito, Domenica Altavilla, Alessandro Antonelli,
Silvia Martina Ferrari, Poupak Fallahi, Domenico Puzzolo and Letteria Minutoli

Chapter 17   **Breast Milk Iodine Concentration is Associated with Infant Growth, Independent of Maternal Weight**.................................229
Lindsay Ellsworth, Harlan McCaffery, Emma Harman, Jillian Abbott and
Brigid Gregg

Permissions

List of Contributors

Index

Preface

Iodine is a mineral found naturally in certain foods. It is a significant component of triiodothyronine and thyroxine, which are known as thyroid hormones. These hormones regulate various significant biochemical reactions, comprising enzymatic activity and protein synthesis, which are important determining factors of metabolic activity. Iodine is a significant component in the development of fetus and infant, production of thyroid hormone, and holds critical nutritional value at all the stages of human life. Lack of iodine rich diet can lead to developmental and functional abnormalities. Severe iodine deficiency can result in preterm delivery, low birth weight, early abortion, hypothyroidism, mental retardation and neuro-cognitive impairment. Iodine is majorly found in sea foods, animal proteins and to certain extent in foods like milk, cereals and bread. This book provides comprehensive insights on iodine and its intake. The readers would gain knowledge that would broaden their perspective regarding this mineral and its health effects.

The information contained in this book is the result of intensive hard work done by researchers in this field. All due efforts have been made to make this book serve as a complete guiding source for students and researchers. The topics in this book have been comprehensively explained to help readers understand the growing trends in the field.

I would like to thank the entire group of writers who made sincere efforts in this book and my family who supported me in my efforts of working on this book. I take this opportunity to thank all those who have been a guiding force throughout my life.

Editor

Vegans, Vegetarians and Omnivores: How Does Dietary Choice Influence Iodine Intake?

Elizabeth R. Eveleigh, Lisa J. Coneyworth, Amanda Avery and Simon J. M. Welham *

Division of Food, Nutrition & Dietetics, School of Biosciences, The University of Nottingham, Sutton Bonington LE12 5RD, UK; elizabeth.eveleigh@nottingham.ac.uk (E.R.E.); lisa.coneyworth@nottingham.ac.uk (L.J.C.); amanda.avery@nottingham.ac.uk (A.A.)

* Correspondence: simon.welham@nottingham.ac.uk

Abstract: Vegan and vegetarian diets are becoming increasingly popular. Dietary restrictions may increase the risk of iodine deficiency. This systematic review aims to assess iodine intake and status in adults following a vegan or vegetarian diet in industrialised countries. A systematic review and quality assessment were conducted in the period May 2019–April 2020 according to Preferred Reporting Items for Systematic Reviews and Meta-Analyses (PRISMA) guidelines. Studies were identified in Ovid MEDLINE, Embase, Web of Science, PubMed, Scopus, and secondary sources. Fifteen articles met inclusion criteria. Participants included 127,094 adults (aged ≥ 18 years). Vegan groups presented the lowest median urinary iodine concentrations, followed by vegetarians, and did not achieve optimal status. The highest iodine intakes were recorded in female vegans (1448.0 ± 3879.0 µg day^{-1}) and the lowest in vegetarians (15.6 ± 21.0 µg day^{-1}). Omnivores recorded the greatest intake in 83% of studies. Seaweed contributed largely to diets of vegans with excessive iodine intake. Vegans appear to have increased risk of low iodine status, deficiency and inadequate intake compared with adults following less restrictive diets. Adults following vegan and vegetarian diets living in countries with a high prevalence of deficiency may be more vulnerable. Therefore, further monitoring of iodine status in industrialised countries and research into improving the iodine intake and status of adults following vegan and vegetarian diets is required.

Keywords: iodine status; iodine intake; iodine deficiency; vegan; vegetarian

1. Introduction

Vegan and vegetarian diets have gained popularity over the past decade. Characteristically, vegans do not consume any animal-derived products including eggs, dairy, meat, and fish. Vegetarians exclude meat and fish but may consume milk and eggs. A subclass of the vegetarian diet may consume fish but not meat, termed pescatarians. Despite these definitions, varying levels of strictness and adherence to dietary restriction exist at the level of the individual [1].

The prevalence of vegetarian and vegan diets differs globally. In developing regions, meat-free diets are traditionally adopted owing to religious, social, ecological, or economic constraints as opposed to personal choice [2]. In industrialised countries, most individuals are afforded the choice of food consumption and level of dietary restriction. Populations in developed countries may adopt these diets for environmental, ethical, religious, health beliefs or social reasons. Presently, well-planned vegan and vegetarian diets have been regarded by the British Dietetic Association and other organizations in industrialised countries to be suitable throughout the lifespan, inclusive of infancy and pregnancy [3–5]. However, concerns have been raised regarding the ability of these diets to adequately provide essential micronutrients, such as iodine [6].

Iodine is an essential micronutrient, required in trace quantities, which is vital for the synthesis of thyroid hormones—triiodothyronine (T3) and thyroxine (T4) [7]. The thyroid hormones are crucial for the regulation of metabolism, growth, and neurological development [8]. Iodine deficiency presents as a spectrum of clinical disorders termed 'iodine deficiency disorders' (IDD's) which occur when recommended intakes are not achieved (150 µg day^{-1}) [8]. These include hypothyroidism, goitre abnormal thyroid nodular pathology, and cretininism in infants born to mothers with a low iodine status during pregnancy and lactation [7,9]. Low iodine intake may be a risk factor for thyroid nodule formation, particularly in females [10,11]. Most nodules are harmless; however, some may result in thyroid dysfunction or malignancy [11]. Excessive iodine intake (>1000 µg day^{-1}) may lead to hyperthyroidism in individuals with preexisting thyroid disease or iodine deficiency [12]. Iodine deficiency is not limited to developing countries—mild–moderate deficiency exists in industrialised nations including Europe, UK, Australia and select populations in the USA [9]. In 2011, iodine nutrition was highlighted as a significant public health concern following estimates indicating that 2 billion people globally were deficient [13]. Recent data collected by the WHO show a global decline in iodine deficiency between 1993 and 2019, suggesting that less than 8.5% of the world's population are affected [14]. However, subgroups of European populations are still at increased risk of iodine deficiency [6].

Iodine deficiency traditionally was assessed by monitoring the prevalence of visible goitre in populations [7]. After the development of newer methods for measuring iodine status, it was recognized that low-level deficiency may be present in industrialised populations not displaying obvious thyroid enlargement [15]. Various biomarkers can be used to estimate population iodine status and intake [15]. Urinary iodine concentration (UIC) is the most common and practical marker [16]. This is because >90% of the iodine ingested from dietary sources is readily excreted in the urine [17]. Spot UIC and 24 h measures can be used to detect and monitor iodine adequacy and deficiency. However, these estimates only correspond to recent intake [16]. Additionally, thyroid function tests are required routinely to detect iodine adequacy in vulnerable populations such as pregnant and/or lactating women and infants [16]. Dietary iodine can be estimated indirectly by UIC or by common dietary assessment methods [15]. Limitations of the methods used must be considered. Biomarkers of status and dietary intake methods are not always the same between studies which adds to the challenge of reliably comparing iodine amid populations [18].

Individuals residing in developing countries, who are reliant on plant-based foods in their diet, have a higher prevalence of iodine deficiency [19]. The bioavailability of iodine from plant sources has been suggested to be determined by rainfall and water collection on crop leaves with much of the iodine within plants not being bioavailable [20]. In industrialised countries where people consume a 'Western diet', the key dietary sources of iodine are bread fortified by iodised salt, cow's milk, and dairy products [21]. Seafood, eggs, and seaweed are also iodine rich but are not regularly consumed [22]. Water and salt iodination strategies are present in most states in the US and select countries in Europe [23,24]. Countries such as the UK have yet to establish a mandatory salt fortification program and despite regular manufacturing of iodised salt, it is not widely available for public purchase [25].

For this reason, individuals who consume diets excluding iodine-rich food, principally dairy, eggs, and/or fish, have increased risk of iodine deficiency [26]. Further complicating this issue is the growing availability and acceptance of plant-based food 'alternatives', regularly consumed by vegans and vegetarians, that naturally have negligible iodine content and are not regularly fortified [27,28]. The size of the plant-based 'alternatives' food market has been reported to have almost doubled between 2014 and 2017 in the UK [29].

Currently, two reviews exist investigating iodine in the diets of vegans and vegetarians, one in 2005, which was updated in 2009 by the same authors [30,31]. The most recent review included eight studies, covering a period between 1981 and 2003, with the conclusion that strict vegans and vegetarians living in Europe have iodine values below recommended levels and are at risk of deficiency. In the years since publication, these diets have become more widely accepted and it is likely that food consumption practices have changed considerably since this last assessment of iodine intake in adults following vegan and vegetarian diets. Given the potential health consequences of iodine deficiency, it is important to re-examine whether adults following either a vegan or vegetarian diet are still at risk of iodine deficiency.

Thus, the aim of this review is to assess the iodine intake and status in adults following a vegan or vegetarian diet in industrialised countries across time. The objectives included (1) evaluation of the methods used to assess iodine; (2) determination of the iodine intake and food consumption in vegan and vegetarian adults; (3) assessment of the iodine status and prevalence of iodine deficiency using urinary iodine concentration (UIC); (4) comparison of the iodine intake, status and prevalence of deficiency between vegans, vegetarians and omnivores; and (5) consideration of gender differences in estimates of iodine nutrition.

2. Materials and Methods

This systematic review was according to the Preferred Reporting Items for Systematic Reviews and Meta-Analyses (PRISMA) checklist [32].

A systematic search of literature was performed from 20 May 2019 to April 2020. Electronic databases (Ovid MEDLINE, Embase, Web of Science, PubMed, and Scopus) were searched using text terms with appropriate truncation, and Medical Subject Headings. Search term sensitivity and relevance of article identification was tested using preliminary searches in Ovid MEDLINE (Supplementary Table S1). All database searches were refined by 'Humans, Adults (aged < 18 years) and English Language'. Identified relevant studies were saved onto EndNoteTM online and duplicates were removed. To limit bias, relevance was confirmed by two investigators. Additional relevant articles were sourced from reference lists of included studies.

The current systematic review addressed study eligibility using the population–intervention–comparison–outcome (PICOS) formulation (Table 1) [33]. Additionally, only articles with full paper availability published in/after 1990 were considered for inclusion.

Table 1. Population–intervention–comparison–outcome (PICOS) criteria for study inclusion and exclusion.

Criteria Category	Inclusion	Exclusion
Population	Adults (aged ≥ 18 y) residing in industrialised nations.	Individuals (aged < 18 y), unless results display separate data; adults residing in developing countries; populations with a high prevalence of thyroid disorders.
Intervention/exposure	Participants with any type of dietary preference or restriction. Voluntary or otherwise.	Use of a dietary grouping without defining diet characteristics.
Comparators	Differing dietary preference or restriction.	None.
Outcome measure	Iodine intake or status measured by UIC or analysis of dietary records.	No analysis of iodine intake or status; use of thyroid measures alone for iodine intake and status.
Study design	Any study design with relevant outcomes.	None.

Data extraction was completed independently. The terms used for data extraction were discussed and finalised by two secondary researchers. A modified version of "Data collection form for intervention review—RCTs and non-RCTs" by The Cochrane Collaboration was used for data extraction [34]. Adaptions considered the characteristics of interest and study design. To permit comparison between groups, 'moderate vegans' were considered as vegetarians. 'Mixed diet' and 'meat eaters' as omnivores and 'living food dieters' as vegans. Due to variation in nomenclature, demi vegetarians will be considered separately. To make comparisons between genders, where possible, data on males and females were extracted separately.

Following data extraction, study quality was critically appraised by one author. Quality was assessed using the National Heart, Lung, and Blood Institute (NHLBI) Quality Assessment Tool for Observational Cohort and Cross-Sectional Studies [35].

According to Guidance for Assessing the Quality of Observational Cohort and Cross-Sectional Studies provided by NHLBI, fixed response was selected for three questions to account for the nature of cross-sectional studies. Exposures and outcomes are measured and assessed during the same timeframe excluding time to see an effect and often lack a follow up, hence questions 6 and 7 would automatically receive a "NO" response. Additionally, question 13 was given a fixed response of "NA"

Assessment of Controlled Intervention Studies, and Matched-Pairs (Case-Control) by The Quality Assessment of Case-Control Studies NHLBI [35]. Assessment was completed by one author and reviewed by another independent assessor prior to agreement (Table 2).

Table 2. NHLBI tool for quality assessment of included studies.

Study, Year	1	2	3	4	5	6	7	8	9	10	11	12	13	14	Rating
Observational Cohort Cross-Sectional Studies															
Alles, 2017 [36]	+	+	+	+	−	−	−	−	+	+	+	−	a	+	Fair
Draper, 1993 [37]	+	−	r	+	−	−	−	+	+	+	+	−	a	−	Fair
Henjum, 2018 [38]	+	+	r	+	−	−	−	+	+	+	+	−	a	+	Good
Krajcovicová-Kudláčková, 2003 [39]	+	−	r	+	−	−	−	+	+	+	+	−	a	−	Fair
Leung, 2011 [40]	+	−	r	+	−	−	−	+	+	+	+	−	a	+	Good
Lightowler, 1998 [41]	+	+	+	+	−	−	−	+	+	+	+	−	a	+	Fair
Lightowler, 2002 [42]	+	+	+	+	−	−	−	−	+	+	+	−	a	+	Good
Nebl, 2019 [43]	+	+	+	+	−	−	−	−	+	+	+	r	a	−	Good
Schüpbach, 2017 [44]	+	−	+	+	−	−	−	+	+	+	+	−	a	+	Good
Sobiecki, 2016 [45]	+	+	+	+	+	−	−	+	+	+	+	−	a	+	Good
Waldmann, 2003 [46]	+	−	+	+	−	−	−	+	+	+	+	−	a	+	Good
Controlled Intervention Studies															
Remer, 1999 [47]	−	?	−	−	−	+	+	+	+	+	+	+	+	+	Good
Case-Control Studies															
Elorinne, 2016 [48]	+	−	+	+	r	+	?	?	−	+	−	+	a	a	Fair
Kristensen, 2015 [49]	+	+	−	−	+	+	?	?	−	+	−	+	a	a	Fair
Rauma, 1994 [50]	+	−	−	+	−	+	?	?	−	+	−	−	a	a	Poor

⊕ +, yes; ● −, no; ⊘ ?, cannot determine; ◐ a, not applicable; ◑ r, not reported; O (outlined), fixed answers according to NHLBI recommendations.

The WHO criteria for assessing the severity of IDD (1994) stratified by median urinary iodine concentration (UIC) was used to assess the relative level of deficiency in each dietary group. According to this classification, the rate of deficiency is described as the percentage of individuals in each group with UIC below <100 or <50 $\mu g\ L^{-1}$, in severe deficiency [6].

Funnel plots were generated for both UIC and dietary iodine intake data. For urinary iodine status, summary values and *number of participants* for each dietary group (Table 3) were used to generate an overall *population mean* value (μ).

$$\text{Population mean } (\mu) = \frac{\sum \text{UIC } values}{total\ number\ of\ participants}$$

Table 3. Iodine status and deficiency in vegans, vegetarians, and omnivores in industrialised countries.

Study, Year	Assessment Method	Dietary Group (n) (Male, Female)	Iodine Status by UIC (µg day⁻¹)	Criteria for Iodine Deficiency Disorders
Elorinne, 2016 [48]	Spot UIC Sandell–Kolthoff method.	Vegan (21) / Omnivore (18)	15.0 (4.6, 21.8) [1,**] / 37.4 (17.7, 86.5) [1]	Severe / Moderate
Henjum, 2018 [38]	Spot UIC.	Vegan (9) / Vegetarian (27)	38.0 [1,**] / [1]	Moderate / Mild
Krajcovicová-Kudláčková, 2003 [39]	24 h UIC Sandell–Kolthoff method.	Vegan (15) (6,9) / Vegetarian (31) (12,19) / Omnivore (Mixed Diet) (35) (15,20)	71.0 (9.0–204.0) [2,**] / 177.0 (44.0–273.0) [2,**] / 210.0 (76.0–423.0) [2]	Mild / Optimal / Optimal with risk of health consequences
Leung, 2011 [40]	Spot UIC spectrophotometry.	Vegan (62) (19,43) / Vegetarian (78) (26,52)	78.5 (6.8–964.7) [2,*] / 147.0 (9.3–778.6) [2]	Mild / Optimal
Lightowler, 1998 [41]	Four 24 h UIC Sandell–Kolthoff method reaction.	Vegan (30) (11,19)	Total, 20.2 [1], M, 16.8 [1], F, 20.5 [1]	Severe-Moderate
Rauma, 1994 [50]	24 h UIC.	Vegan (Living Food Diet) (10) / Omnivore (12)	<450.0 (<200.0–1700.0) [2] / <500.0 (300.0–1200.0) [2]	Optimal with risk of health consequences
Remer, 1999 [47]	Two 24 h UIC.	Vegetarian (6) (3,3) / Omnivore (6) (3,3) / Omnivore (High Protein) (6) (3,3)	36.6 ± 8.8 [3,*] / 50.2 ± 14.0 [3] / 61.0 ± 8 [3]	Moderate / Mild / Mild
Schüpbach, 2017 [44]	Four fasted spot UIC.	Vegan (53) (20,33) / Vegetarian (53) (17,36) / Omnivore (100) (37,63)	56.0 (27.0–586.0) [2,*] / 75.0 (1.0–610.0) [2] / 83.0 (22.0–228.0) [2]	Mild / Mild / Mild

M, male; F, female; [1], median (25th–75th percentile); [2], median (range); [3], mean ± SD; * significantly different between dietary group comparison; $p < 0.05$, ** $p < 0.001$; criteria for iodine deficiency disorders (WHO); severe < 20 µg day⁻¹, moderate 20–49 µg day⁻¹, mild 50–99 µg day⁻¹, adequate 100–199 µg day⁻¹, excessive risk of adverse health consequences ≥ 300 µg day⁻¹.

The standard error for each observation group was generated according to the equation:

$$ SE = SQRT\left(SQRT\left(\mu \times \frac{1 - \mu}{number\ of\ subjects} \right)^2 \right) $$

Confidence limits were generated as indicated below.

$$ 95\%\ CI = \mu \pm (1.96 \times SE) $$
$$ 99.7\%\ CI = \mu \pm (3 \times SE) $$

Confidence limits were generated for each population studied and used to generate funnel plots of UIC or iodine intake shown against study size (Supplementary Figures S1 and S2).

3. Results

The following exclusion of studies qualitative synthesis was completed for fifteen studies. The technique of study selection along with the number of included and excluded studies recorded for this systematic review is shown in the PRISMA 2009 flow diagram (Figure 1) [32].

Fifteen relevant studies were identified examining the iodine intake or status by dietary group Table 4. Consistent with scientific literature, different descriptors and nomenclature were used to define vegetarian diet types (Supplementary Table S3). Three studies used objective assessments to group individuals [43,45,46].

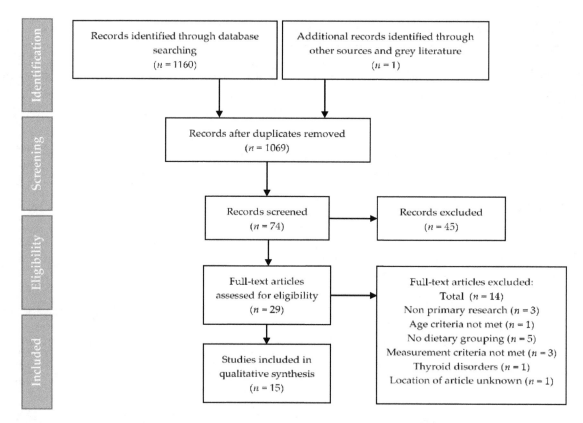

Figure 1. Preferred Reporting Items for Systematic Reviews and Meta-Analyses (PRISMA) flow diagram for included studies.

3.1. Urinary Iodine Status

Eight studies investigated iodine status by urinary iodine concentration (UIC) (Table 3; Figure 2). Four studies measured UIC using spot samples [38,40,44,48]—of which, one study collected multiple fasted samples to determine average values [44].

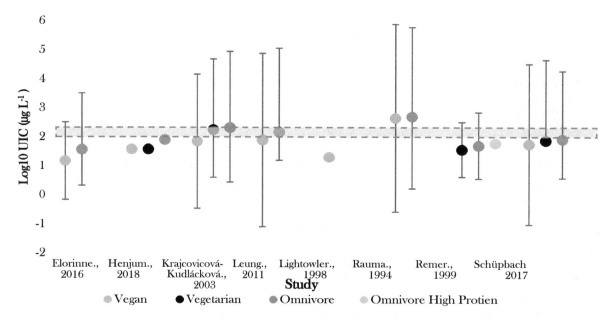

Figure 2. Visual representation of iodine status by median urinary iodine concentration (UIC) for included studies. The shaded grey bar represents the optimal range for iodine status (100–299 µg L^{-1}). Significance values are not presented within this figure. See Table 3.

Table 4. Studies investigating iodine among vegans, vegetarians, and omnivores in industrialised countries.

Study, Year	Study Design	Location	Dietary Groups	Sample (n) (Male, Female)	Method of Dietary Classification	Average Diet Adherence (Years)
Alles, 2017 [36]	Cross-Sectional	France	Vegan	789	Assessed by investigators pre-study	NA
			Vegetarian	2370		
			Omnivore	90,664		
Draper, 1993 [37]	Cross-sectional	London, UK	Vegan	38 (18,20)	Self-reported	1.0
			Lacto-Vegetarian	52 (16,36)		2.0
			Demi-vegetarian	37 (13,24)		5.0–9.0
Elorinne, 2016 [48]	Matched pairs by age and sex	Kuopio, Finland	Vegan	22 (16,6)	Self-reported	8.6
			Omnivore	19 (11,8)		NA
Henjum, 2018 [38]	Cross-Sectional	Norway, eastern and western geographical regions	Vegan	27	Self-reported	NA
			Vegetarian	9		
			Omnivore	367		
Kristensen, 2015 [49]	Matched pairs by age	Denmark	Vegan	75 (36,39)	Self-reported	≤1.0
			Omnivore	1627 (716, 911)		NA
Krajcovicová-Kudláčková, 2003 [39]	Cross-sectional	Slovakia	Vegan	15 (6,9)	Self-reported	9.7
			Vegetarian	31 (12,19)		9.0
			Omnivore (Mixed Diet)	35 (15,20)		NA
Leung, 2011 [40]	Cross-sectional	Boston, Massachusetts	Vegan	63	Self-reported	11.3 ± 11.7 [1]
			Vegetarian	78		5.6 ± 5.7 [1]
Lightowler, 1998 [41]	Cross-sectional	London and surrounding counties, UK	Vegan	30 (11,19)	Self-reported	M, 10.0, F, 9.2
Lightowler, 2002 [42]	Cross-sectional	London and the south-east of England, UK	Vegan	26 (11, 15)	Self-reported	M, 9.9, F, 11.7
Nebl, 2019 [43]	Cross-sectional	Hanover, Germany	Vegan	27 (11,16)	Assessed by investigators pre-study	>2.0
			Vegetarian	25 (10, 15)		>2.0
			Omnivore	27 (10,17)		>3.0
Rauma, 1994 [50]	Matched pairs	Kuopio, Finland.	Vegan (Living Food Diet)	12	Self-reported	6.7 ± 3.8 [1]
			Omnivore	12		NA
Remer, 1999 [47]	Repeated-measures	Germany	Vegetarian (Lacto)	6 (3,3)	Allocated by investigators	0.0
			Omnivore	6 (3,3)		
			Omnivore (High protein)	6 (3,3)		
Schüpbach, 2017 [44]	Cross-sectional	Lausanne and Zurich, Switzerland	Vegan	53 (20,33)	Self-reported	≤1.0
			Vegetarian	53 (17,36)		≤1.0
			Omnivore	100 (37,63)		≤1.0
Sobiecki, 2016 [45]	Cross-sectional	Oxford, UK	Vegan	803	Assessed by investigators pre-study	≤1.0
			Vegetarian	6673		≤1.0
			Pescatarian	4531		≤1.0
			Omnivore (Meat-eaters)	18,244		≤1.0
Waldmann, 2003 [46]	Cross-sectional	Hanover, Germany	Vegan (Strict)	98	Assessed by investigators pre-study	4.3
			Vegan (Moderate)	56		3.4

NA, not assessed; M, male; F, female; [1], mean ± SD.

The lowest median UIC (16.8 μg L^{-1}) was recorded by Lightowler in UK male adults following vegan diets [41]. Rauma [50] reported the highest median UIC (<500.0 μg L^{-1}) in Finish omnivores. Large variation in UIC existed in several studies [40,44,50], with one study showing variation in those following vegan diets between <200 and 1700 μg L^{-1} [50]. The majority (75%) of the recorded values for UIC fell below the expected population mean of 95.6 μg L^{-1} (Supplementary Figure S1) and half of the values fell either on or outside of the 99.7% confidence limit.

In all studies giving intergroup comparisons, the lowest median UIC was recorded for those following vegan diets and the highest for omnivores [38–40,44,47,48,50]. Five out of eight studies recorded median UIC in vegans to be significantly lower than omnivores ($p < 0.005$) [38–40,44,47]. All studies observed UIC in those following vegetarian diets to be higher than vegan diets, yet lower than omnivorous diets [38–40,44,47]. The difference between vegetarian and omnivorous diets was significant in three studies ($p < 0.05$) [38,39,47].

IDD assessment according to the WHO criteria ranged from severe (inadequate) to at 'risk' of adverse health consequences (excess) across studies [51]. Supplementary Table S4 presents national data corresponding to countries of included studies.

Optimal status (100–200 μg L^{-1}) was achieved in vegetarian groups in Slovakia and Boston [39,40]. No adults following vegan diet had median UIC within the optimal range [38–41,44,48,50]. Seven studies observed one or more dietary group below the cut off for optimal population UIC [38–40,42,44,47,48]. Iodine deficiency (mild–severe) (50–99 μg L^{-1}–>20 μg L^{-1}) was recorded in adults following vegan diets in six studies [38–40,42,44,48], vegetarian diets in two studies [44,47], and omnivorous diets in four studies [38,44,47,48].

Those following vegan diets were most frequently seen to exhibit either mild (50–99 μg L^{-1}) or moderate deficiency (20–49 μg L^{-1}) [12,38,39,41,44,48], and in two studies were found to be severely deficient (<20 μg L^{-1}) [40,47]. In one of these studies, >75% of those following vegan diets fell into the severely deficient category [48]. Both those following vegan and vegetarian diets were more commonly observed to be moderately deficient, whilst, conversely, omnivores were found in two studies to exhibit excessive iodine status [39,50]. This was also noted for those following vegan diets in one Finnish study [50].

3.2. Dietary Iodine Intake

Methods for assessing dietary intake are listed in Supplementary Table S5. Ten studies reported estimates for daily iodine intake [36,37,41–43,45–47,49,50]—of which, four studies were investigating iodine specifically [41,42,47,50]. The additional studies investigated other macro- and micronutrient intakes besides iodine (Table 5; Figure 3) [36,37,43,45,46,49].

Table 5. Assessment of dietary iodine intake for vegans, vegetarians, and omnivores in industrialised countries.

Study, Year	Assessment of Dietary Iodine	Criteria for Iodine Intake Used in Study	Dietary Group (N) (Male, Female)	Dietary Iodine Intake (μG Day^{-1})	Contribution of Iodised Salt, Seaweed, and Iodine-Containing Supplements	Meeting Criteria (Y/N)
Allès, 2017 [36]	Three repeated 24 h dietary records.	150 μg day^{-1} RDI for the French population (2001) [52].	Vegan (789) Vegetarian (2370) Omnivore (90,664)	248.3 ± 9.8 (a) [1]; 222.6 ± 5.7 (a) [1]; 180.1 ± 1.1 (a) [1],**	Seaweed, salt, or supplements not measured.	Y Y Y
Draper, 1993 [37]	Three-day weighted food diaries. Analysed using UK Ministry of Agriculture, Fisheries and Food data.	DRV of 140 μg day^{-1} Department of Health (1991) [53].	Vegan (38) (18,20)	M, 98.0 ± 42.0 [2],**; F, 66.0 ± 22.0 [2],**	95% used sea salt or seaweed. 30%–40% consumed food supplements containing seaweed 1–2 days a month. 15.6 μg day^{-1} provided by dietary supplements.	N
			Lacto-Vegetarian (52) (16,36)	M, 216.0 ± 73.0 [2],**; F, 167.0 ± 59.0 [2],**	No iodine provided by salt, seaweed or supplements.	Y
			Demi-Vegetarian (35) (13,24)	M, 253.0 ± 164.0 [2],**; F, 172.0 ± 91.0 [2],**	No iodine provided by salt, seaweed or supplements.	Y
Kristensen, 2015 [49]	Four-day weighed food diary.	150 μg day^{-1} NNR (2012) [54].	Vegan (70) (33,37)	M, 64.0 (43.0–91.0) [3],**; F, 65.0 (54.0–86.0) [3],**	Salt not measured. Three vegans consumed seaweed. 9.0 μg day^{-1} (M) and 6.0 μg day^{-1} (F) was provided by dietary supplements.	N
			Omnivore (1257) (566,691)	M, 213.0 (180.0–269.0) [3]; F, 178.0 (146.0–215.0) [3]	Salt not measured. No iodine provided by seaweed. 107 μg day^{-1} (M) and 78.9 μg day^{-1} (F) was provided by dietary supplements.	Y
Lightowler, 1998 [41]	Four-day weighed food diary with duplicate portion technique.	140 mg day^{-1} RNI Department of Health (1991) [53].	Vegan (30) (11,19)	M, 138.0 ± 149.0 [2]; F, 187.0 ± 246.0 [2]	Salt not measured. Three vegans consumed seaweed, resulting in significantly higher iodine intake ($p < 0.001$) Seaweed consumers were over six times the RNI. Iodine-containing supplements were consumed by five (45%) males and seven females (37%). Providing 54.0 mg day^{-1} on average to the diet.	M, N F, Y
Lightowler, 2002 [42]	Four-day food diaries with duplicate portion technique. Analysed using CompEat 4 software.	140 mg day^{-1} RNI Department of Health (1991) [53].	Vegan (26) (11,15)	Diet Diary M, 42.0 ± 46.0 [2]; F, 1448.0 ± 3879.0 [2]; Duplicate Diary M, 137.0 ± 147.0 [2]; F, 216.0 ± 386.0 [2]	Salt not measured. Two vegans consumed seaweed, resulting in iodine intake to exceed the RNI. Dietary supplement intake was recorded but not included to dietary intake.	Diet Diary M, N F, Y Duplicate Diary M, N F, Y

Table 5. *Cont.*

Study, Year	Assessment of Dietary Iodine	Criteria for Iodine Intake Used in Study	Dietary Group (N) (Male, Female)	Dietary Iodine Intake (µG Day⁻¹)	Contribution of Iodised Salt, Seaweed, and Iodine-Containing Supplements	Meeting Criteria (Y/N)
Nebl, 2019 [43]	Three-day food diaries analysed by PROD16.4®.	200 µg day⁻¹ RV German, Austrian and Swiss Nutrition Societies (2019) [55]	Vegan (27) (10,17)	57.7 (48.4, 67.0) [4],*	Salt or seaweed not measured. No iodine provided by supplements.	N
			Vegetarian (25) (10,15)	61.6 (49.4, 73.7) [4],*		N
			Omnivore (27) (11,16)	88.8 (64.1, 114.0) [4],**		N
Rauma, 1994 [50]	Seven-day food diaries analysed by NUTRICA Finland.	0.1–0.2 mg day⁻¹ RDA (120–200 µg day⁻¹) Committee on Dietary Allowances, Food and Nutrition Board, National Research Council (1989) [56].	Vegan (Living Food Diet) (9)	29.0 ± 18.0 [2]	One participant did not use iodised salt. 25% of daily iodine in vegans was provided by seaweed (estimated >8.0 µg day⁻¹). Four vegans consumed seaweed, resulting in higher intake.	N
Remer, 1999 [47]	Five-day dietary intervention of pre-selected food items representing each diet. Calculated using food tables.	NA	Omnivore (8)	222.0 ± 93.0 [2]		Y
			Vegetarian (Ovo-Vegetarian)(6)	15.6 ± 21.0 [2]	No iodized salt, seaweed or supplements were permitted during the study. All drinks including water were low in iodine and other minerals.	N
			Omnivore (6)	35.2 ± 15.0 [2]		N
			Omnivore (High Protein) (6)	44.5 ± 16.5 [2]		N
Waldmann, 2003 [46]	Pre-study questionnaire identifying regularly consumed foods. Two estimated nine-day FFQs using 7 days of records.	200 mg day⁻¹ RI, German Society of Nutrition (2000) [57]	Vegan (Strict) (98) (48,50)	M, 87.7 ± 30.6 [2] F, 82.1 ± 34.4 [2]	Salt not measured. Seaweed intake not measured. 46% of participants used some form of nutritional supplement. Iodine-specific supplements were not recorded.	N
			Vegan (Moderate) (56) (19,37)	M, 93.7 ± 27.8 [2] F, 78.1 ± 25.6 [2]		N
Sobiecki, 2016 [45]	112-item semi-quantitative FFQ. Analysed based on UK Ministry of Agriculture, Fisheries and Food data.	150 µg day⁻¹ RDA, dietary reference intakes for iodine (2001) [58]	Vegan (803) (269,534)	M, 55.5 ± 40.0 [2] F, 54.1 ± 40.0 [2] Total, 58.5 (a) [2]	Two participants who consumed seaweed had values close to the maximum tolerable daily intake for iodine. Supplement intakes recorded did not specify iodine content.	M, N F, N (a), N
			Vegetarian (6673) (1516,5157)	M, 141.0 ± 77.4 [2] F, 146.1 ± 78.8 [2] Total, 148.1 (a) [2]		M, N F, N (a), N
			Pescatarian (4431) (782,3749)	M, 197.4 ± 84.7 [2] F, 194.8 ± 85.9 [2] Total, 196.8 (a) [2]		Y (a), Y
			Omnivore (Meat-Eaters) (18,244) (3798,14446)	M, 214.3 ± 85.6 [2] F, 213.8 ± 85.2 [2] Total, 212.2 (a) [2]		Y (a), Y

Abbreviations; RDI, Recommended Daily Intake; DRV, Daily Recommended Value; NNR, Nordic Nutrition Recommendations; RNI, Recommended Nutrient Intake; RV, Recommended Value; RDA, Recommended Daily Allowance; RI, Recommended Intake; (a), adjusted by age and sex; [1], mean ± SEM; [2] mean ± SD; [3] , median (25th–75th percentile); [4] , mean (95% CI); * significant difference with other dietary groups; p < 0.005 ** significant difference with other dietary groups; p < 0.001.

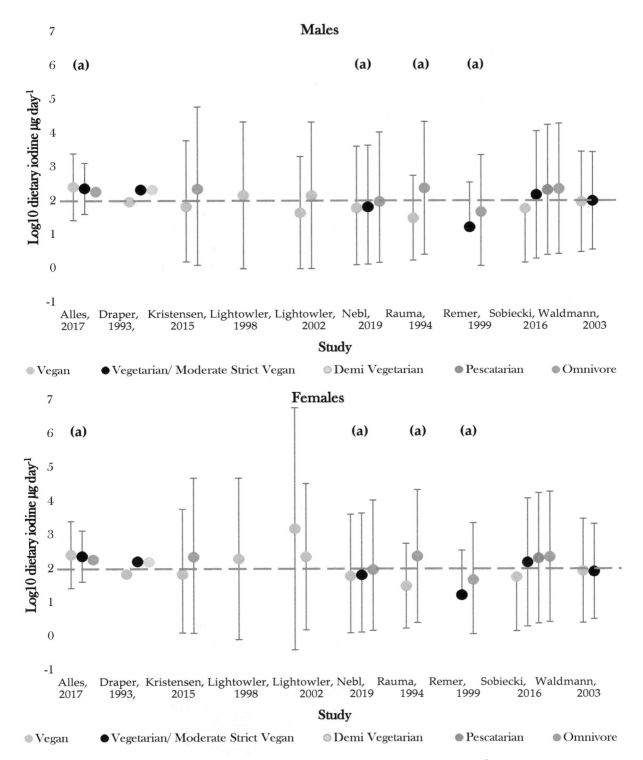

Figure 3. Visual representation of estimated average iodine intake (μg day^{-1}) for included studies. The grey dashed line represents the adequate intake recommended by the WHO of 150 μg day^{-1}. (**a**), mixed gender values. Significance values are not presented within this figure. See Table 5.

The highest daily iodine intake was recorded in females following vegan diets of 1448.0 ± 3879.0; 29.0 ± 18.0 μg day^{-1} [42,50]. The lowest dietary intake was found in those following vegetarian diets of 15.6 ± 21.0 μg day^{-1} [47]. Seven studies assessed iodine intake between vegans and one or more dietary group [36,37,43,45,46,49,50]. Omnivores (male and female) had the highest estimated average intake in 85% of studies [43,45–47,49,50]. Vegan groups tended to have the lowest iodine intake. Males following vegan diets had average intakes lower than all comparative dietary groups in all studies, apart from that conducted by Allès (2017) [36]. Females following vegan diets presented the lowest iodine intake in 75% of studies [37,45,49]. Varied intakes were recorded for moderate vegans, vegetarians, and pescatarians across studies, with estimates ranging between 222.6 ± 1.1 and 15.6 ± 21.0 µg day^{-1} [36,43,47]. The majority of values fell around the expected population mean (184.1 µg day^{-1}), although there was a general tendency for values to be slightly below this level (Supplementary Figure S2).

Recommended criteria for iodine intake varied according to country of study. Comparisons were, therefore, drawn according to recommended intake values denoted by the WHO, with values above 150 µg day^{-1} being classed as adequate [51]. One study recorded estimates above the adequate range for all dietary groups [36]. Omnivores most frequently achieved adequate intake, with only two studies recording intakes below 150 µg day^{-1} for both genders [43,47]. Those following vegan diets most frequently showed dietary iodine inadequacy. Adequate intake was recorded for 44% of female and 66% of mixed gender estimates [36,37,41–43,45,46,49,50]. No groups of males only had intakes above the adequate cut off values [37,41,42,49,50]. Intakes for moderate vegans (vegetarians), vegetarians, and pescatarians were similar between genders and were above adequate in half of studies [36,37,43].

Only four studies investigated the relative consumption of different food groups [36,37,43,46]. None reported the actual contribution of each food group to dietary iodine independent of iodised salt and supplements. However, adults following vegan and vegetarian diets tended to report significantly higher consumption of plant-based food groups (fruit, vegetables, legumes, tubers cereals and grains) [43,46], along with tofu and soya-based products which naturally have a low iodine content. One study reported the consumption of milk alternatives in each dietary group, and vegans had the largest consumption of plant-based milk alternatives [36]. As expected, milk and dairy, egg, and fish consumption was significantly higher ($p < 0.0001$) in vegetarians and omnivores compared to vegans [36,43].

Six studies measured seaweed consumption [37,41,42,45,49,50]. Adults following vegan diets had the greatest seaweed intake, with four studies stating that consumption significantly increased dietary intake such that iodine intake would be considered 'excessive' [37,41,42,49]. Seaweed was not regularly consumed by omnivores and moderate vegans (vegetarians), vegetarians, demi vegetarians or pescatarians [37,45–47,49,50].

Mandatory salt fortification programs were present in three countries of included studies (Table 6) [39,40,49]. Eight studies did not record the contribution of iodised salt to dietary iodine [36,37,41–43,45,46,49].

Table 6. Summary of salt fortification programs present in included studies [59].

Country	Year	Iodate and/or Iodide	Iodine Amount (ppm)	State of Legislation
Boston (U.S.)	1920	Iodide	43	Mandatory
Denmark	1999	Iodide	13	Mandatory
France	1997	Iodide	10–15	Voluntary
Finland	1963	Iodide	25	Voluntary
Germany	1981	Iodate	15–20	Voluntary
Norway	NA	Iodide	5	Voluntary
Slovakia	1966	Iodide	25 ± 10	Mandatory
Switzerland	1922	Both	20–30	Voluntary
UK	NA	Iodide	10–22	Voluntary

Supplement intake was recorded in seven studies [37,41–43,45,46,49]. Two studies did not record iodine-specific supplementation [45,46]. One study prevented supplement intake during the study and another excluded supplement contribution in dietary analysis [42,47].

Three studies recorded supplement intake in adults following vegan diets, contributing between 9.0 and 54.0 µg day^{-1} to dietary intake [37,41,49]. Supplements contributed greater iodine to diets of omnivores (78.9 µg day^{-1}–107.0 µg day^{-1}) [37,49]. No supplement consumption was recorded for moderate vegans (vegetarians), vegetarians, demi vegetarians or pescatarians [37,43,45–47].

4. Discussion

The popularity of vegan and vegetarian diets has increased considerably in the past decade. The prospect of these diets acting as a barrier to adequate iodine nutrition could increase the risk of developing preventable health consequences associated with deficiency and furthering the worldwide public health issue of iodine [60]. Given that these diets are commonly followed by females of childbearing age (16–24 years), lowered dietary iodine intake in these groups could significantly impact future generations and reduce societal productivity [6,61,62].

The present systematic review is the most recent review to evaluate the evidence for iodine intake and status among adults following vegan and vegetarian diets [30]. Our review showed that the discourse has not changed and that adults following a vegan diet, living in industrialised countries, not consuming seaweed or iodine-containing supplements, appear to have increased risk of low iodine status, iodine deficiency and inadequate iodine intake compared to less restrictive dietary groups. Comparison of dietary estimates supports the possibility of a gender difference within vegan groups, as no vegan males achieved adequate intake. Vegetarians or pescatarians are more at risk of low iodine status and intake compared to omnivores but not vegans.

These results are in accordance with the previous review by Fields, Dourson and Borak in 2009 [30], whereby it was concluded that iodine adequacy decreased with increased dietary restriction [30]. However, the previous review did not highlight that some study populations following omnivorous diets also had low iodine status and mild–moderate deficiency [30]. The degree of vulnerability in all dietary groups appears to be impacted by not only individual dietary choices, practices, and restrictions, but country-specific dietary determinants and national food fortification strategies. For this reason, vegans and vegetarians living in industrialised regions where national population iodine measures are below adequate or where dietary intake is insufficient are more susceptible to iodine deficiency. This trend can be observed by comparing median UIC (MUIC) of included studies with the corresponding national data from the country of origin. MUIC tends to closely represent that of omnivorous diets, owing to these practices being the dominant in most industrialised countries.

Vegan and vegetarian MUIC in all studies, apart from that conducted by Rauma (1994), fell below national values [50]. In half of studies, the extent was substantial enough for adults following vegan and vegetarian diets to be classified in a lower deficiency category, according to the WHO criteria, than omnivores and national data—for example, mild (omnivores)–moderate (Vegans and vegetarians) [38–40,48]. This trend can be explained by exploring values determined by Henjum (2018) of non-pregnant young women in Norway [38]. Omnivores in this study presented UIC values concordant with current Norwegian national data (80.0, 75.0 $\mu g \ day^{-1}$), which could be due to efficient data collection of northern, western and eastern regions of Norway [14,38]. As omnivorous diets are the most dominant in industrialised countries, this sample is likely to be representative of the Norwegian population. Omnivorous MUIC and national data are indicative of mild deficiency, whereas for those following vegan and vegetarian diets, MUIC is suggestive of moderate deficiency, therefore indicating that the susceptibility of vegan and vegetarian populations to deficiency is in part dependent on national iodine status.

This trend is not apparent in woman of reproductive age in Switzerland, despite lower observed values in those following vegan diets, as all groups and national data would be classified as mildly deficient [44]. This could be explained by regular consumption of iodized salt in Swiss households, which is greater than 80% [63]. Fortified bread is a significant contributor to dietary iodine and can be consumed by all dietary groups [63]. A reduction or restricted legislation in iodine fortification could increase the risk of iodine deficiency. In Germany, Remer (1999) induced deficiency in vegetarian and omnivorous diets when preventing consumption of fortified and iodinated foods under controlled conditions [47]. In this study, daily iodine intake dropped below requirements required for optimal thyroidal function (50.0–80.0 $\mu g \ day^{-1}$). Disuse or lack of availability of iodine-fortified foods could produce similar consequences.

Shifting legislation reflects changes in iodine status by dietary group over time in Finland from a risk of excess to moderate–severe deficiency in 2016 [48,50]. This is following a reduction in iodised salt consumption possibly influenced by efforts to reduce salt consumption in the general public and replacement of the traditional diet rich in fish and dairy for diets providing improved fruit and vegetable intake [64]. The Finnish Vegan Society was founded in October 1993 [65], a year before Rauma's study was conducted, and food consumption is likely to have changed in this time, as these diets have become widely accepted. Papers published prior to 1990 were excluded, as meat-free diets did not appear in the mainstream until the 1980s, and it is likely that food choices and landscape have changed substantially since this period [66]. Recent studies published after 2010 represent almost half of the included studies which could account for the 'second-wave' vegetarian movement supported today [12,38,43–45,48,49].

Despite the popularity of vegan and vegetarian diets, there is no homogenous term to define these dietary groups, thus questioning the accuracy of group estimates in included studies. Three studies used objective assessments to group individuals by dietary preference [43,45,46]. Self-reported measures are frequently inaccurate at determining dietary preference [30]. Misreporting may additionally be a consequence of misinterpretation of the term "vegetarian" and its associated dietary restrictions or, additionally, over exaggeration of restrictive practices to align with vegetarian ideology [30,67]. Juan, Yamini and Britten (2015) observed errors with adherence to vegetarian diets when investigating food consumption patterns of the U.S. population in the period 2007–2010 [67]. The authors determined that half of those identifying themselves as vegetarian consumed meat, poultry, or seafood and, therefore, would not be described as vegetarian using typical definitions. This issue was discussed previously in the systematic review conducted by Fields, Dourson and Borak, indicating that individual dietary intake based on the description of typical "vegetarian" regimes from self-reports may be inaccurate and indicates that consistent strict dietary adherence in the included studies is likely to be low [30].

The duration of practicing a specific dietary preference must be considered when examining the diets of vegan and vegetarians. Most studies (apart from that conducted in experimental conditions and studies of recreational runners) included participants with 1-year minimum dietary adherence [43,47]. Draper (1993) only recruited participants who had elected to adopt their diets in adulthood and had not grown up as vegetarian [37]. This raises the question as to whether the length of dietary adherence affects iodine measures. Long-term vegetarians could be better at planning their diet adequately if receiving guidance from their parents from a young age or iodine intake could reflect reduced diet diversity and long-term dietary compliance.

Reduced dietary intake for those following vegan diets may reflect difficulties in accurately measuring dietary intake. Intake can be measured using various methods. The "gold standard" for estimating iodine intake is a dietary record or food diary inclusive of one weekend day [17]. Seven included studies followed this methodology, additionally pairing food diaries with weighed or duplicate records [36,37,41–43,47,49]. Food diary measurements reflect recent intake; therefore, 10 days are recommended for iodine to account for food items that are rich in iodine but not regularly consumed [68]. Only two studies collected records exceeding this duration [46,50]. The most frequent length of estimates was 4 days, which is acknowledged as an adequate length to record dietary intake [69]. Duplicate diaries are suitable for valuation of minerals such as iodine [70]. This technique is useful for foods with iodine values not contained within food tables or composition data. For this reason, this technique is useful to assess the dietary iodine of those following vegan diets who may consume foods that are novel or not frequently eaten by the general public.

Two studies used validated FFQs to estimate iodine intake [45,46]. FFQs are often designed to be specific to a nutrient of interest and aim to include food items contributing to intake. Both studies had developed FFQs to address intake of multiple micronutrients and were not iodine specific. As FFQs are a comprehensive list and not all foods can be contained, they are, therefore, limited to the listed items. It is unlikely that these studies addressed foods that largely contribute to iodine intake but are not regularly consumed such as seaweed or novel foods consumed by vegans. In addition, FFQs have been recognised to frequently overestimate iodine intake as supported by previous validation studies [71].

For all studies, estimations of iodine intake were calculated using mean iodine concentration of foods and beverages provided by regional food composition tables or databases and are, therefore, country specific [36,37,41–43,45–47,50]. Estimates based on one summary statistic cannot account for variation in iodine content between food items across time, season, and geographic location—for example, the iodine content of milk, which also varies according to processing and product origin [72]. In vegan adults, the lowest intakes were recorded in Finland (29.0 ± 18.0 µg day^{-1}) [50]. Krajcovicová-Kudláčková (2003) discussed that Finish food tables tended to estimate lower iodine intake compared to British food tables [39], and variation in this case probably represents geographical diversity between countries and food availability. Waldmann (2003) [46] created a database accounting for vegan food items regularly consumed in Germany, thus improving estimates. Four studies were conducted in the 1990s [37,41,47,50]. It is likely that food tables and databases have improved availability of the iodine content of foods. However, these methods lack iodine values for newly consumed food and products, particularly those gaining in popularity such as plant-based alternatives.

Adults following vegan diets had the largest consumption of plant-based milk alternatives. Bath et al. investigated the iodine concentration of milk alternatives available in the UK in 2015 and determined the concentration of unfortified milk-alternative drinks (median 7.3 µg kg^{-1}) to be significantly lower than the dairy milks analysed (median 438.0 µg kg^{-1}) [28]. Those consuming alternative milks may not be aware of the lower contribution of plant-based milks to iodine and need to ensure intake from other sources.

The highest iodine intake was recorded for females following vegan diets, living in London (1448.0 ± 3879.0 µg day^{-1}), whose regular consumption of seaweed increased intakes to over six times the RNI [42]. Five studies recorded seaweed consumption in vegan diets only, observing intakes close to, or over, the maximum tolerant level [37,41,42,46,49]. Seaweed is a naturally rich source of iodine, but the relative content is highly variable and can provide excessive quantities and, therefore, regular consumption is not recommended [73]. Seaweed is not customarily consumed in the Western diet. However, it has recently become popular in UK food products as a whole food and functional ingredient [74]. For example, carrageenan is widely used in newly formulated vegan and vegetarian products. Manufacturers use it to replace gelatine, as it is derived from plant origin [74]. Draper (1993) observed low iodine intakes in adults following vegan diets in London despite 95% recording regular consumption of seaweed or foods containing seaweed powder [37]. While the iodine content of seaweeds is often high, it is not a food that is consumed in large quantities, hence the contribution towards dietary intakes is likely to be small and inconstant [75]. Moreover, iodine content significantly differs between seaweed species consumed [73].

Voluntary fortification is present in most countries [59], yet very few manufacturers add fortified salt to food items and iodinated salt is not easily available to consumers. This appears to be true in the study conducted by Rauma (1994), where only one Finish vegan reported consuming iodised salt regularly [50]. Furthermore, Bath et al. (2013) conducted a shelf survey of five major chain supermarkets in the UK and found that iodized salt was only sold in 42% (32 out of 77) of shops and that the iodine content of fortified salt sold was low (11.5 ± 4.2 µg g^{-1}) [25]. Draper (1993) noted the consumption of 'sea salt' in 95% of UK adults following vegan diets [37]. Although 'sea salt' and other 'specialty' salts such as Himalayan sea salt contain iodine, the concentration is relatively small compared to iodised salts [76]. Additionally, of two studies reporting iodised salt intake [37,50], neither identified having adjusted intakes to account for volatile iodine losses experienced during cooking [77]. Kristensen (2015) attempted to quantify the involvement of iodised salt by measuring reported sodium intake [49]. Despite, the routine uses of iodised salt in Danish households, 55 out of 70 vegans failed to meet dietary recommendations for iodine [49]. Low dietary intake in vegans in this study may be explained by reduced dietary sodium intake reported by vegan participants and infrequent consumption of salt-rich processed food items. Moreover, vegan ready meals are not always readily available from retailers.

Limitations of the study. In addition to the limitations highlighted above, it should be noted that the values recorded in the included studies tended to be skewed below the mean estimated population levels for UIC (Supplementary Figure S1) and intake (Supplementary Figure S2). This would suggest that for most studies, the sample population was not wholly reflective of the general population. This is a challenge for such studies, as the cohort of individuals prepared to participate is often characterised by those with an interest either in their dietary choice or dietary control for health reasons. Accessing the wider public is much more difficult and a challenge that needs to be addressed in future studies. There was some overlap with the previous systematic review, and we found that recent studies investigating iodine nutrition were relatively scarce. Further, it was necessary to combine groups, thereby oversimplifying dietary practice to enable comparison of studies. Lastly, there was a lack of values for contribution of specific food groups (e.g., supplements) and iodised salt.

5. Conclusions

Iodine deficiency remains a public health problem worldwide and is of concern following the "re-emergence" of iodine deficiency, especially in industrialised countries [78]. This review agrees with findings from the previous systematic reviews exploring this topic [30,31], confirming that vegans and vegetarians, living in industrialised countries, not consuming seaweed or iodine-containing supplements, appear to have increased risk of low iodine status, iodine deficiency and inadequate iodine intake compared to adults following less restrictive diets. The evidence suggests that the degree of vulnerability appears to be relative to the prevalence of deficiency at the national level. This review also highlights the variety of methodological issues associated with estimating iodine in unique dietary groups. In conclusion, further monitoring of iodine status in industrialised countries and research into improving the intake and status of vegan and vegetarian diets is required. Efforts need to be made to devise a means of safe iodine consumption whether by fortification of staple foods or iodised salt provision, in addition to information delivery intended for tolerable consumption of seaweed varieties. Lastly, nutrients frequently lacking in vegan and vegetarian diets should be routinely labelled on foods regularly consumed by these groups in order to highlight to those making these purchases that there is a need to consider the levels that are being consumed.

Supplementary Materials:

Figure S1: Funnel plot showing iodide status for individual groups according to number of individuals in each group. For each study, data for urinary iodide concentration (μg L^{-1}) was plotted for omnivores, vegetarians and vegans where provided, against the number of participants in each group. Each data point represents a specific group rather than a specific study. Figure S2 Funnel plot showing iodide consumption for individual groups according to number of individuals in each group. For each study, data for dietary iodide intake (μg Day^{-1}) was plotted for omnivores, vegetarians and vegans where provided, against the Log_{10} of the number of participants in each group. Each data point represents a specific group rather than a specific study. Table S1: Search terms used in the study, Table S2: Quality assessment questions, Table S3: Definitions and characteristics of dietary groups studied in included studies, Table S4: National data corresponding to location of included studies, Table S5:Common methods for assessing Dietary Iodine Intake in Population Studies.

Author Contributions: Conceptualization, E.R.E., L.J.C., and S.J.M.W.; methodology, E.R.E., L.J.C., and S.J.M.W.; formal analysis, E.R.E., and L.J.C.; investigation, E.R.E., L.J.C., and S.J.M.W.; writing—original draft preparation, E.R.E.; writing—review and editing, E.R.E., L.J.C., A.A., and S.J.M.W.; visualization, E.R.E.; supervision, L.J.C., and S.W.; funding acquisition, E.R.E., L.J.C., and S.J.M.W. All authors have read and agreed to the published version of the manuscript.

Acknowledgments: The BBSRC for funding and the Division of Food, Nutrition and Dietetics at The University of Nottingham for backing.

References

1. Phillips, F. Vegetarian nutrition. *Nutr. Bull.* **2005**, *30*, 132–167. [CrossRef]
2. Sebastiani, G.; Herranz Barbero, A. The effects of vegetarian and vegan diet during pregnancy on the health of mothers and offspring. *Nutrients* **2019**, *11*, 557. [CrossRef] [PubMed]
3. British Dietetic Association Confirms Well-Planned Vegan Diets Can Support Healthy Living in People of All Ages. Available online: https://www.bda.uk.com/resource/british-dietetic-association-confirms-well-planned-vegan-diets-can-support-healthy-living-in-people-of-all-ages.html (accessed on 24 February 2020).
4. Vegan Diets: Everything You Need to Know—Dietitians Association of Australia. Available online: https://daa.asn.au/smart-eating-for-you/smart-eating-fast-facts/healthy-eating/vegan-diets-facts-tips-and-considerations/ (accessed on 7 October 2019).
5. Craig, W.J.; Mangels, A.R. American Dietetic Association Position of the American Dietetic Association: Vegetarian diets. *J. Am. Diet Assoc.* **2009**, *109*, 1266–1282. [PubMed]
6. Scientific Advisory Committe on Nutrition Statement on Iodine and Health. 2014. Available online: https://www.gov.uk/government/uploads/system/uploads/attachment_data/file/339439/SACN_Iodine_and_Health_2014.pdf (accessed on 7 October 2019).
7. Eastman, C.J.; Zimmermann, M.B. *The Iodine Deficiency Disorders*, 1st ed.; Feingold, K.R., Anawalt, B., Boyce, A., Chrousos, G., Dungan, K., Grossman, A., Hershman, J.M., Kaltsas, G., Koch, C., Kopp, P., et al., Eds.; Endotext [Internet]: South Dartmouth, MA, USA, 2000.
8. Ahad, F.; Ganie, S.A. Iodine, Iodine metabolism and Iodine deficiency disorders revisited. *Indian J. Endocrinol. Metab.* **2010**, *14*, 13–17. [PubMed]
9. Zimmermann, M.B. Iodine deficiency. *Endocr. Rev.* **2009**, *30*, 376–408. [CrossRef]
10. Zimmermann, M.B. Thyroid gland: Iodine deficiency and thyroid nodules. *Nat. Rev. Endocrinol.* **2014**, *10*, 707–708. [CrossRef]
11. Popoveniuc, G.; Jonklaas, J. Thyroid Nodules. *Med. Clin. N. Am.* **2012**, *96*, 329–349. [CrossRef]
12. Leung, A.M.; Braverman, L.E. Consequences of excess iodine. *Nat. Rev. Endocrinol.* **2014**, *10*, 136–142. [CrossRef]
13. Li, M.; Eastman, C.J. The changing epidemiology of iodine deficiency. *Nat. Rev. Endocrinol.* **2012**, *8*, 434–440. [CrossRef]
14. Iodine Global Network (IGN)—Home. Available online: http://www.ign.org/ (accessed on 13 September 2019).
15. World Health Organization. *Assessment of Iodine Deficiency Disorders and Monitoring their Elimination A Guide for Programme Managers*, 3rd ed.; World Health Organization: Geneva, Switzerland, 2007; pp. 1–60.
16. Pearce, E.N.; Caldwell, K.L. Urinary iodine, thyroid function, and thyroglobulin as biomarkers of iodine status. *Am. J. Clin Nutr.* **2016**, *104*, 898–901. [CrossRef]
17. Serra-Majem, L.; Pfrimer, K.; Doreste-Alonso, J.; Ribas-Barba, L.; Sánchez-Villegas, A.; Ortiz-Andrellucchi, A.; Henríquez-Sánchez, P. Dietary assessment methods for intakes of iron, calcium, selenium, zinc and iodine. *Br. J. Nutr.* **2009**, *102*. [CrossRef] [PubMed]
18. Gunnarsdottir, I.; Dahl, L. Iodine intake in human nutrition: A systematic literature review. *Food Nutr. Res.* **2012**, *56*, 19731. [CrossRef] [PubMed]
19. Fuge, R. Soils and iodine deficiency. In *Essentials of Medical Geology*; Selinus, O., Ed.; Springer: Dordrecht, The Netherlands, 2013; pp. 417–432.
20. Humphrey, O.S.; Young, S.D. Iodine uptake, storage and translocation mechanisms in spinach (*Spinacia oleracea* L.). *Environ. Geochem. Health* **2019**, *41*, 2145–2156. [CrossRef] [PubMed]
21. Zimmermann, M.B. Iodine deficiency in industrialized countries. *Clin. Endocrinol.* **2011**, *75*, 287–288. [CrossRef] [PubMed]
22. Bath, S.; Rayman, M. British Dietetic Association: Iodine Food Fact Sheet. 2016. Available online: https://www.bda.uk.com/resource/iodine.html (accessed on 20 May 2020).
23. Andersson, M.; de Benoist, B.; Delange, F. *Iodine Deficiency in Europe: A Continuing Public Health Problem*, 1st ed.; World Health Organization: Geneva, Switzerland, 2007; pp. 154–196.
24. Gärtner, R. Recent data on iodine intake in Germany and Europe. *J. Trace Elem. Med. Biol.* **2016**, *37*, 85–89. [CrossRef]
25. Bath, S.C.; Button, S.; Rayman, M.P. Availability of iodised table salt in the UK—Is it likely to influence population iodine intake? *Public Health Nutr.* **2014**, *17*, 450–454. [CrossRef]

26. Appleby, P.N.; Thorogood, M. The Oxford Vegetarian Study: An overview. *Am. J. Clin. Nutr.* **1999**, *70*, 525–531. [CrossRef]

27. Elsabie, W.; Aboel Einen, K. Comparative Evaluation of Some Physicochemical Properties for Different Types of Vegan Milk with Cow Milk. *Dairy Sci. Technol.* **2016**, *7*, 457–461. [CrossRef]

28. Bath, S.C.; Hill, S.; Infante, H.G. Iodine concentration of milk-alternative drinks available in the UK in comparison with cows' milk. *Br. J. Nutr.* **2017**, *118*, 525–532. [CrossRef]

29. 52% of UK Meat-Free New Product Launches Are Vegan-Mintel. Available online: https://www.mintel.com/press-centre/food-and-drink/more-than-half-of-all-meat-free-new-product-launches-in-the-uk-carry-a-vegan-claim-1 (accessed on 24 February 2020).

30. Fields, C.; Borak, J. Iodine Deficiency in Vegetarian and Vegan Diets: Evidence-Based Review of the World's Literature on Iodine Content in Vegetarian Diets. In *Comprehensive Handbook of Iodine*, 1st ed.; Elsevier Science Publishing Co.: Amsterdam, The Netherlands, 2009; pp. 521–531.

31. Fields, C.; Dourson, M.; Borak, J. Iodine-deficient vegetarians: A hypothetical perchlorate-susceptible population? *RTP* **2005**, *42*, 37–46. [CrossRef]

32. Moher, D.; Liberati, A. Preferred Reporting Items for Systematic Reviews and Meta-Analyses: The PRISMA Statement—Flow of information through the different phases of a systematic review. *PLoS Med.* **2009**, *6*, e1000097. [CrossRef] [PubMed]

33. Howard, C. Subject & Course Guides: Evidence Based Medicine: PICO. Available online: https://researchguides.uic.edu/c.php?g=252338&p=3954402 (accessed on 13 September 2019).

34. Data extraction forms|Cochrane Developmental, Psychosocial and Learning Problems. Available online: https://dplp.cochrane.org/data-extraction-forms (accessed on 13 September 2019).

35. Study Quality Assessment Tools | National Heart, Lung, and Blood Institute (NHLBI). Available online: https://www.nhlbi.nih.gov/health-topics/study-quality-assessment-tools (accessed on 13 September 2019).

36. Allès, B.; Baudry, J. Comparison of Sociodemographic and Nutritional Characteristics between Self-Reported Vegetarians, Vegans, and Meat-Eaters from the NutriNet-Santé Study. *Nutrients* **2017**, *9*, 1023. [CrossRef] [PubMed]

37. Draper, A.; Lewis, J. The energy and nutrient intakes of different types of vegetarian: A case for supplements? *Br. J. Nutr.* **1993**, *69*, 3–19. [CrossRef] [PubMed]

38. Henjum, S.; Brantsæter, A.L.; Kurniasari, A.; Dahl, L.; Aadland, E.K.; Gjengedal, E.L.F.; Birkeland, S.; Aakre, I. Suboptimal iodine status and low iodine knowledge in young Norwegian women. *Nutrients* **2018**, *10*, 941. [CrossRef]

39. Krajcovicová-Kudláčková, M.; Bucková, K.; Klimes, I.; Seboková, E. Iodine deficiency in vegetarians and vegans. *Ann. Nutr. Metab.* **2003**, *47*, 183–185. [CrossRef]

40. Leung, A.M.; LaMar, A.; He, X.; Braverman, L.E.; Pearce, E.N. Iodine status and thyroid function of Boston-area vegetarians and vegans. *J. Clin. Endocrinol.* **2011**, *96*, 1303–1307. [CrossRef]

41. Lightowler, H.J.; Davies, G.J. Iodine intake and iodine deficiency in vegans as assessed by the duplicate-portion technique and urinary iodine excretion. *Br. J. Nutr.* **1998**, *80*, 529–535. [CrossRef]

42. Lightowler, H.J.; Davies, G.J. Assessment of iodine intake in vegans: Weighed dietary record vs duplicate portion technique. *Eur. J. Clin. Nutr.* **2002**, *56*, 765–770. [CrossRef]

43. Nebl, J.; Schuchardt, J.P.; Wasserfurth, P.; Haufe, S.; Eigendorf, J.; Tegtbur, U.; Hahn, A. Characterization, dietary habits and nutritional intake of omnivorous, lacto-ovo vegetarian and vegan runners—A pilot study. *BMC Nutr.* **2019**, *5*, 51. [CrossRef]

44. Schüpbach, R.; Wegmüller, R.; Berguerand, C.; Bui, M.; Herter-Aeberli, I. Micronutrient status and intake in omnivores, vegetarians and vegans in Switzerland. *Eur. J. Clin. Nutr.* **2017**, *56*, 283–293. [CrossRef]

45. Sobiecki, J.G.; Appleby, P.N.; Bradbury, K.E.; Key, T.J. High Compliance with Dietary Recommendations in a Cohort of Meat Eaters, Fish Eaters, Vegetarians, and Vegans. *Nutr. Res.* **2016**, *36*, 464–477. [CrossRef] [PubMed]

46. Waldmann, A.; Koschizke, J.W.; Leitzmann, C.; Hahn, A. Dietary intakes and lifestyle factors of a vegan population in Germany: Results from the German Vegan Study. *Eur. J. Clin. Nutr.* **2003**, *57*, 947–955. [CrossRef] [PubMed]

47. Remer, T.; Neubert, A.; Manz, F. Increased risk of iodine deficiency with vegetarian nutrition. *Br. J. Nutr.* **1999**, *81*, 45–49. [CrossRef] [PubMed]

48. Elorinne, A.-L.; Alfthan, G.; Erlund, I.; Kivimäki, H.; Paju, A.; Salminen, I.; Turpeinen, U.; Voutilainen, S.; Laakso, J. Food and Nutrient Intake and Nutritional Status of Finnish Vegans and Non-Vegetarians. *PLoS ONE* **2016**, *11*, e0148235. [CrossRef]

49. Kristensen, N.B.; Madsen, M.L.; Hansen, T.H.; Allin, K.H.; Hoppe, C.; Fagt, S.; Lausten, M.S.; Gøbel, R.J.; Vestergaard, H.; Hansen, T.; et al. Intake of macro- and micronutrients in Danish vegans. *Nutr. J.* **2015**, *14*, 115. [CrossRef] [PubMed]

50. Rauma, A.L.; Törmälä, M.L.; Nenonen, M.; Hänninen, O. Iodine status in vegans consuming a living food diet. *Nutr. Res.* **1994**, *14*, 1789–1795. [CrossRef]

51. VMNIS|Vitamin and Mineral Nutrition Information System Urinary Iodine Concentrations for Determining Iodine Status in Populations. Available online: https://www.who.int/vmnis/indicators/urinaryiodine/en/ (accessed on 12 September 2019).

52. Martin, A. The "apports nutritionnels conseillés (ANC)" for the French population. *Reprod. Nutr. Dev.* **2001**, *41*, 119–128. [CrossRef]

53. The Department of Health Dietary Reference Values A Guide. Available online: https://assets.publishing. service.gov.uk/government/uploads/system/uploads/attachment_data/file/743790/Dietary_Reference_Values_-_ A_Guide__1991_.pdf (accessed on 12 September 2019).

54. Nordic Council of Ministers Nordic Nutrition Recommendations 2012 Integrating Nutrition and Physical Activity. Available online: https://norden.diva-portal.org/smash/get/diva2:704251/FULLTEXT01.pdf (accessed on 12 September 2019).

55. Jod. Available online: https://www.dge.de/wissenschaft/referenzwerte/jod/ (accessed on 24 April 2020).

56. National Research Council. *Food and Nutrition Board Recommended Dietary Allowances*; National Academies Press: Washington, DC, USA, 1989; pp. 1–277.

57. German Nutrition Society. *The Nutrition Report 2000*, 2000th ed.; German Nutrition Society: Bonn, Germany, 2000; pp. 1–37.

58. Institute of Medicine (US) Panel on Micronutrients. *Dietary Reference Intakes for Vitamin A, Vitamin K, Arsenic, Boron, Chromium, Copper, Iodine, Iron, Manganese, Molybdenum, Nickel, Silicon, Vanadium, and Zinc*; National Academies Press: Washington, DC, USA, 2001; pp. 1–500.

59. Iodine Global Network (IGN)—Global Iodine Scorecard and Map. Available online: https://www.ign.org/ scorecard.htm (accessed on 20 March 2020).

60. Black, M.M. Micronutrient Deficiencies and Cognitive Functioning. *Nutr. J.* **2003**, *133*, 3927s–3931s. [CrossRef]

61. Zimmermann, M.B. Iodine deficiency and excess in children: Worldwide status in 2013. *Endocr. Pract.* **2013**, *19*, 839–846. [CrossRef]

62. Martinelli, D.; Berkmanienė, A. The Politics and the Demographics of Veganism: Notes for a Critical Analysis. *Int. J. Semiot. Law* **2018**, *31*, 501–530. [CrossRef]

63. Andersson, M.; Aeberli, I.; Wüst, N.; Piacenza, A.M.; Bucher, T.; Henschen, I.; Haldimann, M.; Zimmermann, M.B. The Swiss iodized salt program provides adequate iodine for school children and pregnant women, but weaning infants not receiving iodine-containing complementary foods as well as their mothers are iodine deficient. *J. Clin. Endocrinol. Metab.* **2010**, *95*, 5217–5224. [CrossRef] [PubMed]

64. Nyström, H.F.; Brantsæter, A.L.; Erlund, I.; Gunnarsdottir, I.; Hulthén, L.; Laurberg, P.; Mattisson, I.; Rasmussen, L.B.; Virtanen, S.; Meltzer, H.M. Iodine status in the Nordic countries past and present. *Nutr. Res.* **2016**, *60*, 31969. [CrossRef] [PubMed]

65. International Vegetarian Union—History of IVU. Available online: https://ivu.org/history/ (accessed on 26 September 2019).

66. Leitzmann, C. Vegetarian nutrition: Past, present, future. *Am. J. Clin. Nutr.* **2014**, *100*, 496s–502s. [CrossRef]

67. Juan, W.; Yamini, S.; Britten, P. Food Intake Patterns of Self-identified Vegetarians Among the U.S. Population, 2007–2010. *Procedia Food Sci.* **2015**, *4*, 86–93. [CrossRef]

68. Zimmermann, M.B.; Andersson, M. Assessment of iodine nutrition in populations: Past, present, and future. *Nutr. Rev.* **2012**, *70*, 553–570. [CrossRef]

69. Bingham, S.A.; Cassidy, A.; Cole, T.J.; Welch, A.; Runswick, S.A.; Black, A.E.; Thurnham, D.; Bates, C.; Khaw, K.T.; Key, T.J.A.; et al. Validation of weighed records and other methods of dietary assessment using the 24 h urine nitrogen technique and other biological markers. *Br. J. Nutr.* **1995**, *73*, 531–550. [CrossRef]

70. DAPA Measurement Toolkit. Available online: https://dapa-toolkit.mrc.ac.uk/diet/objective-methods/ duplicate-diets (accessed on 26 September 2019).

71. Rasmussen, L.B.; Ovesen, L.; Bülow, I.; Jørgensen, T.; Knudsen, N.; Laurberg, P.; Perrild, H. Evaluation of a semi-quantitative food frequency questionnaire to estimate iodine intake. *Eur. J. Clin. Nutr.* **2001**, *55*, 287–292. [CrossRef]

72. O'Kane, S.M.; Pourshahidi, L.K.; Mulhern, M.S.; Weir, R.R.; Hill, S.; O'Reilly, J.; Kmiotek, D.; Deitrich, C.; Mackle, E.M.; Fitzgerald, E.; et al. The effect of processing and seasonality on the iodine and selenium concentration of cow's milk produced in Northern Ireland (NI): Implications for population dietary intake. *Nutrients* **2018**, *10*, 287. [CrossRef]

73. Yeh, T.S.; Hung, N.H.; Lin, T.C. Analysis of iodine content in seaweed by GC-ECD and estimation of iodine intake. *J. Food Drug Anal.* **2014**, *22*, 189–196. [CrossRef]

74. Bouga, M.; Combet, E. Emergence of Seaweed and Seaweed-Containing Foods in the UK: Focus on Labeling, Iodine Content, Toxicity and Nutrition. *Foods* **2015**, *4*, 240–253. [CrossRef]

75. Lightowler, H.J. Assessment of Iodine Intake and Iodine Status in Vegans. In *Comprehensive Handbook of Iodine*; Elsevier Inc.: Amsterdam, The Netherlands, 2009; pp. 429–436.

76. Dasgupta, P.K.; Liu, Y.; Dyke, J.V. Iodine nutrition: Iodine content of iodized salt in the United States. *Environ. Sci. Technol.* **2008**, *42*, 1315–1323. [CrossRef] [PubMed]

77. Rana, R.; Raghuvanshi, R.S. Effect of different cooking methods on iodine losses. *J. Food Sci. Technol.* **2013**, *50*, 1212–1216. [CrossRef] [PubMed]

78. Rayman, M.P.; Bath, S.C. The new emergence of iodine deficiency in the UK: Consequences for child neurodevelopment. *Ann. Clin. Biochem.* **2015**, *52*, 705–708. [CrossRef] [PubMed]

2

Iodine Intake in Norwegian Women and Men:
The Population-Based Tromsø Study 2015–2016

**Ahmed A Madar [1],*, Espen Heen [1]◉, Laila A Hopstock [2], Monica H Carlsen [3] and
Haakon E Meyer [1,4]**

[1]   Department of Community Medicine and Global Health, Institute of Health and Society, University of Oslo,
      0318 Oslo, Norway; e.k.heen@medisin.uio.no (E.H.); h.e.meyer@medisin.uio.no (H.E.M.)
[2]   Department of Community Medicine, Faculty of Health Sciences, UiT The Arctic University of Norway,
      9037 Tromsø, Norway; laila.hopstock@uit.no
[3]   Department of Nutrition, Institute of Basic Medical Sciences, University of Oslo, 0318 Oslo, Norway;
      m.h.carlsen@medisin.uio.no
[4]   Division of Mental and Physical Health, Norwegian Institute of Public Health, 0213 Oslo, Norway
*   Correspondence: a.a.madar@medisin.uio.no

Abstract: Ensuring sufficient iodine intake is a public health priority, but we lack knowledge about the status of iodine in a nationally representative population in Norway. We aimed to assess the current iodine status and intake in a Norwegian adult population. In the population-based Tromsø Study 2015–2016, 493 women and men aged 40–69 years collected 24-h urine samples and 450 participants also completed a food frequency questionnaire (FFQ). The 24-h urinary iodine concentration (UIC) was analyzed using the Sandell–Kolthoff reaction on microplates followed by colorimetric measurement. Iodine intake was estimated from the FFQ using a food and nutrient calculation system at the University of Oslo. The mean urine volume in 24 h was 1.74 L. The median daily iodine intake estimated (UIE) from 24-h UIC was 159 µg/day (133 and 174 µg/day in women and men). The median daily iodine intake estimated from FFQ was 281 µg/day (263 and 318 µg/day in women and men, respectively). Iodine intake estimated from 24-h UIC and FFQ were moderately correlated (Spearman rank correlation coefficient r = 0.39, $p < 0.01$). The consumption of milk and milk products, fish and fish products, and eggs were positively associated with estimated iodine intake from FFQ. In conclusion, this shows that iodine intake estimated from 24-h UIC describes a mildly iodine deficient female population, while the male population is iodine sufficient. Concurrent use of an extensive FFQ describes both sexes as iodine sufficient. Further studies, applying a dietary assessment method validated for estimating iodine intake and repeated individual urine collections, are required to determine the habitual iodine intake in this population.

Keywords: 24-h iodine; urinary iodine excretion; food frequency questionnaire; population-based studies; adult; iodine intake

1. Introduction

Iodine is an essential trace element and it is required for the production of thyroid hormones (thyroxine and triiodothyronine) which are essential for regulation of energy metabolism in adults [1]. Too little and too much iodine can both increase the risk of thyroid dysfunction, and iodine deficiency can lead to a variety of health consequences known as iodine deficiency disorders (IDDs) [2]. Globally, before 1990, only a few countries were iodine sufficient, but comprehensive progress has been made since the primary intervention strategy for IDD control, i.e., universal salt iodization was adopted in 1993 [3,4]. Despite this global progress, recently, Europe has been one of the regions in the world where mild iodine deficiency has been most prevalent [5–9].

In Norway, IDD used to be endemic, but fortification of animal fodder since the early 1950s (2 mg of iodine per kilogram) contributed to the elimination of goiter and the prevention of IDD due to consumption of milk and dairy products [10]. Since then, milk, dairy products, fish, and fish products have been the main sources of iodine in the diet of Norwegians, contributing about 80% of the total iodine intake [11,12]. Although iodized salt is an important source of iodine in many countries, iodine fortification is only permitted in table salt (five milligrams of iodine per kilogram) in Norway. Furthermore, in recent years, consumption of milk and seafood has decreased [13]. A reduction of iodine content in milk has also been reported, linked to changed composition of cow fodder and possibly less use of iodophors for cleaning milk teats [14].

For many years, Norway has been considered to be an iodine-sufficient country, but recent findings have confirmed inadequate iodine intake among subgroups including pregnant and lactating women, vegans, and certain immigrant groups [9,15–17].

The World Health Organization (WHO) recommends regular mapping of iodine status in the population to counteract iodine deficiency, and the Norwegian Nutrition Council has recently recommended systematic monitoring of iodine status in the Norwegian population [1,18].

The recommended daily intake (RDI) of iodine in the Nordic countries (NNR12) is 150 μg/day for adults [18], and the estimated average requirement (EAR) is 100 μg/day, in line with the WHO guideline [19]. Around 90% of iodine intake is believed to be excreted via urine within 24 h, and the median urinary iodine concentration (UIC) is currently the most practical method for assessing the overall iodine status in a population [20]. However, UIC cannot be used to quantify the proportion of individuals with iodine deficiency or iodine excess. Calculating iodine intake from diet and dietary iodine supplements might provide a more complete understanding of habitual (long-term) iodine intake in the population. The WHO recommends a median UIC of at least 100 μg/L to prevent IDD in the general population [1]. In addition, no more than 20% of the UIC samples should be lower than 50 μg/L and a median UIC higher than 600 μg/L is defined as 'excessive iodine intake [21].

For ensuring adequate iodine intake in all groups of the population, the Norwegian Nutrition Council has recently recommended universal salt iodization [18]. However, knowing that iodine deficiency and excess iodine both have adverse health consequences, it is important to monitor the iodine status in the population.

By drawing from the population-based Tromsø Study, the aim of the present study was to assess the current iodine status and intake in a Norwegian adult population.

2. Materials and Methods

The Tromsø Study is a population based, prospective, multipurpose study consisting of seven repeated surveys conducted from 1974 to 2016 (Tromsø 1–Tromsø 7), inviting whole birth cohorts and random samples of the inhabitants in the Tromsø Municipality, Northern Norway. Data collection included questionnaires and interviews, biological sampling, and clinical examinations. Tromsø is situated ~400 km north of the Arctic Circle, and has approximately 76,000 inhabitants. The seventh survey (Tromsø 7) was carried out during 2015–2016 and all 32,591 inhabitants aged 40 years and above were invited. A total of 21,083 women and men participated (65%) [22]. After excluding participants with self-reported heart failure, stroke, liver disease, participants who had started treatment with diuretics during the preceding two weeks, or with conditions making it difficult to collect urine (e.g., poor general health condition), a random subsample of 608 participants aged 40–69 years was invited for a 24-h urine collection substudy. Of these, 496 (82%) responded and collected urine. There were no statistically significant differences in body mass index (BMI) or education level between those collecting and not collecting urine. Three participants with undetermined urine volume were excluded from the analyses. Thus, a total of 493 participants were included in urine analyses.

2.1. Data Collection

2.1.1. Twenty-Four-Hour Urine Collection

As previously reported [23], the participants were instructed (oral and written) to collect all urine during a 24-h period and record the first and last urination time points, as well as any missed voids or other irregularities. The participants should void their bladder in the first morning of collection and discard this urine, and then collect all urine until and including the morning void of the day after. After returning the 24-h urine specimens, the containers were well stirred, and the volume was read and recorded. Urine samples were extracted and stored at −20 °C until analysis.

2.1.2. Questionnaires and Measurements

Information about education level and smoking habits was collected from questionnaires. Height and weight were measured in light clothing and without footwear.

To collect dietary data, an extensive previously validated FFQ [24], developed at the University of Oslo (UiO), was used to assess food and nutrient intake during the last year. The questionnaire included measures on frequency and amount of food intake, in addition to open questions. The FFQ was handed out to all Tromsø 7 participants at the examination site and could be completed at the examination site or at home and returned by mail with a prepaid envelope. Estimations of intakes of energy, food, and macro- and micronutrients intake was performed at UiO using the food composition database software system Kostberegningssystemet (KBS, version 7.3), database version AE14, based on the Norwegian Food Composition Tables from 2014 and 2015 [25]. The estimations of iodine intake were done in the AE18 food composition database. Detailed descriptions of the Tromsø 7 FFQ data collection and processing are presented elsewhere [26].

The FFQ was designed to assess habitual diet the preceding year. Frequencies of intake ranged from never, per month, per week, to several times a day, varying with the type of food item in question. Amounts were given in household measures, units of liter, deciliter, a piece, a slice, etc., or as portion sizes. Questions about supplement use were included.

Among the 493 participants included in the urine analysis (see above), 450 participants completed the FFQ and were included in this analysis.

2.2. Urine Analysis

Urine iodine analyses were done at the Hormone Laboratory, Oslo University Hospital, Norway. The UIC was measured colorimetrically using the Sandell–Kolthoff's reaction based on the catalytic effect of iodine on the redox reaction between arsenic and cerium after ammonium persulfate digestion of the samples. Intra- and inter-assay coefficients of variation (CVs) were 8%. The Hormone Laboratory is accredited as a testing laboratory by Norwegian Accreditation according to the standard NS-EN ISO/IEC 17025, with Registration number TEST 099.

Daily urinary iodine excretion (UIE) was calculated using the following formula:

$$\text{24-h UIE (μg/day)} = \text{UIC (μg/L)} \times \text{24-h urine volume (L).} \tag{1}$$

Daily iodine intake (g/day) was estimated using the following formula [20]:

$$\text{Daily 24-h UIE (μg/day)}/0.83. \tag{2}$$

This is based on an estimate of 92% bioavailability and 90% excretion of iodine in an ordinary diet where iodine is in the form of salt and also protein bound.

The median UIC of the participants was compared with the iodine status criteria developed by the WHO, UNICEF, and International Council for the Control of Iodine Deficiency Disorders (ICCIDD) for adults [1].

2.3. Ethics

The study adhered to the tenets of the Declaration of Helsinki and the Norwegian Data Protection Authority. The Regional Committee of Medical and Health Research Ethics North approved Tromsø 7 (REK 2014/940). This substudy was approved by the Regional Committee of Medical and Health Research Ethics (REK 2016/1795). All participants gave written informed consent.

2.4. Statistical Analysis

Analysis of the data was performed using IBM SPSS statistical software (V.22 SPSS Inc., Chicago, IL, USA). Descriptive statistics are presented as mean with standard deviation (SD) and as medians, with 25th and 75th percentiles for variables that were not normally distributed. To compare variables, relevant statistics such as independent samples t-test, Mann–Whitney U Test, and Spearman correlation analysis and regression models were performed. p-values < 0.05 were considered to be statistically significant.

For the comparisons of iodine intake estimated from 24-h urine and FFQ, we used Spearman's correlation coefficient. Bland–Altman plots with limits of agreement were constructed to evaluate whether the difference between estimated iodine intake from 24-h urine and FFQ varied across the mean iodine intake from the two methods and the agreement between the two methods. Two influential points were excluded when testing correlations (extreme outliers that completely changed the direction of the line and gave inflated limits of agreement). We performed additional analysis excluding those who reported that their urine collection was incomplete, completed less than 90% of the FFQ, and participants having very high or low total energy intake (the 1% highest and 1% lowest), in total 190 participants, leaving 303 participants for sensitivity analysis.

3. Results

3.1. Participant Characteristics

The study sample consisted of 493 participants (51% women) with a mean age of 56 years, mean BMI around 27 kg/m^2, and more than 50% had tertiary education (Table 1).

The total mean 24-h creatinine concentration was 9.7 (SD 4.1) mmol/L; men had higher creatinine value than women (11.7 (SD 5.4) and 7.9 (SD 4.6), respectively) ($p < 0.01$).

Table 1. Characteristics of the women and men who collected 24-h urine in the Tromsø Study 2015–2016 ($n = 493$).

	All	Women	Men
Gender, n	493	252	241
Age, years	56 (8.4)	57 (8.4)	55 (8.4)
Primary education (up to 10 yrs.), %	20.4 (100)	21.5 (54)	19.2 (46)
Secondary education (up to 13 yrs.), %	28.3 (139)	27.1 (68)	29.6 (71)
Tertiary education (university), %	51.3 (252)	51.4 (129)	51.2 (123)
Body mass index, kg/m^2	27.2 (4.3)	27.5 (3.7)	26.8 (4.7)

Values are mean (standard deviations) or percentages (numbers). yrs, years.

3.2. Iodine Excretion and Estimated Iodine Intake

The median (25th and 75th percentiles) 24-h urine volume for the study population was 1.69 L (1.3, 2.20) and was not statistically different between women and men ($p = 0.06$) (Table 2). The total 24-h median UIC (25th and 75th percentiles) in all participants was 88 μg/L (38, 100), and 63 and 100 μg/L in women and men, respectively, ($p = 0.14$) (Table 2). Around 16% of the participants (23 and 8% of women and men, respectively) had UIC values below 50 μg/L, while 1.4% had UIC > 600 μg/L.

Table 2. Median and interquartile ranges of 24-h urine volume, 24-h urine iodine concentration (UIC), 24-h iodine excretion (UIE), and 24-h iodine intake by sex and age stratification in men and women aged 40–69 years in the Tromsø Study 2015–2016.

	Total Population	Women (n = 252)			Men (n = 241)		
	All (40–69 Years (n = 493))	All (n = 252)	40–54 Years (n = 112)	55–69 Years (n = 140)	All (n = 241)	40–54 Years (n = 90)	55–69 Years (n = 151)
24-h urine volume (L)							
Mean (SD)	1.74 (0.59)	1.77 (0.60)	1.74 (0.62)	1.79 (0.58)	1.67 (0.57)	1.64 (0.61)	1.70 (0.55)
Median (25th, 75th) *	1.69 (1.31, 2.20)	1.80 (1.29, 2.30)	1.73 (1.24, 2.35)	1.80 (1.36, 2.32)	1.62 (1.27, 2.10)	1.53 (1.13, 2.21)	1.65 (1.32, 2.01)
24-h UIC (µg/L)							
Median (25th, 75th)	88 (50, 125)	63 (50, 100)	63 (38, 100)	75 (50, 113)	100 (63, 150)	88 (63, 125)	100 (63, 153)
24-h UIE (µg/day) #							
Mean (SD)	199 (545)	182 (724)	222 (1079)	150 (116)	214 (247)	150 (96)	253 (297)
Median (25th, 75th) *	132 (87, 200)	111 (78, 170)	102 (79, 149)	117 (75, 184)	145 (108, 234)	132 (95, 176)	168 (113, 265)
24-h iodine intake (µg/day) †							
Mean (SD)	241.6 (670)	222.5 (890)	271.6 (1327)	183.2 (141)	261.6 (302)	182.9 (117)	308.5 (364)
Median (25th, 75th) *	158.9 (106, 245)	133.2 (93, 205)	122.8 (95, 182)	141.1 (91, 223)	174.4 (129, 284)	159.3 (114, 216)	202.9 (135, 321)

* 25th percentile and 75 percentile, # 24-h iodine excretion (µg/day) = UIC (µg/L) × 24-h urine volume (L/day) and † 24-h iodine intake, estimated from 24-h UIE divided by intake/excretion ratio of 0.83.

The median (25th and 75th percentiles) UIE for the study population was 132 (87, 200) µg/day. Men had higher UIE values than women ($p < 0.01$).

The median daily iodine intake for the study population estimated from UIE (on the basis that 83% of ingested iodine is excreted) was 158.9 µg/day (174 in men and 133 µg/day in women, $p < 0.001$) and did not differ significantly with respect to BMI or education levels.

Median iodine intake (estimated from UIE) was significantly higher in men aged 55–69 years as compared with men aged 40–54 years ($p < 0.001$), but no significant age difference was found in women ($p = 0.14$).

3.3. Estimated Iodine Intake from Diet and Supplements (FFQ)

Overall, the estimated daily iodine intake of the 450 participants who completed the FFQ ranged from 38 to 1165 µg/day with a median (25th, 75th percentiles) iodine intake of 281 µg/day (212.5, 378.5). Men had significantly higher iodine intake than women ($p < 0.001$) (Table 3). The iodine intake was still higher among men after adjusting for energy intake (data not shown).

Table 3. Estimated daily habitual iodine intake (µg/day) from food frequency questionnaire in men and women aged 46–69 years, Tromsø Study 2015–2016.

Subgroup	n	Mean (SD)	Median (P25, P75) *
All (40–69 years)	450	314.3 (157.1)	281 (212.5, 378.5)
Women	234	288.1 (142.9)	263 (200, 355.3)
40–54 years	102	271.6 (151.9)	244 (186.5, 328.3)
55–69 years	132	300.8 (142.9)	278.5 (216.3, 371.3)
Men	216	342.7 (166.7)	317.5 (228.3, 407.5)
40–54 years	80	304.6 (133)	295 (215.8, 367.8)
55–69 years	136	365.2 (189.6)	329 (246.3, 447.3)

* 25th and 75th percentile.

In women, 10.7% had iodine intake below the recommended daily intake (150 µg/day), while only 4% had intake below the EAR (100 µg/day) and the proportion of upper intake levels (UL > 600) of iodine intake was 3%.

In men, 7.9% had iodine intake below the recommended daily, almost no men had intake below the EAR intake, while 7.8% had excessive intake.

The estimated iodine intake was significantly higher in the older age group, both in men ($p = 0.01$)) and in women ($p = 0.02$). Iodine intake did not differ significantly with respect to education levels or BMI in men and women.

3.4. Sources of Iodine

Table 4 shows intake of typical iodine source food groups in the study population.

The intake of dairy products and fish was higher among men than women ($p < 0.001$), but there were no differences in egg consumption.

In women, there was a moderate correlation between total iodine intake estimated from diet and intake of milk and milk products (Spearman rank correlation coefficient, r = 0.49, $p < 0.01$), and the Spearman rank correlation coefficient between iodine intake and fish and fish product, and eggs was r = 0.65 ($p < 0.01$) and r = 0.23 ($p < 0.01$), respectively.

In men, the correlation between total iodine intake estimated from diet and intake of milk and milk products was r = 0.47 ($p < 0.01$), intake of fish showed a correlation of r = 0.68 ($p < 0.01$), and intake of eggs showed a correlation of r = 0.17 ($p = 0.01$).

Table 4. Estimated mean intake of dairy products, fish, and eggs among men and women aged 46–69 years, Tromsø Study 2015–2016.

	N	Dairy (g) (Min–Max)	Fish (g) (Min–Max)	Eggs (g) (Min–Max)
All (40–69 yrs)	450	496.6 (0–3061)	119.3 (0–606)	27.1 (0–234)
Women	234	422.6 (0–1957)	108.2 (0–606)	28.3 (0–234)
40–54 (yrs)	102	412.8 (0–1957)	92.1 (0–606)	32.9 (0–234)
55–69 (yrs)	132	430.1 (30–1657)	120.6 (0–375)	24.7 (0–233)
Men	216	576.0 (16–3016)	131.2 (0–489)	25.8 (0–186)
40–54 (yrs)	80	596.7 (16–3061)	107.9 (0–360)	28.0 (0–101)
55–69 (yrs)	136	563.8 (26–1919)	144.9 (10–489)	24.4 (0–186)

Min, Minimum; Max, maxium. yrs, years.

3.5. Supplements

Around 13% ($n = 64$) of the participants reported taking multivitamin and mineral supplements. Among these, 61% ($n = 39$) took the supplements daily. The estimated median iodine intake from diet was 448 µg/day among daily users of dietary supplements, and significantly different ($p < 0.001$) from the median 270 µg/day among no supplement users ($n = 396$).

The median intake of iodine in female ($n = 24$) and male ($n = 15$) daily supplement users was 415 and 488 µg/day, respectively. The median iodine intake was higher in the older age group (490 and 383 µg/day, respectively).

3.6. Relationship between the Two Methods for Estimating Iodine Intake

Among the 450 participants who completed the FFQ and provided a 24-h urine sample, the median iodine intake calculated from the FFQ was significantly higher than the iodine intake estimated from the UIE ($p < 0.001$).

In all participants combined, there was a moderate correlation between total iodine intake estimated from the FFQ and the UIE (Spearman rank correlation coefficient, r = 0.39, $p < 0.01$). The correlation was r = 0.30 ($p < 0.01$) and r = 0.39 ($p < 0.01$) in women and men, respectively.

The differences between paired estimates from UIE and FFQ are plotted against the mean values of the paired estimates (Bland–Altman plot).

The Bland–Altman plots showed that the FFQ overestimated the intake of iodine as compared with the UIE, and that the differences between the methods increased with increasing intakes. The mean differences were 119 (SD 162) µg/day in women and 87 (SD 280) µg/day in men (Figure 1A,B).

3.7. Sensitivity Analyses

In subanalysis, excluding those who reported that their urine collection was incomplete or completed less than 90% of the FFQ, and participants having very high or low total energy intake (the 1% highest and 1% lowest), we found that the estimated intake of iodine, calculated from 24-h urine excretion or the FFQ, was not significantly different from the whole sample (before exclusion). For women, the median daily iodine intake calculated from the UIE was 133.2 and 138.4 µg/day before and after exclusion, respectively. The corresponding figures in men were 174.4 versus 179.5 µg/day. Furthermore, the median daily iodine intake estimated from the FFQ was 263 and 262 µg/day in women and 317.5 and 305 µg/day in men, before and after exclusion, respectively. The median energy intake for women and men was 8.6 and 10.7 MJ/day before exclusion ($n = 450$) and 8.9, and 10.4 MJ/day after exclusion ($n = 303$).

(A)

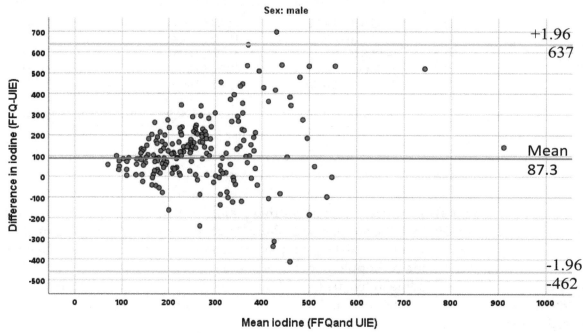

(B)

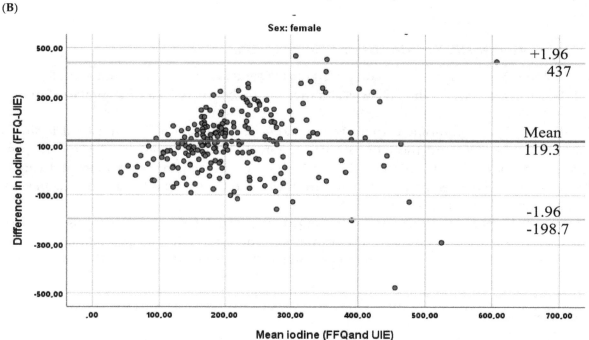

Figure 1. Bland–Altman plot, mean iodine intake estimated from 24 h-urine and the FFQ versus the difference between the methods (FFQ-UIE), in men (**A**) and women (**B**), The vertical line indicates mean difference in iodine intake estimates (red line), with the representation of the limits of agreement (green lines), from −1.96 SD to +1.96 SD.

4. Discussion

In the present study, iodine intake was assessed both by 24-h UIE and by using a FFQ in an adult population aged 40 to 69 years living in Tromsø, Norway. The median iodine intake estimated from 24-h UIE was 159 µg/day (174 and 133 µg/day in men and women, respectively) and, from the FFQ, the median iodine intake was 281 µg/day (317 and 263 µg/day in men and women, respectively). The iodine intake estimated from 24-h UIC describes a mildly iodine deficient female population, while the iodine intake findings based on these two methods indicate that the adult male study population have iodine intake within recommended values.

Inadequate iodine status has been documented in different groups in Norway and in other Nordic countries, mainly pregnant and lactating women [5,15–17], but studies in a representative adult population is still lacking in Norway. However, our findings are in line with what has been found in a recent study on iodine intake in Norway with a convenience sample [9].

4.1. Variation in Iodine Intake by Gender, Age, and Education

The median energy intakes in women and men of 8.6 and 10.7 MJ/day, respectively, are similar to what was observed previously in other Norwegian population-based studies [12,27].

An average higher iodine intake is expected in men as compared with women, because men have higher food and energy intake. In our study, men had 25% higher energy intake and around 20% higher iodine intake as compared with women, even when adjusting for energy intake. These different intakes between men and women are in agreement with earlier studies that showed a low iodine intake among women in Norway [12] and in Switzerland [28].

Compared with the findings from other Norwegian dietary surveys among adult men and women, our population had a relatively higher median intake of iodine [12,29]

Iodine estimated from the FFQ and UIE was significantly higher in men aged 55–69 as compared with those 49–54 years, but this age difference was not found in women. Although a lower intake of iodine among younger women has previously been reported in Norway [29], the reason for our findings is not clear. One explanation can be the small spread in age in this group. The same tendency of age and gender difference in iodine intake, although not significant, have been documented in the Danish population [30]. Furthermore, as previously documented, the iodine intake was not related to education level [31,32].

4.2. Iodine Intake as Compared with Recommendations

To our knowledge, this is the first population-based study among healthy adults in Norway to evaluate how iodine intake estimated from FFQ compares with iodine intake estimated by 24-h urinary iodine excretion.

According to the WHO criteria (assuming that a single 24-h UIC value in reality is the mean of a number of spot urine samples from an individual), iodine deficiency is defined as a population median UIC below 100 μg/L. The UIC, in this study, was 63 and 100 μg/L in women and men, respectively, indicating that iodine nutrition is not likely to be a problem for men but denotes an iodine deficiency among women. Apparently, the proportion of UIC values <50 μg/L was 23% for women, which is above the recommendation that no more than 20% of the participants should be below 50 μg/L. Even when adjusted for the potential dilution effect from large urine volumes of about 1.8 L in women to the normalized mean volume of 1.5 L, the median UIC (76 μg/L) is still below the current WHO criteria [33].

The median UIC among men in this study was higher as compared with Somali immigrant men living in Oslo, who had a 24-h UIC of 63 μg/L, but similar in women [31]. The 24-h UIC in our population was closer to that reported for adults in Norway [9] and in Switzerland [28].

The distribution of intake, calculated from FFQ, was also assessed to determine the proportion of the population below estimated average requirements (EAR) using the EAR cut-point approximation [34]. Around 4% of women and almost none of men had intakes below the EAR of 100 μg/day, indicating adequate iodine intake in men, and very close to adequate intake in women; expecting 2.5% of the population below the cut-off at sufficiency.

Although the results showed a correlation between the two methods, the estimated iodine intake calculated from FFQ was much higher as compared with iodine estimated from UIE. The FFQ dietary assessment of iodine intake aims to measure the average long-term iodine intake from the total habitual diet. Dietary assessment using FFQs largely depends on the participants memory and perceptions [35].

As with all self-reporting dietary data, the present dietary assessment can be affected by an external bias caused by social desirability and memory lapses [36]. The findings also illustrate that the two methods cannot be used interchangeably (Figure 1).

The higher iodine intake, estimated from FFQ analysis in the present study, may at least partly be explained by an over-reporting of healthy food, such as fish intake. The iodine content of the main dietary sources in Norway is well characterized, but for other food groups the food composition data may introduce more uncertainty. In addition, the iodine content in otherwise comparable foods may vary, due to natural variation in soil, water, fertilizers and the use of iodine enrichment. Similar discrepancies of iodine intake estimated from UIC and FFQ methods have been reported [30,37,38].

The large spread in the individual urine volumes in this study is supported by data from other studies [39,40]. Although the participants were informed not to change their daily routines and habits during the urine collection, we are not sure whether our findings represent the habitual urinary volume excretion, or whether participants changed their habits and routines, for example stayed home the day they were collecting urine and therefore drank more fluids. However, excluding persons who stated that they did not collect urine samples fully, hardly affected our results.

4.3. Study Limitations and Strengths

The main strength of this study was the randomly selected sample from a population-based study with high participation, the iodine intake estimated from both FFQ and 24-h urinary iodine excretion, and urine samples being analyzed in one batch. Twenty-four-hour urinary iodine excretion is the most reliable biochemical marker for assessing iodine status. Other strengths in this study was that the data collection was conducted during nine months (August 2015–April 2016), although it did not include the summer months when milk and milk products have a lower iodine concentration than during winter months due to increased use of fortified cattle feed during the winter period [41].

The main limitation of this study is due to day-to-day variation, because the 24-h urine was collected only once, whereas multiple measurements is optimal. Another limitation is the risk of selection bias common in population-based studies, which cannot be ruled out. In addition, the attendance was rather high in the Tromsø Study as compared to many other population-based studies. A comparison between responders and non-responders randomly invited for this substudy showed no statistically significant differences in education levels or BMI. Finally, the FFQ data are self-reported, and thus there is a risk of bias resulting in over-reporting of healthy food such as fish. The other limitation is that the study does not include adults in the age group 18–39 years.

5. Conclusions

The current study on a healthy adult population in Norway shows that iodine intake estimated from 24-h UIC and its derivative measures, describes a mildly iodine deficient female population, while the male population is iodine sufficient. Concurrent use of an extensive FFQ describes both sexes as iodine sufficient.

Further studies, applying a dietary assessment method validated for estimating iodine intake and repeated individual urine collections, are required to determine the habitual iodine intake in this population.

Author Contributions: Performed data analysis and prepared the manuscript, A.A.M.; Methodology, L.A.H., M.H.C., E.H. and H.E.M. All authors critically reviewed the draft, contributed to the interpretation of the findings and approved the final version of the manuscript. All authors have read and agreed to the published version of the manuscript.

Abbreviations

EAR   Estimated Average Requirements
FFQ   Food frequency questionnaire
IDD   Iodine deficiency disorders
RDI   Recommended daily intake
UIC   Urinary iodine concentration
UIE   Urinary iodine excretion
TSH   Thyroid stimulating hormone

References

1. World Health Organization (WHO); United Nations Children's Fund (UNICEF); International Council for Control of Iodine Deficiency Disorders (ICCIDD). *Assessment of the Iodine Deficiency Disorders and Monitoring Their Elimination*, 3rd ed.; World Health Organitzation: Geneva, Switzerland, 2007.
2. Hetzel, B.S. Iodine deficiency disorders (IDD) and their eradication. *Lancet* **1983**, *2*, 1126–1129. [CrossRef]
3. Aburto, N.J.; Abudou, M.; Candeias, V.; Wu, T. *Effect and Safety of Salt Iodization to Prevent Iodine Deficiency Disorders: A Systematic Review with Meta-Analyses*; WHO: Geneva, Switzerland, 2014.
4. Andersson, M.; Karumbunathan, V.; Zimmermann, M.B. Global iodine status in 2011 and trends over the past decade. *J. Nutr.* **2012**, *142*, 744–750. [CrossRef] [PubMed]
5. Nystrom, H.F.; Brantsaeter, A.L.; Erlund, I.; Gunnarsdottir, I.; Hulthen, L.; Laurberg, P.; Mattisson, I.; Rasmussen, L.B.; Virtanen, S.; Meltzer, H.M. Iodine status in the Nordic countries-past and present. *Food Nutr. Res.* **2016**, *60*, 31969. [CrossRef] [PubMed]
6. Lazarus, J.H. Iodine status in europe in 2014. *Eur. Thyroid J.* **2014**, *3*, 3–6. [CrossRef]
7. Mian, C.; Vitaliano, P.; Pozza, D.; Barollo, S.; Pitton, M.; Callegari, G.; di Gianantonio, E.; Casaro, A.; Nacamulli, D.; Busnardo, B.; et al. Iodine status in pregnancy: Role of dietary habits and geographical origin. *Clin. Endocrinol.* **2009**, *70*, 776–780. [CrossRef]
8. Alvarez-Pedrerol, M.; Ribas-Fito, N.; Garcia-Esteban, R.; Rodriguez, A.; Soriano, D.; Guxens, M.; Mendez, M.; Sunyer, J. Iodine sources and iodine levels in pregnant women from an area without known iodine deficiency. *Clin. Endocrinol.* **2010**, *72*, 81–86. [CrossRef]
9. Brantsaeter, A.L.; Knutsen, H.K.; Johansen, N.C.; Nyheim, K.A.; Erlund, I.; Meltzer, H.M.; Henjum, S. Inadequate Iodine Intake in Population Groups Defined by Age, Life Stage and Vegetarian Dietary Practice in a Norwegian Convenience Sample. *Nutrients* **2018**, *10*, 230. [CrossRef]
10. Frey, H.; Tangen, T.; Lovik, J.; Thorsen, R.K.; Sand, T.; Rosenlund, B.; Kornstad, L. Endemic goiter no longer exists in the community of Modum. *Tidsskr. Nor. Laegeforen.* **1981**, *101*, 1184–1186.
11. Dahl, L.; Meltzer, H.M. The Iodine Content of Foods and Diets: Norwegian Perspectives. In *Comprehensive Handbook of Iodine*; Preedy, V.R., Burrow, G.N., Watson, R.R., Eds.; Academic Press: London, UK, 2009; pp. 345–352.
12. Totland, T.H.; Melnæs, B.K.; Lundberg-Hallén, N.; Helland-Kigen, K.M.; Lund-Blix, N.A.; Myhre, J.B.; Johansen, A.M.W.; Løken, E.B.; Andersen, L.F. *Norkost 3 En Landsomfattende Kostholdsundersøkelse Blant Menn og Kvinner i Norge i Alderen 18-70 år, 2010–11*; Helsedirektoratet: Oslo, Norway, 2012.
13. Norwegian Directorate of Health. *Utviklingen i Norsk Kosthold 2015*; IS-2382; Helsedirektoratet: Oslo, Norway, 2015. Available online: https://wwwhelsedirektoratetno/rapporter/utviklingen-i-norsk-kosthold (accessed on 5 September 2020). (In Norwegian)
14. Troan, G.; Dahl, L.; Meltzer, H.M.; Abel, M.H.; Indahl, U.G.; Haug, A.; Prestløkken, E. A model to secure a stable iodine concentration in milk. *Food Nutr. Res.* **2015**, *59*, 29829. [CrossRef]
15. Brantsaeter, A.L.; Abel, M.H.; Haugen, M.; Meltzer, H.M. Risk of suboptimal iodine intake in pregnant Norwegian women. *Nutrients* **2013**, *5*, 424–440. [CrossRef]
16. Henjum, S.; Lilleengen, A.M.; Aakre, I.; Dudareva, A.; Gjengedal, E.L.F.; Meltzer, H.M.; Brantsæter, A.L. Suboptimal Iodine Concentration in Breastmilk and Inadequate Iodine Intake among Lactating Women in Norway. *Nutrients* **2017**, *9*, 643. [CrossRef] [PubMed]
17. Garnweidner-Holme, L.; Aakre, I.; Lilleengen, A.M.; Brantsaeter, A.L.; Henjum, S. Knowledge about Iodine in Pregnant and Lactating Women in the Oslo Area, Norway. *Nutrients* **2017**, *9*, 493. [CrossRef] [PubMed]

18. Meltzer, H.M.; Torheim, L.E.; Brantsæter, A.L.; Madar, A.; Abel, M.H.; Dahl, L. *Risiko for Jodmangel i Norge—Identifisering av et Akutt Behov for Tiltak*; Nasjonalt råd for Ernæring: Oslo, Norway, 2016. Available online: http://wwwernaeringsradetno/wp-content/uploads/2016/06/IS-0591_RisikoForJodmangeliNorgepdf (accessed on 2 July 2020). (In Norwegian)

19. World Health Organization (WHO). *Urinary Iodine Concentrations for Determining Iodine Status in Populations*; (WHO/NMH/NHD/EPG/131); World Health Organization: Geneva, Switzerland, 2013.

20. Zimmermann, M.B.; Andersson, M. Assessment of iodine nutrition in populations: Past, present, and future. *Nutr. Rev.* **2012**, *70*, 553–570. [CrossRef]

21. Ministers NCo. *Nordic Nutrition Recommendations 2012*, 5th ed.; Nordic Council of Ministers: Copenhagen, Denmark, 2012.

22. Tromsøundersøkelsen. Om Tromsøundersøkelsen 2017. Available online: https://uitno/forskning/forskningsgrupper/sub?p_document_id=367276&sub_id=377965 (accessed on 15 August 2020).

23. Meyer, H.E.; Johansson, L.; Eggen, A.E.; Johansen, H.; Holvik, K. Sodium and Potassium Intake Assessed by Spot and 24-h Urine in the Population-Based Tromso Study 2015–2016. *Nutrients* **2019**, *11*, 1619. [CrossRef]

24. Medin, A.C.; Carlsen, M.H.; Hambly, C.; Speakman, J.R.; Strohmaier, S.; Andersen, L.F. The validity of a web-based FFQ assessed by doubly labelled water and multiple 24-h recalls. *Br. J. Nutr.* **2017**, *118*, 1106–1117. [CrossRef]

25. Matportalen. Old tables—The Norwegian Food Compostion Table 2015. Matportalen no. 2015. Available online: https://wwwmatportalenno/verktoy/the_norwegian_food_composition_table/old_tables (accessed on 15 August 2020).

26. Lundblad, M.W.; Andersen, L.F.; Jacobsen, B.K.; Carlsen, M.H.; Hjartaker, A.; Grimsgaard, S.; Hopstock, L.A. Energy and nutrient intakes in relation to National Nutrition Recommendations in a Norwegian population-based sample: The Tromso Study 2015-16. *Food Nutr. Res.* **2019**, *63*. [CrossRef]

27. Johansson, L.; Solvoll, K.N. *Landsomfattende Kostholdsundersøkelse Blant Menn og Kvinner i Alderen 16-79 år (National Dietary Survey Among Males and Females, 16–79 Years)*; National Nutrition and Physical Education Council: Oslo, Norway, 1999.

28. Haldimann, M.; Bochud, M.; Burnier, M.; Paccaud, F.; Dudler, V. Prevalence of iodine inadequacy in Switzerland assessed by the estimated average requirement cut-point method in relation to the impact of iodized salt. *Public Health Nutr.* **2015**, *18*, 1333–1342. [CrossRef]

29. Carlsen, M.H.; Andersen, L.F.; Dahl, L.; Norberg, N.; Hjartaker, A. New Iodine Food Composition Database and Updated Calculations of Iodine Intake among Norwegians. *Nutrients* **2018**, *10*, 930. [CrossRef]

30. Rasmussen, L.B.; Ovesen, L.; Bulow, I.; Jorgensen, T.; Knudsen, N.; Laurberg, P.; Pertild, H. Dietary iodine intake and urinary iodine excretion in a Danish population: Effect of geography, supplements and food choice. *Br. J. Nutr.* **2002**, *87*, 61–69. [CrossRef]

31. Madar, A.A.; Meltzer, H.M.; Heen, E.; Meyer, H.E. Iodine Status among Somali Immigrants in Norway. *Nutrients* **2018**, *10*, 305. [CrossRef] [PubMed]

32. Katagiri, R.; Asakura, K.; Uechi, K.; Masayasu, S.; Sasaki, S. Iodine Excretion in 24-hour Urine Collection and Its Dietary Determinants in Healthy Japanese Adults. *J. Epidemiol.* **2016**, *26*, 613–621. [CrossRef] [PubMed]

33. Censi, S.; Manso, J.; Barollo, S.; Mondin, A.; Bertazza, L.; De Marchi, M.; Mian, C. Changing Dietary Habits in Veneto Region over Two Decades: Still a Long Road to Go to Reach an Iodine-Sufficient Status. *Nutrients* **2020**, *12*, 2399. [CrossRef] [PubMed]

34. Institute of Medicine. *Dietary Reference Intakes for Vitamin A, Vitamin K, Arsenic, Boron, Chromium, Copper, Iodine, Iron, Manganese, Molybdenum, Nickel, Silicon, Vanadium, and Zinc*; National Academy Press: Washington, DC, USA, 2001.

35. Biro, G.; Hulshof, K.F.; Ovesen, L.; Amorim Cruz, J.A. Selection of methodology to assess food intake. *Eur. J. Clin. Nutr.* **2002**, *56* (Suppl. 2), S25–S32. [CrossRef] [PubMed]

36. Althubaiti, A. Information bias in health research: Definition, pitfalls, and adjustment methods. *J. Multidiscip. Healthc.* **2016**, *9*, 211–217. [CrossRef] [PubMed]

37. Xu, C.; Guo, X.; Tang, J.; Guo, X.; Lu, Z.; Zhang, J.; Bi, Z. Iodine nutritional status in the adult population of Shandong Province (China) prior to salt reduction program. *Eur. J. Nutr.* **2016**, *55*, 1933–1941. [CrossRef] [PubMed]

38. Bath, S.C.; Sleeth, M.L.; McKenna, M.; Walter, A.; Taylor, A.; Rayman, M.P. Iodine intake and status of UK women of childbearing age recruited at the University of Surrey in the winter. *Br. J. Nutr.* **2014**, *112*, 1715–1723. [CrossRef] [PubMed]

39. Fitzgerald, M.P.; Stablein, U.; Brubaker, L. Urinary habits among asymptomatic women. *Am. J. Obstet. Gynecol.* **2002**, *187*, 1384–1388. [CrossRef] [PubMed]

40. Perucca, J.; Bouby, N.; Valeix, P.; Bankir, L. Sex difference in urine concentration across differing ages, sodium intake, and level of kidney disease. *Am. J. Physiol. Regul. Integr. Comp. Physiol.* **2007**, *292*, R700–R705. [CrossRef]

41. Dahl, L.; Opsahl, J.A.; Meltzer, H.M.; Julshamn, K. Iodine concentration in Norwegian milk and dairy products. *Br. J. Nutr.* **2003**, *90*, 679–685. [CrossRef]

3

Low-Salt Intake Suggestions in Hypertensive Patients do not Jeopardize Urinary Iodine Excretion

Natale Musso *[ID], Lucia Conte, Beatrice Carloni, Claudia Campana, Maria C. Chiusano and Massimo Giusti

Centre for Secondary Hypertension, Unit of Clinical Endocrinology, Department of Internal Medicine, University of Genoa Medical School, IRCCS Ospedale Policlinico San Martino, 16132 Genova, Italy; luciaconte88@hotmail.it (L.C.); beatrice.carloni@gmail.com (B.C.); claudiadindon@hotmail.it (C.C.); mcristinachiusano@libero.it (M.C.C.); magius@unige.it (M.G.)
* Correspondence: natale.musso@hsanmartino.it

Abstract: A low-sodium diet is an essential part of the treatment of hypertension. However, some concerns have been raised with regard to the possible reduction of iodine intake during salt restriction. We obtained 24-h urine collections for the evaluation of iodine (UIE) and sodium excretion (UNaV) from 136 hypertensive patients, before and after 9 ± 1 weeks of a simple low-sodium diet. Body mass index (BMI), blood pressure (BP), and drug consumption (DDD) were recorded. Data are average $\pm$ SEM. Age was 63.6 ± 1.09 year. BMI was 25.86 ± 0.40 kg/m^2 before the diet and 25.38 ± 0.37 kg/m^2 after the diet ($p < 0.05$). UNaV decreased from 150.3 ± 4.01 mEq/24-h to 122.8 ± 3.92 mEq/24-h ($p < 0.001$); UIE decreased from 186.1 ± 7.95 µg/24-h to 175.0 ± 7.74 µg/24-h (p = NS); both systolic and diastolic BP values decreased (by 6.15 ± 1.32 mmHg and by 3.75 ± 0.84 mmHg, respectively, $p < 0.001$); DDD decreased (ΔDDD 0.29 ± 0.06, $p < 0.05$). UNaV and UIE were related both before ($r = 0.246$, $p = 0.0040$) and after the diet ($r = 0.238$, $p = 0.0050$). UNaV and UIE were significantly associated both before and after the diet ($p < 0.0001$ for both). After salt restriction UIE showed a non-significant decrease remaining in an adequate range. Our dietary suggestions were aimed at avoiding preserved foods, whereas the cautious use of table salt was permitted, an approach which seems safe in terms of iodine intake.

Keywords: blood pressure; dietary sodium; hypertension; iodine; salt

1. Introduction

A low-salt diet constitutes a standard approach to the treatment of hypertensive patients [1–4]. Salt is the fundamental source of dietary sodium, an excess of which is linked to hypertension and cardiovascular diseases [5–7]. While reducing excess dietary sodium is universally acknowledged to be a favorable step in the reduction of cardiovascular risk [1–4], the recommendation of a low-sodium approach in the general population is still controversial [8]. Recently, a J-shaped curve linking sodium intake to cardiovascular events has been proposed [9,10], pointing to a possible risk induced by a decreased sodium intake in the general population. However, these data have been disputed [11].

In Italy iodine supplementation was first undertaken in 1921 and iodized salt was introduced by regulatory authorities in 1924 [12]. Since then, substantial progress has been made in the struggle against iodine deficiency [13]. Nevertheless a mild insufficiency persists [14] and only recently (Law n.55/2005) was a nationwide salt iodization program implemented [15].

The main concern raised by the reduction of sodium intake regards the possible deficiency of iodine intake during a low-sodium diet [16]. In hypertensive patients in whom iodine status (IS) has been evaluated by 24-h urinary iodine excretion (UIE) or by spot urine iodine concentration (UIC), or by anamnestic instruments such as 24-h dietary recalls or food frequency questionnaires (FFQ), no general consensus has emerged [17,18]. This may partly stem from the different methods employed, the greatest limitation being associated with anamnestic evaluation [19] and with the variability of spot urine measurements versus the gold standard of UIE [20,21]. Another issue concerns the general approach of studies in which sodium and iodine intake have been evaluated, in accordance with an observational protocol, whereby it is assumed that patients displaying a reduction in urinary sodium excretion are following a low-sodium diet, while those displaying no reduction are not [22,23]. Few intervention studies have shown adequate levels of iodine intake after salt restrictions [24,25].

An additional problem arises from the type of population examined. As a general rule, when an iodine-sufficient population is studied, patients on a low-sodium diet show reduced UIC/UIE, but no substantial change in IS [26]. When iodine-deficient patients follow a low-sodium diet, IS worsens [17,27].

In Italy, these concerns have already been raised [28]. Iodine deficiency leads to endemic goiter and cretinism, because iodine is essential for the synthesis of thyroid hormones. In our country public committees were appointed since the first half of the XIX century, for the identification of areas of endemic goiter and endemic cretinism, mostly in the north-western and insular areas [15]. Since then, many epidemiological evidences showed that iodine deficiency is present in mountain as well as in coastal regions [15]. Although our district, the Liguria Region, is situated in a country of mild iodine deficiency, it has recently become iodine-sufficient [29].

The aim of the present study was to evaluate the modification of UIE induced by a proposed low-sodium diet in hypertensive patients. Urinary iodine excretion and 24-h urinary sodium excretion (UNaV) were measured by standard methods before and after the administration of a dietary protocol.

2. Materials and Methods

In a larger cohort of 291 hypertensive patients [30], we obtained a 24-h urine collection (above at least 700 mL) from 157 patients for UIE and UNaV evaluation (basal value: time t0), together with BMI and blood pressure (BP) measurements. A low-sodium diet was then proposed. After 9 ± 1 weeks (mean $\pm$ SD) we repeated the 24-h urine collection (time t2), BMI recording, and BP measurements.

The low-sodium diet prescribed by a dietitian was based on simple recommendations printed on a single A4 sheet of paper [30]. Patients were advised to avoid salty foods, ice-cream, cheese, and cured meats, such as bacon, ham, sausages, and so on. Low-sodium bottled water was recommended. The patients were also asked to switch from regular bread to salt-free bread, which is commonly available in Italy. Table salt itself was not banned, although limited use was suggested [30].

Twenty-four hour urines were collected in accordance with a standard protocol: after the first morning void (to be discarded) patients were requested to record the time and to collect every subsequent void until the same time the following day, when they had to collect the content of the last void. All patients received written and verbal instructions, together with the appropriate urine containers.

Blood pressure was measured by means of a semi-automated repeated-measures method (HEM 907 BP monitor, OMRON, Kyoto, Japan) as previously described [30] both at t0 and at t2. Blood pressure was measured three times at each visit and the last value (BP3) was considered for analysis. Body weight and BMI were obtained both at t0 and at t2. Anti-hypertensive drugs (as defined daily doses-DDD following the WHO definitions) [31] were recorded both at t0 and at t2. Halfway between the two visits, patients were suggested to have their BP evaluated by their general practitioner (who was aware of the study but blind to the results), which adjusted their drug treatment, if necessary [30].

UNaV was measured by an AutoAnalyzer (COBAS 8000 Roche/Hitachi with an ISE module; Roche Diagnostics, Indianapolis, IN, USA), while urinary iodine was measured by means of a current commercial colorimetric method (Celltech, Turin, Italy) all CVs are below 8%.

All patients were on anti-hypertensive drug treatment. Patients on thyroid hormones, amiodarone or with a recent history of contrast-media exposure were excluded. Patients unable or unwilling to provide two (t0 and t2) 24-h urine collections (i.e., those with less than 700 mL of urines and/or violation of void collection), or with concomitant diseases such as congestive heart failure, atrial fibrillation, renal failure, diabetes, electrolyte abnormalities, secondary hypertension, or goiter were deemed ineligible.

Finally, 136 patients, who had successfully provided 24-h urine collections twice in a two months period, were selected. Neither FFQ nor 24-h dietary recalls were used. The study population consisted of Caucasian Europeans, 98%, and Latin Americans, 2%. Of the 136 patients, 84 (61.76%) claimed to use iodized table salt routinely, in agreement with our national data [15]. All subjects gave their informed consent for inclusion before they participated in the study. The study was conducted in accordance with the Declaration of Helsinki, and the protocol was approved by the Ethics Committee of our Hospital.

Statistics

Statistical analysis was performed using a commercial software package: PRISM 7.0 (Graph Pad Software, La Jolla, CA, USA). Paired Student's *t*-test, non-parametric analysis (Mann-Whitney, or *t*-test with Welch correction, followed by F-test to compare variances), repeated-measures ANOVA followed by multiple-comparison Newman-Keuls post-test, Kruskal-Wallis test (with Dunn's multiple comparison test), one-way ANOVA followed by Bartlett's test for equal variances, linear regression analysis, Fisher's exact test and Chi-square test were carried out. The significance cut-off was set at $p < 0.05$.

3. Results

Data are reported throughout as average ± SEM unless otherwise stated.

Patients were 83 females and 53 males. Their mean age was 63.6 ± 1.09 year.

Our intervention consisted of proposing a simple low-sodium protocol. The time-span between the administration of the dietary protocol (visit at time t0) and the final visit (time t2) was 9 ± 0.12 weeks:

- BMI was 25.86 ± 0.40 kg/m^2 before the dietary suggestions (visit t0) and 25.38 ± 0.37 kg/m^2 afterwards (visit t2) (*t*-test and repeated-measures ANOVA and Newman-Keuls post-test, $p < 0.05$).
- UNaV decreased from 150.3 ± 4.01 mEq/24-h at visit t0 to 122.8 ± 3.92 mEq/24-h at visit t2 (repeated-measures ANOVA and post-test, $p < 0.001$).
- Both systolic and diastolic BP values decreased significantly from visit t0 to visit t2 (by 6.15 ± 1.32 mmHg and by 3.75 ± 0.94 mmHg, respectively. ANOVA and post-test, $p < 0.001$) (Figure 1).
- Drug consumption also decreased from visit t0 to visit t2 (ΔDDD 0.29 ± 0.06, *t*-test, $p < 0.05$).
- Median UIE global values were 184.2 µg/24-h (lower and upper 95% CI 170.3 and 201.9) at t0, and 162.0 µg/24-h (lower and upper 95% CI 159.6 and 190.3) at t2.
- Median UIE values in females were 178.2 µg/24-h (lower and upper 95% CI 163.0 and 204.3) at t0, and 153.7 µg/24-h (lower and upper 95% CI 151.3 and 188.5) at t2.
- Median UIE values in males were 188.0 µg/24-h (lower and upper 95% CI 164.9 and 215.2) at t0, and 170.0 µg/24-h (lower and upper 95% CI 155.9 and 210.5) at t2. One way ANOVA (F = 0.6105, *R* square 0.006788) showed non-significant differences between UIE values in males vs. females both before and after the diet period ($p = 0.6087$). Bartlett's test for equal variances gave non-significant results (Bartlett's statistics 1.449, $p = 0.6940$, Newman-Keuls multiple comparison test $p > 0.05$).
- UIE was below 100 µg/24-h in 28 patients before the suggested diet, and in 28 patients thereafter (Fisher's exact test: $p = $ NS; Chi-square, df: 0.0, 1; $p = $ NS).
- UIE decreased from 186.1 ± 7.95 µg/24-h at visit t0, to 175.0 ± 7.74 µg/24-h at visit t2 (repeated-measures ANOVA and post-test, $p = $ NS). Furthermore, these data were reanalyzed with non-parametric tests (Mann-Whitney, or Welch correction, $t = 1.002$, df = 269, 95% C.I. −10.67 to +32.97), to avoid distributional assumptions (again, differences were non-significant: $p = 0.2737$ to $p = 0.3173$). A possible UIE variability induced by the dietary suggestions was challenged with an

F test to compare variances before and after the observation period. F test showed non-significant differences (F, DFn, Dfd, 1057, 135, 135; $p = 0.7484$).

- Significant relationships were found between UNaV and UI both before the administration of the protocol, at visit t0 ($r = 0.246$, $p = 0.004$) (Figure 2) and after, at visit t2 ($r = 0.238$, $p = 0.005$) (Figure 3).
- UNaV and UIE were significantly associated both before and after the dietary suggestions (Chi-square test; df at t0 75.55, 1; df at t2 205.6, 1; $p < 0.0001$ for both).

-

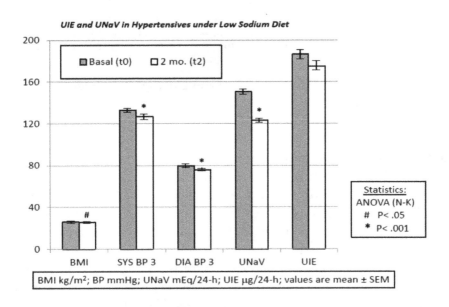

Figure 1. Main Data. $n = 136$ pts, 83 females and 53 males. ANOVA followed by Newman-Keuls post-test for repeated measures. Data are reported as mean and SD.

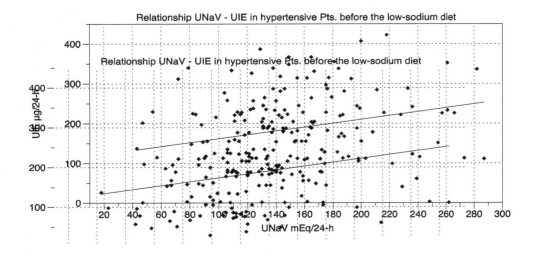

Figure 2. Relationship between UNaV (mEq/24-h) and UIE (g/24-h) before the diet period (time t0). Statistics: $r = 0.246$; $p = 0.004$.

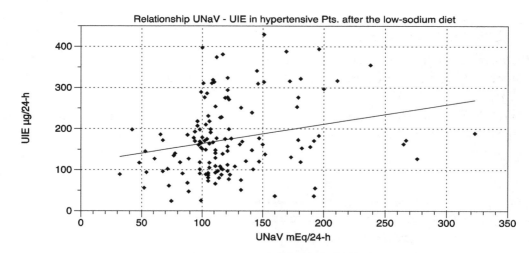

Figure 3. Relationship between UNaV (mEq/24-h) and UIE (µg/24-h) after the diet period (time t2). Statistics: $r = 0.238$; $p = 0.005$.

4. Discussion

The proposed low-sodium diet induced a significant reduction in UNaV, BMI, BP, and DDD in our patients. Urinary iodine excretion showed a small, non-significant decrease.

We did not monitor the actual diet in our patients, because of the inherent limits of FFQ and 24-h recall methods [19]. Instead, we relied on the UNaV, which is usually considered the gold standard for the assessment of the sodium content of a diet [19]. Similarly, we relied on the UIE as a reference index of iodine intake [20,21].

In our patients we did not evaluate urinary creatinine excretion, which is of limited value as a measure of the completeness of 24-h collection [32,33], because of the high variability of creatinine in urine, with a reported SD as high as 29 to 79% of the mean [32,34], with sensitivity and specificity for identifying incomplete collections as low as 6% and 57%, respectively [35]. Instead, we relied on the total 24-h urine volumes, with a high cut-off of 700 mL [30].

In our patients, the decrease in UNaV after the dietary suggestions was paralleled by significant improvements in BMI and BP values, with an additional significant decrease in drug consumption.

Our patients seemed to follow our suggestions, apparently reducing their sodium intake from (150.3 mEq × 23 =) 3.46 g/day, which is equivalent to 8.78 g/day of salt, to (122.8 mEq × 23 =) 2.82 g/day, which is equivalent to 7.17 g/day of salt. This small but significant decrease, albeit lower than that suggested in the Guidelines [1–4], yielded a significant improvement in our patients' BP values (even more important in light of their reduced drug intake), once again displaying the favorable effect of a low-sodium approach to arterial pressure control.

This effective UNaV reduction did not appear to affect UIE, which showed a non-significant reduction from 186.1 to 175.0 µg/24-h. The approximate iodine intake thus decreased from (186.1/0.92 =) 202.3 µg/day, to (175.0/0.92 =) 190.2 µg/day [25,36].

The number of iodine-deficient patients (UIE below 100 µg/24-h) did not change from the basal observation to the final visit (28/136 to 28/136, i.e., 20.59%).

Our data agree with previously published findings, which indicate that reducing sodium consumption in an iodine-sufficient population does not compromise iodine intake [26]. In our hypertensive patients, a successful intervention (in the form of dietary salt intake suggestions) was followed by favorable effects in terms of UNaV, BMI, and BP reduction (even with a reduction in the need for drugs).

Our instructions do not appear to induce a substantial nor significant decrease in iodine intake, and the number of iodine-deficient subjects did not change substantially, nor significantly (actually, it did not change at all). Differences between females and males were non-significant.

In Italy, the primary source of salt is not processed or canned food (the use of which remains negligible), nor the amount of salt added at the table or during cooking; rather, it is constituted by three categories of food: bread, cheese, and cured meats [37]. The aim of our dietary suggestions was to reduce sodium intake, while minimizing the iodine decrease. On our market, sales of iodized table salt have risen to a current level of the 60% [15]. Although our district, the Liguria Region, has recently achieved iodine sufficiency, Italy (as noted in the Introduction) suffers from mild iodine deficiency [29]. This situation is reflected in our data, which showed average iodine sufficiency (average UIE 186.1 µg/24-h, median UIE 184.2 µg/24-h; lower and upper 95% CI 170.3 and 201.9 before the dietary suggestions), but with 20% of iodine-deficient subjects (UIE < 100 µg/24-h). Efforts to reduce salt intake in our country must take this fragile IS into account. This is why our suggestions were aimed at reducing the main sources of salt (bread, cheese, and cured meats), whereas table salt was not banned; we therefore managed not to cut a possible main source of iodine.

The fact that UNaV and UIE were significantly related and associated, both before and after the administration of the diet protocol, suggests a possible common source of both sodium and iodine; given that the three salty foods had been excluded from the dietary protocol, this common source was presumably table salt. Our results support this view: the non-significant decrease in UIE seen in our patients seems to fit in with the current low use of iodized salt (3–8%) by the Italian food industry [28], with the implication that table salt remains the main source of iodine in our country [28].

5. Conclusions

In an area of iodine sufficiency, albeit in a mild iodine-deficient country, where table salt is the main source of iodine, a low-sodium approach which primarily limits the salty foods (instead of a "no salt added" suggestion) seems safe in terms of iodine intake, and does not worsen the IS.

Author Contributions: Conceptualization: M.G. and N.M.; Methodology: N.M., B.C., M.C.C.; Investigation and Data Curation: N.M., B.C., C.C., M.C.C.; Formal Analysis and Writing-Original Draft Preparation: N.M., L.C., M.G.; Writing-Review and Editing: N.M.; Supervision: M.G.

References

1. James, P.A.; Oparil, S.; Carter, B.L.; Cushman, W.C.; Dennison-Himmelfarb, C.; Handler, J.; Lackland, D.T.; LeFevre, M.L.; MacKenzie, T.D.; Ogedegbe, O.; et al. 2014 Evidence-Based Guideline for the Management of High Blood Pressure in Adults: Report From the Panel Members Appointed to the Eighth Joint National Committee (JNC 8). *JAMA* **2014**, *311*, 507–520. [CrossRef] [PubMed]
2. Van Horn, L.; Carson, J.A.S.; Appel, L.J.; Burke, L.E.; Economos, C.; Karmally, W.; Lancaster, K.; Lichtenstein, A.H.; Johnson, R.K.; Thomas, R.J.; et al. Recommended dietary pattern to achieve adherence to the American Heart Association/American College of Cardiology (AHA/ACC) Guidelines: A scientific statement from the American Heart Association. *Circulation* **2016**, *134*, e505–e529. [CrossRef] [PubMed]
3. Whelton, P.K.; Carey, R.M.; Aronow, W.S.; Casey, D.E., Jr.; Collins, K.J.; Dennison Himmelfarb, C.; DePalma, S.M.; Gidding, S.; Jamerson, K.A.; Jones, D.W.; et al. 2017 ACC/AHA/AAPA/ABC/ACPM/AGS/APhA/ASH/ASPC/NMA/PCNA Guideline for the Prevention, Detection, Evaluation, and Management of High Blood Pressure in Adults. *Hypertension* **2018**. [CrossRef]
4. Williams, B.; Mancia, G.; Spiering, W.; Agabiti Rosei, E.; Azizi, M.; Burnier, M.; Clement, D.L.; Coca, A.; de Simone, G.; Dominiczak, A.; et al. 2018 ESC/ESH Guidelines for the management of arterial hypertension. *Eur. Heart J.* **2018**, *39*, 3021–3104. [CrossRef] [PubMed]
5. Strazzullo, P.; D'Elia, L.; Kandala, N.B.; Cappuccio, F.P. Salt intake, stroke, and cardiovascular disease: Meta-analysis of prospective studies. *BMJ* **2009**, *339*, b4567. [CrossRef] [PubMed]
6. He, F.J.; MacGregor, G.A. Salt reduction lowers cardiovascular risk: Meta-analysis of outcome trials. *Lancet* **2011**, *378*, 380–382. [CrossRef]

7.   Taylor, R.S.; Ashton, K.E.; Moxham, T.; Hooper, L.; Ebrahim, S. Reduced dietary salt for the prevention of cardiovascular disease: A meta-analysis of randomized controlled trials (Cochrane review). *Am. J. Hypertens.* **2011**, *24*, 843–853. [CrossRef] [PubMed]

8.   Bram, B.; Huang, X.; Cupples, W.A.; Hamza, S.M. Understanding the two faces of low-salt intake. *Curr. Hypertens. Rep.* **2017**, *19*, 49. [CrossRef] [PubMed]

9.   Graudal, N.; Jurgens, G.; Baslund, B.; Alderman, M.H. Compared with usual sodium intake, low- and excessive-sodium diets are associated with increased mortality: A meta-analysis. *Am. J. Hypertens.* **2014**, *27*, 1129–1137. [CrossRef] [PubMed]

10.   O'Donnell, M.; Mente, A.; Rangarajan, S.; McQueen, M.J.; Wang, X.; Liu, L.; Yan, H.; Lee, S.F.; Mony, P.; Devanath, A.; et al. Urinary sodium and potassium excretion, mortality, and cardiovascular events. *N. Engl. J. Med.* **2014**, *371*, 612–623. [CrossRef] [PubMed]

11.   Oparil, S. Low sodium intake-Cardiovascular health benefit or risk? *N. Engl. J. Med.* **2014**, *371*, 677–679. [CrossRef] [PubMed]

12.   Kimball, O.P. Endemic goiter and public health. *Am. J. Public Health Nations Health* **1928**, *18*, 587–601. [CrossRef] [PubMed]

13.   Bath, S.C. The challenges of harmonising the iodine supply across Europe. *Lancet Diabetes Endocrinol.* **2017**, *5*, 411–412. [CrossRef]

14.   Lazarus, J.H. Iodine status in Europe in 2014. *Eur. Thyroid J.* **2014**, *3*, 3–6. [CrossRef] [PubMed]

15.   Olivieri, A.; Di Cosmo, C.; De Angelis, S.; Da Cas, R.; Stacchini, P.; Pastorelli, A.; Vitti, P. Regional Observatory for Goiter Prevention. The way forward in Italy for iodine. *Minerva Med.* **2017**, *108*, 159–168. [PubMed]

16.   World Health Organization. *Salt Reduction and Iodine Fortification Strategies in Public Health*; World Health Organization: Geneva, Switzerland, 2014.

17.   Tayie, F.A.; Jourdan, K. Hypertension, dietary salt restriction and iodine deficiency among adults. *Am. J. Hypertens.* **2010**, *23*, 1095–1102. [CrossRef] [PubMed]

18.   Pearce, E.N.; Andersson, M.; Zimmermann, M.B. Global iodine nutrition: Where do we stand in 2013? *Thyroid* **2013**, *23*, 523–528. [CrossRef] [PubMed]

19.   McLean, R.M.; Farmer, V.L.; Nettleton, A.; Cameron, C.M.; Cook, N.R.; Campbell, N.R.C.; TRUE Consortium. Assessment of dietary sodium intake using food frequency questionnaires and 24-hour urinary sodium excretion: A systematic literature review. *J. Clin. Hypertens.* **2017**, *19*, 1214–1230. [CrossRef] [PubMed]

20.   Ji, C.; Lu, T.; Dary, O.; Legetic, B.; Campbell, N.R.; Cappuccio, F.P. Systematic review of studies evaluating urinary iodine concentration as a predictor of 24 hour urinary iodine excretion for estimating population iodine intake. *Rev. Panam. Salud Publica* **2015**, *38*, 73–81. [PubMed]

21.   Conkle, J.; van der Haar, F. The use and interpretation of sodium concentrations in casual (spot) urine collections for population surveillance and partitioning of dietary iodine intake sources. *Nutrients* **2017**, *9*, 7. [CrossRef] [PubMed]

22.   Charlton, K.E.; Jooste, P.L.; Steyn, K.; Levitt, N.S.; Ghosh, A. A lowered salt intake does not compromise iodine status in Capetown, South Africa, where salt iodization is mandatory. *Nutrition* **2013**, *29*, 630–634. [CrossRef] [PubMed]

23.   Ahn, J.; Lee, J.H.; Lee, J.; Baek, J.Y.; Song, E.; Oh, H.S.; Kim, M.; Park, S.; Jeon, M.J.; Kim, T.Y.; et al. Association between urinary sodium levels and iodine status in Korea. *Korean J. Int. Med.* **2018**. [CrossRef] [PubMed]

24.   Simpson, F.O.; Thaler, B.I.; Paulin, J.M.; Phelan, E.L.; Cooper, G.J. Iodide excretion in a salt-restriction trial. *N. Z. Med. J.* **1984**, *97*, 890–893. [PubMed]

25.   He, F.J.; Ma, Y.; Feng, X.; Zhang, W.; Lin, L.; Guo, X.; Zhang, J.; Niu, W.; Wu, Y.; MacGregor, G.A. Effect of salt reduction on iodine status assessed by 24 hour urinary iodine excretion in children and their families in northern China: A substudy of a cluster randomised controlled trial. *BMJ Open* **2016**, *6*, e011168. [CrossRef] [PubMed]

26.   Vega-Vega, O.; Fonseca-Correa, J.I.; Mendoza-De la Garza, A.; Rincon-Pedrero, R.; Espinosa-Cuevas, A.; Baeza-Arias, Y.; Dary, O.; Herrero-Bervera, B.; Nieves-Anaya, I.; Correa-Rotter, R. Contemporary dietary intake: Too much sodium, not enough potassium, yet sufficient iodine: The SALMEX Cohort study. *Nutrients* **2018**, *10*, 816. [CrossRef] [PubMed]

27.   Charlton, K.; Ware, L.J.; Baumgartner, J.; Cockeran, M.; Schutte, A.E.; Naidoo, N.; Kowal, P. How will South Africa's mandatory salt reduction policy affect its salt iodisation programme? A cross-sectional analysis from the WHO-SAGE Wave 2 Salt & Tobacco study. *BMJ Open* **2018**, *8*, e020404. [PubMed]

28. Pastorelli, A.A.; Stacchini, P.; Olivieri, A. Daily iodine intake and the impact of salt reduction on iodine prophylaxis in the Italian population. *Eur. J. Clin. Nutr.* **2015**, *69*, 211–215. [CrossRef] [PubMed]

29. Monitoring of the Nationwide Program of Iodine Prophylaxis in Italy. Available online: http://old.iss.it/binary/publ/cont/14_6_web.pdf (accessed on 15 August 2018).

30. Musso, N.; Carloni, B.; Chiusano, M.C.; Giusti, M. Simple dietary advice reduces 24-hour urinary sodium excretion, blood pressure, and drug consumption in hypertensive patients. *J. Am. Soc. Hypertens.* **2018**, *12*, 652–659. [CrossRef] [PubMed]

31. WHO Collaborating Centre for Drug Statistics Methodology. *Guidelines for ATC Classification and DDD Assignment*; Norwegian Institute of Public Health: Oslo, Norway, 2017.

32. Greenblatt, D.J.; Ransil, B.J.; Harmatz, J.S.; Smith, T.W.; Duhme, D.W.; Koch-Weser, J. Variability of 24-hour urinary creatinine excretion by normal subjects. *J. Clin. Pharmacol.* **1976**, *16*, 321–328. [CrossRef] [PubMed]

33. Sawant, P.D.; Kumar, S.A.; Wankhede, S.; Rao, D.D. Creatinine as a normalization factor to estimate the representativeness of urine sample. Intra-subject and inter-subject variability studies. *Appl. Radiat. Isot.* **2018**, *136*, 121–126. [CrossRef] [PubMed]

34. Murakami, K.; Sasaki, S.; Takahashi, Y.; Uenishi, K.; Watanabe, T.; Kohri, T.; Yamasaki, M.; Watanabe, R.; Baba, K.; Shibata, K.; et al. Sensitivity and specificity of published strategies using urinary creatinine to identify incomplete 24-h urine collection. *Nutrition* **2008**, *24*, 16–22. [CrossRef] [PubMed]

35. John, K.A.; Cogswell, M.E.; Campbell, N.R.; Nowson, C.A.; Legetic, B.; Hennis, A.J.M.; Patel, S.M. Accuracy and usefulness of select methods for assessing complete collection of 24-hour urine: A systematic review. *J. Clin. Hypertens.* **2016**, *18*, 456–467. [CrossRef] [PubMed]

36. Nath, S.K.; Moinier, B.; Thuillier, F.; Rongier, M.; Desjeux, J.F. Urinary excretion of iodide and fluoride from supplemented food grade salt. *Int. J. Vitam. Nutr. Res.* **1992**, *62*, 66–72. [PubMed]

37. WHO-Salt Reduction. Available online: https://www.who.int/news-room/fact-sheets/detail/salt-reduction (accessed on 15 August 2018).

4

Iodine Status Assessment in South African Adults According to Spot Urinary Iodine Concentrations, Prediction Equations and Measured 24-h Iodine Excretion

Karen E. Charlton [1,2,*] (iD), Lisa J. Ware [3,4] (iD), Jeannine Baumgartner [5], Marike Cockeran [6], Aletta E. Schutte [3,7] (iD), Nirmala Naidoo [8] and Paul Kowal [8,9]

[1] School of Medicine, University of Wollongong, Wollongong 2500, New South Wales, Australia
[2] Illawarra Health and Medical Institute, University of Wollongong, Wollongong 2500, New South Wales, Australia
[3] Hypertension in Africa Research Team (HART), North-West University, Potchefstroom 2531, North West Province, South Africa; lisa.jayne.ware@gmail.com (L.J.W.); alta.schutte@nwu.ac.za (A.E.S.)
[4] MRC/Wits Developmental Pathways for Health Research Unit, University of the Witwatersrand, Johannesburg 2193, Gauteng, South Africa
[5] Centre of Excellence for Nutrition (CEN), North-West University, Potchefstroom 2531, North West Province, South Africa; jeannine.baumgartner@nwu.ac.za
[6] Statistical Consultation Services, North-West University, 11 Hoffman Street, Potchefstroom; Private Bag X6001, Potchefstroom 2520, North West Province, South Africa; Marike.Cockeran@nwu.ac.za
[7] MRC Research Unit for Hypertension and Cardiovascular Disease, North-West University, Potchefstroom 2531, North West Province, South Africa
[8] World Health Organization (WHO), Avenue Appia 20, CH-1211 Geneva 27, Switzerland; naidoon@who.int (N.N.); kowalp@who.int (P.K.)
[9] Research Centre for Generational Health and Ageing, University of Newcastle, Newcastle 2308, New South Wales, Australia
* Correspondence: karenc@uow.edu.au

Abstract: The iodine status of populations is conventionally assessed using spot urinary samples to obtain a median urinary iodine concentration (UIC) value, which is assessed against standard reference cut-offs. The assumption that spot UIC reflects daily iodine intake may be flawed because of high day-to-day variability and variable urinary volume outputs. This study aimed to compare iodine status in a sample of South African adults when determined by different approaches using a spot urine sample (median UIC (MUIC), predicted 24 h urinary iodine excretion (PrUIE) using different prediction equations) against measured 24 h urinary iodine excretion (mUIE). Both 24 h and spot urine samples were collected in a subsample of participants (n = 457; median age 55 year; range 18–90 year) in the World Health Organization Study on global AGEing and adult health (SAGE) Wave 2 in South Africa, in 2015. Kawasaki, Tanaka, and Mage equations were applied to assess PrUIE from predicted urinary creatinine (PrCr) and spot UIC values. Adequacy of iodine intake was assessed by comparing PrUIE and mUIE to the Estimated Average Requirement of 95 µg/day, while the MUIC cut-off was <100 µg/L. Bland Altman plots assessed the level of agreement between measured and predicted UIE. Median UIC (130 µg/L) indicated iodine sufficiency. The prediction equations had unacceptable bias for PrUIE compared to measured UIE. In a sample of adult South Africans, the use of spot UIC, presented as a group median value (MUIC) provided similar estimates of inadequate iodine status, overall, when compared to EAR assessed using measured 24 h iodine excretion (mUIE). Continued use of MUIC as a biomarker to assess the adequacy of population iodine intake appears warranted.

Keywords: iodine; median urinary concentration; 24 h urine collection; prediction equations; agreement; estimated average requirement

1. Introduction

Iodine deficiency is the largest preventable cause of brain damage and mental impairment worldwide. Populations that consume diets that contain small amounts of fish and seafood, moderate to low quantities of milk and dairy products, and include locally produced fruits and vegetables grown in iodine-poor soils are likely to be iodine deficient. For this reason, in order to prevent iodine deficiency disorders, the World Health Organization (WHO) recommends universal salt iodization (USI), where all salt for human and animal consumption is iodized [1].

Three quarters of the world's population in 2016, in a total of 130 countries, was estimated to use iodized salt [2,3]. The 2016 global estimate of iodine nutrition, based on surveys of school-age children conducted between 2002 and 2016, showed that iodine intake is insufficient in 15 countries, sufficient in 102, and excessive in 10 countries [4,5]. This represents a halving of the number of countries with insufficient iodine intake over five years, from 32 in 2011 [6] to 15 countries in 2016 [4], and reflects continuing progress to improve the coverage of iodized salt at a national level.

Children born to women who are iodine deficient are at risk of impaired psychomotor development and behavioral problems [7]. Even mild iodine deficiency in pregnancy is associated with learning deficits in offspring at age 8–9 year [8], which persist through to adolescence, despite adequate iodine exposure during early childhood.

Monitoring and surveillance of iodine status is routinely conducted in many countries and reported against a global iodine scorecard [9]. Approximately 90% of dietary iodine is excreted in the urine, therefore, the most commonly used biomarker of iodine intake is urinary iodine concentration (UIC) in collections of casual or spot urine samples for the assessment of median UIC (MUIC) in a population group [10]. This is the method recommended by the WHO/ICCIDD (International Council for Control of Iodine Deficiency Disorders), with iodine sufficiency indicated if the MUIC for a non-pregnant population exceeds 100 µg/L, and if no more than 20% of the population have a urinary iodine concentration below 50 µg/L [1]. The iodine scorecard, published periodically by the Iodine Global network, collates country-level data of MUIC in both school-age children and in women of a reproductive age. Adequate iodine intake in school-age children corresponds to median UIC values in the range of 100–299 µg/L, while for pregnant women the range indicating adequacy is 150–249 µg/L [1]. In the absence of recent national surveys, sub-national UIC surveys are included in the scorecard, but those data should be interpreted with caution [6].

The recommended method of assessing success or failure of fortification programmes in correcting iodine deficiency, while avoiding excess, is determined by assessing MUIC every five years in school-aged children (6–12 year). This indicator is also included in the battery of measures used to capture various aspects of food insecurity, as recommended by the Committee on World Food Security (CFS) [11]. The choice of indicators, including for iodine, was based on both expert judgment and the availability of data with sufficient coverage to enable comparisons across regions and over time. Under the food security pillar of "utilisation", nutritional indicators include: The prevalence of inadequate iodine intakes using MUIC, along with the prevalence of stunting, wasting, and underweight in children; underweight in adults; anaemia in pregnancy and children; population-level vitamin A deficiency; and improved access to sanitation and clean water.

Use of MUIC, as a measure of population-level iodine status, is based on the assumption that daily urinary excretion of iodine closely reflects iodine intake in non-pregnant populations. The other assumption is that a spot urine collection reflects urinary excretion over the entire day [9]. It is well documented that UIC should not be used to assess iodine status in individuals because of its high intra- and inter-individual variation [12–15]. A 13-month longitudinal study of 16 healthy men living in an area of mild to moderate iodine deficiency has provided information on the number of spot urine samples needed to estimate the iodine level in a population. To obtain a MUIC with 95% confidence within a precision range of either 10% or 5%, urine samples are needed from 125 and 500 individuals, respectively. For an individual, to obtain an iodine value within a precision range of $+/- 20\%$, 12 or more repeated spot urine samples are required [16]. Other authors have demonstrated that 10 repeat collections are required for urinary iodine from either spot samples or 24-h samples to provide a reliable estimate of individual iodine status in women [13].

The assumption that MUIC reflects daily iodine intake may be flawed because of high day-to-day variability and variable urinary volume outputs. The aim of this study was to compare iodine status in a sample of South African adults, recruited countrywide, when determined by different approaches using a spot urine sample (median UIC (MUIC) and predicted 24 h urinary iodine excretion (PrUIE) using different prediction equations) compared to measured 24 h urinary iodine excretion (mUIE).

2. Materials and Methods

The study sample is from a nested tobacco and salt sub-study included in the World Health Organization Study on global AGEing and adult health (WHO SAGE) [17]. WHO SAGE is a multinational cohort study examining the health and wellbeing of adult populations and the ageing process. Two waves of this longitudinal study have been completed in China, Ghana, India, Mexico, Russia, and South Africa [18]. In total, 42,464 respondents were recruited across the six countries for Wave 1 (2007–2010), including 4223 respondents in South Africa (9% 18–49 years; 40% 50–59 years; 51% 60+ years). Respondents were recruited from selected probability sampled enumeration areas (EAs) using a multi-stage cluster sampling strategy, with stratification by province, residence, and race. Urine capture was included as part of the SAGE South Africa Wave 2 data collection. The Wave 2 data collection sampling strategy in South Africa (2015) was designed to follow up on Wave 1 households where possible, accounting for attrition with systematic random sampling of new households. This process uses EA aerial photographic maps on which dwellings are clearly visible and, starting at a random point on the periphery of the EA, follows pre-determined routes.

During Wave 2 data collection, 20 survey teams (one nurse and three interviewers per team) simultaneously collected data and samples from respondents across all provinces in the country over a five-month period. Respondents that were recruited to provide urine samples ($n = 1200$) were from the first households visited within each EA, as a means to simplify logistics and reduce sample transit time to the central Durban laboratory. Inclusion criteria for urine collection were: Respondent must be part of the WHO SAGE cohort, with no indication of urinary incontinence or any other condition that could impede 24-h urine collection; and, if female, not menstruating, pregnant, or breastfeeding on the day of collection.

All survey teams were trained with support from the WHO Geneva. As part of the larger survey, anthropometry, household and individual questionnaires, blood sampling, blood pressure (BP), and physical function tests were completed, as described previously in SAGE Wave 1 [18]. Interviewers spoke the respondents' home languages, with consent forms available in the most widely spoken languages for each area. All respondents provided written informed consent prior to taking part in the study. The study complies with the ethical principles for medical research involving human subjects as per the Declaration of Helsinki [19]. The WHO Ethics Review Committee approved the study [RPC149]. Local ethical approval was obtained from the North-West University Human Research Ethics Committee (Potchefstroom, South Africa), and the University of the Witwatersrand Human Research Ethics Committee (Johannesburg, South Africa).

2.1. Urine collection

The protocol used for collection of the 24-h urine samples followed the WHO/PAHO (Pan American Health Organization) guidelines [20]. Respondents were requested to collect all urine produced over 24 h, excluding the first pass of urine on day 1, but including the first urine of the following morning (day 2), in a 5-L plastic container, with 1 g thymol as a preservative. The spot sample was collected without preservative from the second urine passed on day 1 (marking the start of the 24-h collection) and decanted into three 15 ml Porvair tubes (Porvair Sciences, Leatherhead, UK and kept in a cool box powered by the fieldwork vehicles. The 24-h sample volumes were recorded upon collection the next morning and any aliquots generated thereafter (4 × Porvair tubes), with all samples then shipped to the laboratory maintaining the cold chain. Thymol, a crystalline natural derivative of the Thyme plant, has been shown to prevent changes in urinary creatinine, sodium, and potassium concentrations for up to five days [21]. Even though there is no evidence that the addition of preserving substances, such as thymol, affect urinary iodine concentrations [22], we undertook testing to examine the influence of adding thymol or HCl to urine samples ($n = 20$) on urinary iodine concentrations. The results indicated no significant or relevant (below assay coefficient of variation) differences when compared to samples without added preservatives (results not shown here). Incomplete 24-h urine collections were assumed if: Total volume ≤300 mL; or creatinine excretion ≤4 mmol/day (women) or ≤6 mmol/day (men) [23].

2.2. Urine Analysis

Samples from spot and 24 h urine for iodine analysis were stored at −20 °C and batch analysed using the Sandell-Kolthoff method with ammonium persulfate digestion and microplate reading [24] at the North-West University Centre of Excellence for Nutrition. The spot and 24 h urine samples from a single participant were analysed within the same assay to exclude inter-assay variation. The laboratory participates successfully in the Program to Ensure the Quality of Urinary Iodine Procedures (EQUIP, U.S. Centres for Disease Control and Prevention, Atlanta GA, USA) [25], and internal quality control samples (two different levels) were analysed with each assay.

2.3. Comparison of Measured UIE with MUIC and Predicted UIE Using Spot Iodine Concentrations

An electronic data capture system was used during face-to-face interviews. SPSS version 24 was used for statistical analysis (IBM Corporation, New York, NY, USA). Categorical data frequencies were examined using the Pearson Chi-Square and Fisher's Exact tests. Visual inspection of histograms confirmed a non-Gaussian data distribution so that the Mann-Whitney U and Kruskal-Wallis tests were used to compare group distributions and Spearman's Rho for correlations. In order to obtain predicted UIE values based on spot UIC concentrations, an estimation of 24 h urinary volume is required. Creatinine concentration serves as a surrogate for the state of concentration or dilution of the urine, varying inversely with urine volume. We used three different published equations based on age, weight, and height to calculate the predicted 24 h urinary creatinine excretion (PrCr): (1) The Tanaka equation [26]; (2) the Kawasaki equation [27]; and (3) an adapted Mage equation [28] (Table 1). The predicted 24 h creatinine excretion, calculated using each of these equations, was then used to determine the predicted 24 h iodine excretion [PrUIE] as follows: PrUIE = [(spot iodine (μg/L)/spot creatinine) × PrCr]. Differences between the measured UIE (24 h urinary volume (L) × aliquot of iodine from 24 h collection (μg/L)) and PrUIE were assessed using the non-parametric independent samples Mann-Whitney U test. To investigate whether spot UIC can be used to estimate mUIE, agreement between the predicted UIEs from spot urine samples using the different formulas and the measured UIE was assessed using Bland-Altman plots and assessment of limits of agreement (LOA). The LOA approach provides an informative analysis of reliability, including information about the magnitude of errors between methods. The 95% LOA represents a range of values within which, 95% of all differences between methods are expected to fall. Using the standard deviation (sd) of differences between methods, the 95% LOA were calculated for each of the three PrUIEs as mean agreement ±1.96 (sd diff). Both mUIE and PrUIE values were transformed to their natural logarithms (ln) before analyses because of the skewness in distributions. These are reported as the antilogarithm of the difference i.e. the geometric mean of the mUIE/PrUIE ratios and the antilogarithms of the LOA, which provide an interval within which 95% of the ratios lie [29]. For example, mean agreement of 100% suggests exact agreement, whereas mean agreement of 80% indicates that the PrUIE underestimates mUIE by 20%, on average. In the case of LOA values of 40–200%, this would suggest that 95% of PrUIE estimates are between 60 % underestimation and twofold overestimation, compared to mUIE value.

Table 1. Prediction equations used to estimate 24 h urinary creatinine excretion (PrCr).

Equation for Estimating Predicted 24 h Creatinine Excretion	Notes	Reference
Pr24hCr (mg/day) = (−2.04 × age (year)) + (14.89 × weight (kg)) + (16.14 × height (cm)) − 2244.45.	Developed in 591 Japanese adults aged 20–59 year	Tanaka, T.; Okamura, T.; Miura, K.; Kadowaki, T.; Ueshima, H.; Nakagawa, H.; Hasimoto, T. A simple method to estimate populational 24-hour urinary sodium and potassium excretion using a casual urine specimen. *J. Hum. Hypertens* **2002**, *16*, 97–103. [26]
Pr24hCr (mg/day) for men = (12.63 × age (year)) + (15.12 × weight (kg)) + (7.39 × height (cm)) − 79.9 Pr24hCr (mg/day) for women = (−4.72 × age (year)) + (8.58 × weight (kg)) + (5.09 × height (cm)) − 74.5	Equation for predicted 24-h urine creatinine excretion developed in a study of 256 male and 231 female participants aged 20–79 year [30] and validated in 20 male and 27 female Japanese and foreign (including 16 American) subjects.	Kawasaki, T.; Itoh, K.; Uezono, K.; Sasaki, H. A simple method for estimation of 24 h urinary sodium and potassium excretion from second morning voiding urine specimens in adults. *Clin. Exp. Pharmacol. Physiol.* **1993**, *20*, 7–14. [27]
Pr24hCr (mg/day) for men = 0.00179 × (140 − age (year)) − (weight (kg)$^{1.5}$ × height (cm)$^{0.5}$) × (1 + 0.18 × A × (1.366–0.0159 × BMI (kg/m^2)) Pr24hCr (mg/day) for women = 0.00163 × (140 − age (year)) × (weight (kg)$^{1.5}$ × height (cm)$^{0.5}$) × (1 + 0.18 × A × (1.429–0.0198 × BMI (kg/m^2)), where A is African American or black race = 1, other race = 0.	The Mage equation was developed to predict urine pesticide and chemical exposure with NHANES urine specimens. Equation for predicted 24-h urine creatinine excretion developed in a separate study [31] of 249 men in Canada with corrections based on the relative amounts of fat and muscle mass in women and differences in muscle mass by race and BMI.	Mage, D.T.; Allen, R.H.; Kdali, A. Creatinine corrections for estimating children's and adult's pesticide intake doses in equilibrium with urinary pesticide and creatinine concentrations. *J. Expo. Sci. Environ. Epidemiol.* **2008**, *18*, 360–368. [28] Huber, D.R.; Blount, B.C.; Mage, D.T.; Letkiewicz, F.J.; Kumar, A.; Allen, R.H. Estimating perchlorate exposure from food and tap water based on US biomonitoring and occurrence data. *J. Expo. Sci. Environ. Epidemiol.* **2011**, *21*, 395–407. [32]

Table adapted from Cogswell et al. (2013) [33].

Pr24hCr (mg/d) for women = 0.00163 3 (140 2 age (year)) 3 (weight (kg)$^{1.5}$ 3 height (cm)$^{0.5}$) 3 (1 + 0.18 3 A 3 (1.429–0.0198 3 BMI (kg/m^2)), A median UIC (MUIC) of <100 μg/L indicates a population-level deficiency (there is no reference range for individuals) [34]. The EAR cut point approach, recommended by Zimmerman [35], was applied in order to assess the proportion of participants that would be considered to have an inadequate iodine status. This was applied to both the measured and predicted UIE values to provide information about potential bias in assessing the proportion of people with inadequate intakes of iodine if using the spot UIC values to estimate PrUIE. To convert urinary excretion values to estimated daily iodine intake (μg/day), both mUIE and PrUIE were divided by 0.92 to account for the 92% of dietary iodine that is absorbed [35]. The proportion of the population that had iodine intakes below the Estimated Average Requirement of 95 μg/day was compared across the measured and predicted values generated by the three equations. We further compared the proportion of subjects who would be considered iodine deficient (or insufficient iodine intake) based on the MUIC, predicted 24 h UIE (PrUIE), and measured 24 h UIE (mUIE) using respective cut-offs to determine whether MUIC over or underestimates iodine deficiency in a population. Iodine intake (μg/day) was also calculated using the IOM equation of ((UIC (μg/ L)/0.92) × (0.0009 L per h per kg × 24 × weight (kg))) [36] where 0.92 refers to 92% bioavailability and 0.0009 L per h per kg refers to the excreted urine volume from studies in children.

3. Results

Characteristics of the study cohort by sex are shown in Table 2. More women than men were included and the median age was 52 (IQR 24) years, with 65% of the sample being older than 50 years. The Cohens Kappa statistic for inter-rater agreement between 24 h UIE and PrUIE using the Tanaka, Kawasaki and Mage equations indicated poor agreement (0.351, 0.324, and 0.309, respectively; all $p < 0.001$) [31] (Table 3). According to 24 h UIE, 41.1% of participants had an estimated daily iodine intake below the EAR, which differed significantly from estimates using PrUIE calculated using the Tanaka, Kawasaki, and Mage equations (39.3%, 41.3%, and 49.4%, respectively; all $p < 0.05$) (Table 4). Comparing only the subsample of subjects with PrUIE calculated from Mage equations ($n = 428$), the median PrUIE remained similar to the larger sample ($n = 454$), described in Table 4 (130 (139) and 123 (137) for the Tanaka and Kawasaki equations, respectively). The sensitivity of the equations to detect iodine intakes below the EAR of 95 µg/day was 59.9%, 60.4%, and 68.2%, for the Tanaka, Kawasaki. and Mage, respectively. Specificity to detect 24 h iodine intakes above the EAR of was 75%, 72%, and 63.6%, respectively.

The IOM weight-based equation [37], used to estimate the proportion of participants with dietary intakes below the EAR of 95 µg/day, identified only 34.7% of those categorised as such using measured 24 h UIE (X^2 test; $p < 0.0001$).

Table 2. Characteristics of the study cohort by sex, WHO Study on global AGEing and adult health (SAGE) South Africa Wave 2 (2015).

	All $n = 457$	Men $n = 109$	Women $n = 348$	p Value
Age (years)	52 (24)	50 (23)	54 (23)	0.072
Aged over 50 years, n (%)	298 (65)	63 (58)	235 (68)	0.066
Ethnicity, n (%) Black African Coloured, mixed race Indian White	315 (73) 70 (16) 36 (8) 10 (2)	77 (73) 16 (15) 7 (7) 5 (5)	238 (73) 54 (17) 29 (9) 5 (2)	0.248
Rural, n (%)	131 (29)	31 (28)	100 (29)	0.926
Education (years)	9 (5)	10 (4)	8 (6)	0.001
Currently employed, n (%)	83 (31)	37 (51)	46 (23)	<0.001
BMI kg/m^2	29.2 (9.1)	25.7 (7.3)	30.3 (9.3)	<0.001
Waist to height ratio, mean ± SD	0.58 ± 0.13	0.53 ± 0.11	0.60 ± 0.13	<0.001
Never used alcohol, n (%)	287 (81)	59 (63)	228 (88)	<0.001
Spot urinary cotinine (ng/mL)	19.1 (753)	19 (843)	19 (725)	0.867
Median UIC (µg/L)	130 (129)	149 (124)	121 (131)	0.102
UIC < 100 µg/L, n (%)	181 (39.5)	38 (34.9)	143 (41.0)	0.255
UIC < 50 µg/L, n (%)	70 (15.3)	14 (12.8)	56 (16.1)	0.450
Spot urinary iodine per creatinine (µg/g)	102 (103)	102 (106)	102 (99)	0.305
24-h urinary volume (mL/day)	1400 (1390)	1450 (1350)	1370 (1430)	0.929
24-h urinary iodine (mUIE) (µg/day)	124 (134)	137 (190)	119 (121)	0.010

All data is shown as median (IQR, interquartile range) unless otherwise indicated. Hypertensive categorised as BP ≥ 140/90 mmHg or previous diagnosis; Tobacco use/exposure identified by urinary cotinine analysis; BMI, body mass index; UIC, spot Urinary Iodine Concentration; mUIE, measured 24 h Urinary Iodine Excretion. Continuous median variables compared using Independent Samples Mann-Whitney U test and mean values with independent t-test; categorical variables compared using the Pearson Chi-Square and Fisher's Exact Test.

Table 3. Agreement between measured (mUIE) and Predicted (PrUIE) urinary iodine excretion using prediction equations (*n*).

	mUIE †			
	Below EAR (<95 µg/day)	**Above EAR (>=95 µg/day)**	**Total**	***Kappa* Statistic *p* Value**
Tanaka PrUIE				
Below EAR	112	67	179 (39.3%)	0.351
Above EAR	75	201	276 (60.7%)	<0.001
Total	187 (41.1%)	268 (58.9%)	455	
Kawasaki PrUIE				
Below EAR	113	75	188 (41.3%)	0.324
Above EAR	74	193	267 (58.7%)	<0.001
Total	187 (41.1%)	268 (58.9%)	455	
Mage PrUIE				
Below EAR	120	92	212 (49.4%)	0.309
Above EAR	56	161	217 (50.6%)	<0.001
Total	176 (41.0%)	253 (59.0%)	429	

† Daily iodine intake assumed as 24 h UIE (µg/day)/0.92 to account for bioavailability. PrUIE, Predicted Urinary Iodine Excretion (µg/day); EAR, Estimated Average Requirement (µg/day); mUIE, measured 24 h Urinary Iodine Excretion (µg/day).

Table 4. Difference between measured and predicted 24 h urinary iodine excretion (UIE), SAGE South Africa Wave 2 (2015).

Prediction Equation	*n*	Median (IQR)	Median (IQR) Difference †	Mann Whitney Test *p* Value	Spearman Correlation Coefficient *p* Value	EAR ‡ Below (%)
Mage equation (µg/day)						
mUIE	428	124 (137)	17.8 (108)	0.000	0.402	49.5 *
PrUIE		105 (117)			0.000	
Tanaka equation (µg/day)						
mUIE	454	124 (136)	−3.2 (117)	0.399	0.413	39.3 *
PrUIE		130 (136)			0.000	
Kawasaki equation (µg/day)						
mUIE	454	124 (136)	4.1 (110)	0.443	0.425	41.3 *
PrUIE		122 (131)			0.000	

PrUIE, Predicted Urinary Iodine Excretion (µg/day); mUIE, measured 24 h Urinary Iodine Excretion (µg/day). † mUIE minus PrUIE; ‡ EAR = 95 µg/day. Percentage below EAR is shown for each of the equations (X^2 test compared to mUIE (41%); * $p < 0.001$). Mage n is lower as equation requires additional data on ethnicity (*n* = 26 with missing ethnicity data).

Bland Altman plots are shown in Figure 1a–c for natural logarithmic (ln) transformed values of predicted and measured UIE. Mean differences between values and limits of agreement (LOA) are presented as as the anti-log of the arithmetic mean of the ln-transformed values (i.e., the geometric mean). Thus, differences between PrUIE and mUIE were as follows: Tanaka: 68% (LOA 12–380%); Kawasaki: (71% (13–391%); and Mage: 83% (11–605%). The Mage equation (Figure 1c) had the widest LOA, but all three equations had unacceptably wide LOAs, indicating poor agreement with mUIE.

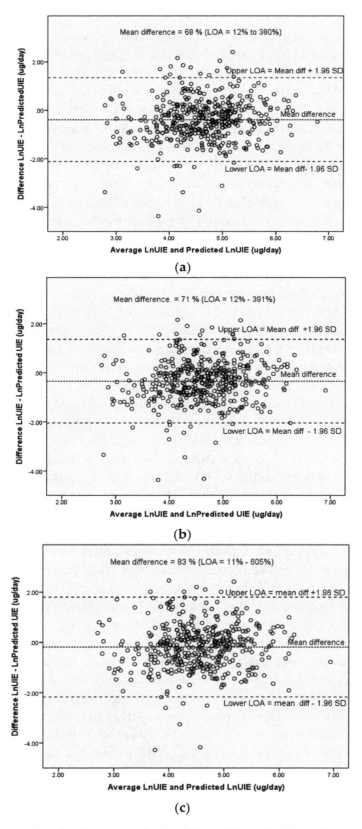

Figure 1. Bland Altman plots for the mean of natural logarithmic (Ln) transformed measured 24 h UIE and Ln transformed predicted UIE against the difference between ln transformed measured 24 h UIE and predicted UIE, using the following equations: (**a**) Tanaka; (**b**) Kawasaki; and (**c**) Mage equations; LOA = Limits of Agreement (Ln mean difference between measured and predicted UIE +/− 1.96 SD; shown as antilog or geometric mean, expressed as a ratio of difference between predicted UIE and measured 24 h UIE).

4. Discussion

The purpose of the current study was to assess the degree to which a spot urinary iodine concentration could be used as a proxy for measured 24 h urinary iodine excretion, for the purpose of assessing the adequacy of dietary iodine intake. The use of spot UIC values to indicate suboptimal iodine status (39% with MUIC <100 µg/L) provided a similar estimate to 24 h UIE (41% <EAR of 95 µg/day) at the group level. The use of spot UIC values in prediction equations to estimate 24 h UIE in this sample of South African adults provided a reasonable estimate of the prevalence of insufficient intakes below the EAR of 95 µg/day. For predicted 24 h UIE, based on spot UIC concentrations, all three prediction equations resulted in average under-estimations, ranging from 17% to 32 % for the different equations, with accompanying unacceptably wide limits of agreement. The difficulty of deciding on clinically relevant acceptable limits of agreement has previously been discussed by various authors [37,38]. In the case of iodine, for populations where intakes may be inadequate and where the consequences of inadequacy have serious impacts on health outcomes, such as in the case of pregnant women, more stringent cut-offs for determining acceptable limits of agreement may be warranted.

Our data suggests that spot UIC values provide an acceptable indication of population level deficiency, as compared to the EAR cutpoint method using measured 24 h UIE. Complex prediction equations applied to spot UIC values offered no greater accuracy and, rather, introduced major bias. Our findings are in contrast to those reported by Perrine et al. (2014) [39] in a study of younger healthy adults aged 18–39 years, in which UIC provided a reasonable estimate of 24-h UIE when prediction equations were used to determine 24-h urinary creatinine excretion.

Despite serious bias in predicted UIE, we did not find this bias to be systematic at higher levels of UIE. This is important in iodine replete populations that have been exposed to a well-functioning iodine fortification programme for some years and that may be at risk of potentially adverse excessive levels. A recent study of South African infant-mother pairs found that 21% of households consumed salt iodized above the upper level of 65 ppm and that the median UIC in the infants aged 2–4 months was more than three times higher than the WHO UIC threshold [40]. It is noteworthy that most recent estimates (2016) indicate that 10 countries have median urinary iodine concentration (MUIC) values considered to be in the excessive range (MUIC > 300µg/L) [4,5]. High iodine intakes are associated with iodine-induced hyperthyroidism and autoimmune thyroid disease [41,42], but there is a lack of consensus regarding the iodine intake that constitutes an adverse risk to health as indicated by a wide range in tolerable upper levels between countries. The WHO has expressed a cautious approach regarding upper levels, stating that a daily intake higher than 500 mg per day in pregnancy and lactation and more than 180 mg per day in children younger than two years is not necessary because it may, theoretically, be associated with impaired thyroid function [43].

As daily creatinine excretion is fairly constant at about one gram per day in healthy, well-nourished adults, it has been proposed that expression of UIC per gram of creatinine approximates the value in a 24-h collection and reduces variation due to hydration status [44]. However, malnourished populations with low protein intakes tend to have more variable daily creatinine excretion that is often lower than one gram per day [45]. In these settings, expressing the UIE as mg iodine/g creatinine may introduce greater, rather than less, variation. In our sample, dietary protein intake data was not available to test this hypothesis and the lack of reference values for UIC expressed as per gram of creatinine limits further interpretation.

While the use of spot urine samples to monitor the iodine status of a population is widely accepted, there is potential for error in using the current MUIC reference cut-offs of <100 µg/L to indicate iodine deficiency in adults. The original MUIC reference cut-off values were determined based on a daily urinary volume of 1 L (as would be the case for school aged children), such that the UIC would approximate the UIE. However, in adults, who tend to have urine volumes that approximate 1.5 L/day [46], the UIC in µg/L is not equivalent to the 24 h UIE, expressed as µg/24 h. Based on the expected adult urine volume, UIC (µg/L) in spot samples could be expected to be about 60–65% of the amount excreted in 24 h [35]. Therefore, in adults, a UIE of 100 µg/24 h corresponds to a UIC of approximately 60–70 μg/L and this has been proposed by Zimmermann and Andersson (2012) [35] as being a more appropriate cut-off to indicate deficiency in adults. The Estimated Average Intake (EAR) value for iodine has been derived from balance studies and from studies measuring the daily iodine uptake, accumulation, and turnover in the thyroid gland using radioactive iodine in euthyroid adult subjects. These studies indicate that, to achieve iodine balance, the daily iodine intake (EAR) must be sufficient to enable the thyroid to turn over 95 mg iodine per day to maintain euthyroidism [36].

The large variation in a single spot urine iodine sample from day to day within individuals increases the spread of the distribution [16,47] so that it does not reflect the range of long-term or 'usual' iodine status around the median in a population. There are various available methods to reduce or remove the effects of measurement error due to the intra-individual variation that results from collecting a single-spot urine sample in population survey data. One method is to collect repeat samples over multiple days and average the data for each participant, but this substantially increases costs and logistics when conducting a national survey. Another method is to apply a correction factor to the distribution [47,48]. This requires estimation of a correction factor by collecting multiple samples from a representative subset of the survey population. Our group previously applied this method to three repeated UIC measures in a sample of healthy older Australians in the period prior to the introduction of mandatory iodine fortification [49]. After statistical adjustment for intra-individual variation, the proportion with UIC <50 μg/L reduced from 33% to 19%, while the proportion with UIC ≥100 μg/L changed from 21% to 17%, and the 95th centile for UIC decreased from 176 to 136 μg/L.

The EAR cut point method proposed by Zimmermann and Anderson (2012) [35] has been widely applied as an evaluation tool for nutrient intakes of groups [50,51] and to define the optimal fortification level of nutrients in foods [52]. The EAR cut-point method can be used to estimate the prevalence of iodine deficiency based on UIC distributions. The population distribution of UICs is typically skewed towards lower intakes, with a scattered tail of high intakes because of wide day-to-day variability in intakes. Assuming an adequate sample size of the group to account for inter-individual variation in the population distribution of UIC, it is possible to adjust the distribution to account for intra-individual variation using the National Cancer Institute or other similar statistical approaches [53,54]. This requires two or more repeated spot urine samples from the same individual in a subset of the study population in order to adjust the intake distribution closer to the mean. The Institute of Medicine suggest that daily iodine intake can be estimated using the weight-based equation: ((UIC (μg/L)/0.92) × (0.0009 L per h per kg × weight (kg))) [36]. In this equation, 0.92 refers to 92% bioavailability and 0.0009 L per h per kg refers to the excreted urine volume from studies in children. The estimated iodine intakes are adjusted for intra-individual variability and, thereafter, the proportion of individuals below the EAR (95 μg/day) can be ascertained to estimate the prevalence of iodine deficiency.

In our sample of adult South Africans intra-individual variability could not be assessed as only a single spot and 24 h urine sample was collected from each individual. Konig et al. (2011) [15] have reported a trend for higher intra-individual variation for spot UIC (38%) compared to measured 24 h urinary iodine excretion (32%) and this warrants further consideration. Other limitations include the sample population not being nationally representative as it was biased towards older adults aged more than 50 years, as well as the time of day for spot urine collection not being recorded and the lack of dietary intake data. Additionally, no information was collected on thyroid disorders nor on the use of thyroid medications in the SAGE sample. Therefore, we were unable to consider this in the selection criteria. It is, however, unlikely that many participants would have been diagnosed with thyroid disorders or taking medication for these conditions, since management of the condition on the continent is inadequate [55]. Strengths of the study design include a relatively large sample from all regions of the country, including inland, coastal, and mountainous regions. Furthermore, all analysis was conducted in one central laboratory, with quality control according to the CDC-EQUIP protocol (Ensuring the Quality of Iodine Procedures (EQUIP), Centers for Disease Control and Prevention) [21].

5. Conclusions

In a sample of adult South Africans, iodine status, assessed using median urinary iodine concentration at the group level, closely approximates urinary iodine excretion from 24 h urine collections. The use of complex prediction equations that incorporate spot UIC does not appear to offer additional accuracy in assessing population iodine deficiency. Continued use of the pragmatic collection of spot urine samples to assess population iodine status is supported.

Author Contributions: Authors' contributions were as follows: K.E.C., and P.K. designed research; N.N. was responsible for sampling, L.J.W. implemented research; J.B. analysed iodine samples; M.C., L.J.W., and K.E.C. analysed data; K.E.C., L.J.W., J.B., A.E.S., M.C., and P.K. wrote the paper; K.E.C. takes responsibility for the contents of this article. All authors read and approved the final manuscript.

Acknowledgments: The authors thank all respondents for contributions and acknowledge Stephen Rule, Robin Richards, and Godfrey Dlulane of Outsourced Insight who were subcontracted to conduct the surveys and coordinate data collection within South Africa.

References

1.   World Health Organization. *Assessment of Iodine Deficiency Disorders and Monitoring Their Elimination: A Guide for Programme Managers*, 3rd ed.; WHO: Geneva, Switzerland, 2007.

2.   UNSCN. *Universal Salt Iodisation*; LavenhamPress: UK, 2007. United Nations System Standing Committee on Nutrition (SCN). No. 35. Available online: https://www.unscn.org/web/archives_resources/files/scnnews35.pdf (accessed on 30 January 2018).

3.   UNICEF. The State of the World's Children. Available online: https://www.unicef.org/sowc2016/ (accessed on 12 January 2018).

4.   IGN. Global Iodine Nutrition Scorecard 2016. Available online: http://www.ign.org/cmdata/Scorecard_2016_SAC_PW.pdf (accessed on 12 January 2018).

5.   Gizak, M.; Gorstein, J.; Andersson, M. Epidemiology of iodine deficiency. In *Iodine Deficiency Disorders and Their Elimination*; Springer: Berlin, Germany, 2017; pp. 29–43.

6.   Andersson, M.; Karumbunathan, V.; Zimmermann, M.B. Global iodine status in 2011 and trends over the past decade. *J. Nutr.* **2012**, *142*, 744–750. [CrossRef] [PubMed]

7.   Delange, F. The role of iodine in brain development. *Proc. Nutr. Soc.* **2000**, *59*, 75–79. [CrossRef] [PubMed]

8.   Hynes, K.L.; Otahal, P.; Hay, I.; Burgess, J.R. Mild iodine deficiency during pregnancy is associated with reduced educational outcomes in the offspring: 9-year follow-up of the gestational iodine cohort. *J. Clin. Endocrinol.* **2013**, *98*, 1954–1962. [CrossRef] [PubMed]

9.   Iodine Global Network. *Global Scorecard of Iodine Nutrition in 2017 in the General Population and in Pregnant Women (pw)*; IGN: Zurich, Switzerland, 2017.

10.   Ma, Z.F.; Skeaff, S.A. Assessment of population iodine status. In *Iodine Deficiency Disorders and Their Elimination*; Pearce, E.N., Ed.; Springer: Cham, Switzerland, 2017; pp. 15–28.

11.   FAO. Food Security Indicators. Available online: http://www.fao.org/economic/ess/ess-fs/ess-fadata/en/#.WoJVGq6WaUl (accessed on 13 February 2018).

12.   Rasmussen, L.B.; Ovesen, L.; Christiansen, E. Day-to-day and within-day variation in urinary iodine excretion. *Eur. J. Clin. Nutr.* **1999**, *53*, 401–407. [CrossRef] [PubMed]

13. Rasmussen, L.B.; Ovesen, L.; Bülow, I.; Jørgensen, T.; Knudsen, N.; Laurberg, P.; Perrild, H. Dietary iodine intake and urinary iodine excretion in a Danish population: Effect of geography, supplements and food choice. *Br. J. Nutr.* **2002**, *87*, 61–69. [CrossRef] [PubMed]

14. Als, C.; Helbling, A.; Peter, K.; Haldimann, M.; Zimmerli, B.; Gerber, H. Urinary iodine concentration follows a circadian rhythm: A study with 3023 spot urine samples in adults and children. *J. Clin. Endocrinol. MeTable* **2000**, *85*, 1367–1369. [CrossRef]

15. König, F.; Andersson, M.; Hotz, K.; Aeberli, I.; Zimmermann, M.B. Ten repeat collections for urinary iodine from spot samples or 24-hour samples are needed to reliably estimate individual iodine status in women. *J. Nutr.* **2011**, *141*, 2049–2054. [CrossRef] [PubMed]

16. Andersen, S.; Karmisholt, J.; Pedersen, K.M.; Laurberg, P. Reliability of studies of iodine intake and recommendations for number of samples in groups and in individuals. *Br. J. Nutr.* **2008**, *99*, 813–818. [CrossRef] [PubMed]

17. Charlton, K.; Ware, L.J.; Menyanu, E.; Biritwum, R.B.; Naidoo, N.; Pieterse, C.; Madurai, S.L.; Baumgartner, J.; Asare, G.A.; Thiele, E. Leveraging ongoing research to evaluate the health impacts of South Africa's salt reduction strategy: A prospective nested cohort within the who-sage multicountry, longitudinal study. *BMJ Open* **2016**, *6*, e013316. [CrossRef] [PubMed]

18. Kowal, P.; Chatterji, S.; Naidoo, N.; Biritwum, R.; Fan, W.; Ridaura, R.L.; Maximova, T.; Arokiasamy, P.; Phaswana-Mafuya, N.; Williams, S. Data resource profile: The World Health Organization Study on Global Ageing and Adult Health (SAGE). *Int. J. Epidemiol.* **2012**, *41*, 1639–1649. [CrossRef] [PubMed]

19. World Medical Association. *World Medical Association Declaration of Helsinki Ethical Principles for Medical Research Involving Human Subjects*; World Medical Association: Ferney-Voltaire, France, 2013.

20. Wang, S.M.; Fu, L.J.; Duan, X.L.; Crooks, D.R.; Yu, P.; Qian, Z.M.; Di, X.J.; Li, J.; Rouault, T.A.; Chang, Y.Z. Role of hepcidin in murine brain iron metabolism. *Cell. Mol. Life Sci.* **2010**, *67*, 123–133. [CrossRef] [PubMed]

21. Nicar, M.J.; Hsu, M.C.; Johnson, T.; Pak, C.Y. The preservation of urine samples for determination of renal stone risk factors. *Lab. Med.* **1987**, *18*, 382–384. [CrossRef] [PubMed]

22. Sullivan, K.M.; May, S.; Maberly, G. *Urinary Iodine Assessment: A Manual on Survey and Laboratory Methods*; Program Against Micronutrient Malnutrition: Atlanta, GA, USA, 2000.

23. Stolarz-Skrzypek, K.; Kuznetsova, T.; Thijs, L.; Tikhonoff, V.; Seidlerová, J.; Richart, T.; Jin, Y.; Olszanecka, A.; Malyutina, S.; Casiglia, E. Fatal and nonfatal outcomes, incidence of hypertension, and blood pressure changes in relation to urinary sodium excretion. *JAMA* **2011**, *305*, 1777–1785. [CrossRef] [PubMed]

24. Ohashi, T.; Yamaki, M.; Pandav, C.S.; Karmarkar, M.G.; Irie, M. Simple microplate method for determination of urinary iodine. *Clin. Chem.* **2000**, *46*, 529–536. [PubMed]

25. Caldwell, K.L.; Makhmudov, A.; Jones, R.L.; Hollowell, J.G. Equip: A worldwide program to ensure the quality of urinary iodine procedures. *Accreditat. Qual. Assur.* **2005**, *10*, 356–361. [CrossRef]

26. Tanaka, T.; Okamura, T.; Miura, K.; Kadowaki, T.; Ueshima, H.; Nakagawa, H.; Hashimoto, T. A simple method to estimate populational 24-h urinary sodium and potassium excretion using a casual urine specimen. *J. Hum. Hypertens.* **2002**, *16*, 97–103. [CrossRef] [PubMed]

27. Kawasaki, T.; Itoh, K.; Uezono, K.; Sasaki, H. A simple method for estimating 24 h urinary sodium and potassium excretion from second morning voiding urine specimen in adults. *Clin. Exp. Pharmacol. Physiol.* **1993**, *20*, 7–14. [CrossRef] [PubMed]

28. Mage, D.T.; Allen, R.H.; Kodali, A. Creatinine corrections for estimating children's and adult's pesticide intake doses in equilibrium with urinary pesticide and creatinine concentrations. *J. Expo. Sci. Environ. Epidemiol.* **2008**, *18*, 360–368. [CrossRef] [PubMed]

29. Bland, J.M.; Altman, D.G. Measuring agreement in method comparison studies. *Stat. Methods Med. Res.* **1999**, *8*, 135–160. [CrossRef] [PubMed]

30. Cockcroft, D.W.; Gault, H. Prediction of creatinine clearance from serum creatinine. *Nephron* **1976**, *16*, 31–41. [CrossRef] [PubMed]

31. Fleiss, J.L. *Statistical Methods for Rates and Proportions*, 2nd ed.; John Wiley: New York, NY, USA, 1981; ISBN 0-471-26370-2.

32. Huber, D.R.; Blount, B.C.; Mage, D.T.; Letkiewicz, F.J.; Kumar, A.; Allen, R.H. Estimating perchlorate exposure from food and tap water based on us biomonitoring and occurrence data. *J. Expo. Sci. Environ. Epidemiol.* **2011**, *21*, 395–407. [CrossRef] [PubMed]

33. Cogswell, M.E.; Wang, C.-Y.; Chen, T.-C.; Pfeiffer, C.M.; Elliott, P.; Gillespie, C.D.; Carriquiry, A.L.; Sempos, C.T.; Liu, K.; Perrine, C.G. Validity of predictive equations for 24-h urinary sodium excretion in adults aged 18–39 y. *Am. J. Clin. Nutr.* **2013**, *98*, 1502–1513. [CrossRef] [PubMed]

34. Delange, F.; de Benoist, B.; Burgi, H. Determining median urinary iodine concentration that indicates adequate iodine intake at population level. *Bull. World Health Organ.* **2002**, *80*, 633–636. [PubMed]

35. Zimmermann, M.B.; Andersson, M. Assessment of iodine nutrition in populations: Past, present, and future. *Nutr. Rev.* **2012**, *70*, 553–570. [CrossRef] [PubMed]

36. Trumbo, P.; Yates, A.A.; Schlicker, S.; Poos, M. Dietary reference intakes: Vitamin A, Vitamin K, arsenic, boron, chromium, copper, iodine, iron, manganese, molybdenum, nickel, silicon, vanadium, and zinc. *J. Am. Diet. Assoc.* **2001**, *101*, 294–301. [CrossRef]

37. Lombard, M.J.; Steyn, N.P.; Charlton, K.E.; Senekal, M. Application and interpretation of multiple statistical tests to evaluate validity of dietary intake assessment methods. *Nutr. J.* **2015**, *14*, 40. [CrossRef] [PubMed]

38. Batterham, M.J.; Van Loo, C.; Charlton, K.E.; Cliff, D.P.; Okely, A.D. Improved interpretation of studies comparing methods of dietary assessment: Combining equivalence testing with the limits of agreement. *Br. J. Nutr.* **2016**, *115*, 1273–1280. [CrossRef] [PubMed]

39. Perrine, C.G.; Cogswell, M.E.; Swanson, C.A.; Sullivan, K.M.; Chen, T.-C.; Carriquiry, A.L.; Dodd, K.W.; Caldwell, K.L.; Wang, C.-Y. Comparison of population iodine estimates from 24-hour urine and timed-spot urine samples. *Thyroid* **2014**, *24*, 748–757. [CrossRef] [PubMed]

40. Osei, J.; Andersson, M.; van der Reijden, O.; Dold, S.; Smuts, C.M.; Baumgartner, J. Breast-milk iodine concentrations, iodine status, and thyroid function of breastfed infants aged 2–4 months and their mothers residing in a south african township. *J. Clin. Res. Pediatr. Endocrinol.* **2016**, *8*, 381–391. [CrossRef] [PubMed]

41. Pedersen, I.B.; Knudsen, N.; Carlé, A.; Vejbjerg, P.; Jørgensen, T.; Perrild, H.; Ovesen, L.; Rasmussen, L.B.; Laurberg, P. A cautious iodization programme bringing iodine intake to a low recommended level is associated with an increase in the prevalence of thyroid autoantibodies in the population. *Clin. Endocrinol.* **2011**, *75*, 120–126. [CrossRef] [PubMed]

42. Bürgi, H. Iodine excess. *Best Pract. Res. Clin. Endocrinol. Metab.* **2010**, *24*, 107–115. [CrossRef] [PubMed]

43. Andersson, M.; De Benoist, B.; Delange, F.; Zupan, J. Prevention and control of iodine deficiency in pregnant and lactating women and in children less than 2-years-old: Conclusions and recommendations of the technical consultation. *Public Health Nutr.* **2007**, *10*, 1606–1611. [PubMed]

44. Vejbjerg, P.; Knudsen, N.; Perrild, H.; Laurberg, P.; Andersen, S.; Rasmussen, L.B.; Ovesen, L.; Jørgensen, T. Estimation of iodine intake from various urinary iodine measurements in population studies. *Thyroid* **2009**, *19*, 1281–1286. [CrossRef] [PubMed]

45. Bourdoux, P. Evaluation of the iodine intake: Problems of the iodine/creatinine ratio-comparison with iodine excretion and daily fluctuations of iodine concentration. *Exp. Clin. Endocrinol. Diabetes* **1998**, *106*, S17–S20. [CrossRef] [PubMed]

46. Manz, F.; Johner, S.A.; Wentz, A.; Boeing, H.; Remer, T. Water balance throughout the adult life span in a german population. *Br. J. Nutr.* **2012**, *107*, 1673–1681. [CrossRef] [PubMed]

47. Armstrong, B.K.; White, E.; Saracci, R. *Principles of Exposure Measurement in Epidemiology*; Monographs in Epidemiology and Biostatistics; Oxford University Press: New York, NY, USA, 1992; Volume 1.

48. Dyer, A.R.; Shipley, M.; Elliott, P.; Group, I.C.R. Urinary electrolyte excretion in 24 hours and blood pressure in the intersalt study: I. Estimates of reliability. *Am. J. Epidemiol.* **1994**, *139*, 927–939. [CrossRef] [PubMed]

49. Charlton, K.E.; Batterham, M.J.; Buchanan, L.M.; Mackerras, D. Intraindividual variation in urinary iodine concentrations: Effect of adjustment on population distribution using two and three repeated spot urine collections. *BMJ Open* **2014**, *4*, e003799. [CrossRef] [PubMed]

50. De Lauzon, B.; Volatier, J.; Martin, A. A Monte Carlo simulation to validate the EAR cut-point method for assessing the prevalence of nutrient inadequacy at the population level. *Public Health Nutr.* **2004**, *7*, 893–900. [CrossRef] [PubMed]

51. Ribas-Barba, L.; Serra-Majem, L.; Román-Vinas, B.; Ngo, J.; García-Álvarez, A. Effects of dietary assessment methods on assessing risk of nutrient intake adequacy at the population level: From theory to practice. *Br. J. Nutr.* **2009**, *101*, S64–S72. [CrossRef] [PubMed]

52. Allen, L.H.; De Benoist, B.; Dary, O.; Hurrell, R.; Organization, W.H. *Guidelines on Food Fortification with Micronutrients*; World Health Organization: Geneva, Switzerland, 2006.

53. Murphy, S.P.; Barr, S.I. Practice paper of the American Dietetic Association: Using the Dietary Reference Intakes. *J. Am. Diet. Assoc.* **2011**, *111*, 762–770. [PubMed]

54. Murphy, S.P.; Barr, S.I.; Poos, M.I. Using the new dietary reference intakes to assess diets: A map to the maze. *Nutr. Rev.* **2002**, *60*, 267–275. [CrossRef] [PubMed]

55. Ogbera, A.O.; Kuku, S.F. Epidemiology of thyroid diseases in Africa. *Indian J. Endocrinol. Metab.* **2011**, *15*, S82–S88. [CrossRef] [PubMed]

56. Study on Global AGEing and Adult Health (SAGE). Available online: http://apps.who.int/healthinfo/systems/surveydata/index.php/catalog/sage/about (accessed on 6 June 2018).

5

Iodine and Pregnancy—A Qualitative Study Focusing on Dietary Guidance and Information

Maria Bouga ⓘ, **Michael E. J. Lean and Emilie Combet** * ⓘ

Human Nutrition, School of Medicine, College of Medical, Veterinary and Life Sciences, 10–16 Alexandra Parade, University of Glasgow, Glasgow G31 2ER, UK; mairabouga@gmail.com (M.B.); mike.lean@glasgow.ac.uk (M.E.J.L.)
* Correspondence: emilie.combetaspray@glasgow.ac.uk

Abstract: Iodine is essential for thyroid hormones synthesis and normal neurodevelopment; however, ~60% of pregnant women do not meet the WHO (World Health Organization) recommended intake. Using a qualitative design, we explored the perceptions, awareness, and experiences of pregnancy nutrition, focusing on iodine. Women in the perinatal period (n = 48) were interviewed and filled in a food frequency questionnaire for iodine. Almost all participants achieved the recommended 150 μg/day intake for non-pregnant adults (99%), but only 81% met the increased demands of pregnancy (250 μg/day). Most were unaware of the importance, sources of iodine, and recommendations for iodine intake. Attitudes toward dairy products consumption were positive (e.g., helps with heartburn; easy to increase). Increased fish consumption was considered less achievable, with barriers around taste, smell, heartburn, and morning sickness. Community midwives were the main recognised provider of dietary advice. The dietary advice received focused most often on multivitamin supplements rather than food sources. Analysis highlighted a clear theme of commitment to change behaviour, motivated by pregnancy, with a desired focus on user-friendly documentation and continued involvement of the health services. The study highlights the importance of redirecting advice on dietary requirements in pregnancy and offers practical suggestions from women in the perinatal period as the main stakeholder group.

Keywords: iodine; pregnancy; qualitative research; awareness; perceptions; nutrition

1. Introduction

Iodine is key for synthesis of the thyroid hormones, which play a vital role in normal brain development in fetal and postnatal life. Iodine deficiency (ID) during pregnancy (defined as a median population urinary iodine concentration (UIC) of less than 150 μg/L) or neonatal life (<100 μg/L) [1] is the most preventable cause of brain retardation for the infant [2]. The consequences of ID range from subtle loss of intelligence quotient (IQ) to cretinism. Recent evidence indicates that there is mild iodine insufficiency in the United Kingdom (UK) and several other European countries (Finland, Italy, Latvia), with limited insight into the consequences of this insufficiency for children's cognitive development (e.g., reduced verbal IQ, poorer educational attainment, reduced reading speed) [3,4].

ID is a global issue [2], not limited to developing countries or high-altitude areas where endemic cretinism was classically found. Based on the 2017 International Council for the Control of Iodine Deficiency Disorders (ICCIDD) global map and scorecard of ID, Europe has a high number of countries where iodine intakes are of concern, including Denmark, Estonia, Finland, Ireland, Italy, Lithuania, and the UK. Women in the UK have been shown, in national and sub-national studies, to be iodine insufficient at a population level [5–7]. The UK Reference Nutrient Intake for adults is 140 μg/day and the recommended level of intake according to the WHO/United Nations Children's

Fund (UNICEF)/ICCIDD is 150 µg/day [2], which is not met by schoolgirls in the UK (68% below threshold) [7]. After conception, the WHO recommendation rises to 250 µg/day, which is only met by 40% of pregnant women [8]. The European Food Safety Authority (EFSA) recently proposed a new reference value for adequate intake for pregnancy (200 µg/day). In the UK, there is no proposed increment for iodine intake during pregnancy and lactation.

Although recommendations focus on daily consumption, adequate status may also be achieved through intermittently greater intakes, to reach an average intake that meets the recommended intake. Iodine is stored in the thyroid (~75% of the total body iodine −15–20 mg), and daily usage from the thyroid store is estimated to 60–80 µg in non-pregnant adults [9].

The main dietary sources of iodine in the UK are dairy and seafoods, which together make up 13% of energy intake in adult women [10]. Recommended intakes could potentially be met by consuming two portions of white sea fish per week, in addition to the equivalent of two glasses of milk (as drinks, or in cereals for example), a yoghurt, and a cheese serving per day. However, many women avoid these foods and lack knowledge and know-how to include them in their diet. Including milk in the diet is the factor that contributes most toward iodine status, as found in a Danish study with more than 4500 participants [11]. Rasmussen et al. [11] showed that the risk of a low iodine intake is higher in those whose diets do not include at least 0.5 L milk per day and 200 g of fish per week. Stricter forms of the vegetarian diet, which excludes fish and seafood products consumption, are also associated with a higher risk of iodine insufficiency, based on measured urinary iodine excretion [12]. Although seaweed is an acceptable food for vegetarians, it is not widely consumed, and 25% of vegetarians and 80% of vegans have an insufficient iodine status compared to 9% of non-vegetarians [13,14]. Vegans also have been shown to have a lower urinary iodine excretion compared to vegetarians (78.5 µg/L vs. 147 µg/L, $p < 0.01$) [15].

The consequences of an iodine insufficient population include personal and societal costs. The absence of prophylactic fortification in the UK, combined with the low knowledge and awareness of iodine nutrition, has led to iodine insufficiency becoming a serious public health concern. In a recent meta-analysis, ID children aged five years and under had a 6.9 to 10.2 lower IQ compared to iodine replete children [16]. In the Mother and Child Cohort Study (MoBa) study, a recent large prospective cohort study in Norway, children born from mothers who consumed insufficient iodine from foods during pregnancy have significantly higher attention-deficit/hyperactivity disorder symptom scores [17]. The cost effectiveness of iodine supplementation in pregnancy has been modelled, suggesting a saving of £199 in healthcare costs and £4476 societal costs for an increase of 1.22 IQ points per offspring [18].

There is a sustained debate on the ethical implications of a randomised controlled trial of iodine supplementation in pregnancy, in parallel with concerns over the adverse effects of salt and the conflicted message that salt iodisation would convey [19,20]. There are a range of other strategies to tackle iodine insufficiency, including updating dietary recommendations, introducing mandatory salt fortification, and new nutritional education strategies aiming to increase awareness and promote iodine rich foods [21,22]. In a UK survey, over half of mothers (55%) could not identify correct sources of iodine, commonly mistaking salt (21%) and vegetables (54%) as iodine-rich foods. Moreover, healthcare professionals could not recognise iodine-rich foods either [23]. Most women (87%) reported willingness to modify their dietary behavior, if they received information related to the importance of iodine in pregnancy [8].

To find an effective way to address iodine insufficiency, there is a need to explore the current level of awareness about iodine in pregnancy and related dietary recommendations. Few studies in the UK have explored the level of knowledge and awareness of iodine [8,24] and highlighted the need to understand in-depth the perceptions of women in relation to dietary guidance, the way these are provided, and the most endorsed approach for provision of such recommendations.

This qualitative study is articulated around three main research questions, engaging stakeholders to canvass current perceptions and experiences of dietary guidance and recommendations relating to iodine in pregnancy:

1. What is the current perceived level and quality of dietary guidance received by expectant mothers and new mothers?
2. What are the perceived barriers to increasing or maintaining an adequate intake of dairy and seafood pre-conception and during pregnancy/lactation?
3. What would be the most effective delivery of dietary guidance to expectant and new mothers?

2. Materials and Methods

2.1. Study Design and Choice of Methods

A cross-sectional design was used to explore stakeholders' experiences, views, and attitudes. Participants' perceptions, opinions, beliefs, and attitudes were captured through interviews, either face-to-face or by phone. Topic guides included elements relevant to the Health Belief Model [25]. A food frequency questionnaire (FFQ) (validated for iodine-rich food intake [26]) was used to explore demographic characteristics, iodine intake, and practices related to pregnancy. The qualitative approach was chosen as it provides a better understanding and allows the exploration of issues that have not been deeply investigated by existing quantitative research [27]. It aims to give voice to people talking about their beliefs and expectations, instead of focusing on a range of pre-determined questions in semi-quantitative surveys [28].

2.2. Subjects

Recruitment took place from May to December 2015 in a community setting, by snowball sampling. Women were recruited through social media, fora, online advertisement, and by word of mouth. Participants were provided with the study information and gave informed consent.

The inclusion criteria were English-speaking women (fluency level sufficient to follow an active conversation), of childbearing age, living in the UK, having a baby (younger than two years old), being pregnant, or planning to start a family. There were no further restrictions in terms of selection.

2.3. Questionnaire

Socio-demographic characteristics were recorded in the first part of the questionnaire, including smoking status (those answering "yes" to the question "Are you currently a smoker?" were categorised as smokers), use of medication, and self-reported anthropometric measures (pre-pregnancy weight, current weight, height). Education level was categorised as school level (School certificate, standard grade/GCSE (General Certificate of Secondary Education), Highers/A levels), college level (HND (Higher National Diplomas)/HNC (Higher National Certificates), NVQs (National Vocational Qualifications), other higher education diploma), undergraduate degree (Bachelor degree), and postgraduate degree (Master's Degree, Ph.D.). To assess iodine intake with minimal participant burden, we used our previously validated short FFQ which captures the intake frequencies of iodine-rich foods in eight categories (i.e., milk, oil-rich fish, white sea fish, other seafood, cheese (hard and soft), yoghurts, milk or cream-based puddings, cheese-based dishes) [26]. Participants were categorised according to their iodine needs: participants with "increased demands" (250 μg/day, pregnant and breastfeeding) and "basic demands" (normal adult demands, 150 μg/day). Questions on nutrients' awareness, iodine confidence, and dietary changes during pregnancy (increased, decreased, or maintained intake of a list of foods) were also included as part of the questionnaire, as previously described [8].

2.4. Interviews

All interviews were conducted by the same researcher either in person or over the phone. Participants were already in possession of the study information sheet and had provided informed consent. Prior to the start of the interview, the overall process was explained again, and participants were notified that interviews would get recorded.

A narrative focusing on current barriers to adequate dairy, seafood, and ultimately iodine intake, as well as desired content and mode of delivery for dietary guidance/recommendation, was obtained through interviews with the recruited participants. Outcome measures were qualitative and analysed using thematic analysis.

Interviews were structured and followed a topic guide based around the Health Belief Model:

1. Form of dietary guidance received before pregnancy/during pregnancy/lactation.
2. The role of received dietary guidance in shaping food choices.
3. The perceived recommended levels of intake for iodine in pregnancy.
4. Knowledge on how the recommended intake of 250 µg per day iodine in pregnancy can be met.
5. Barriers and facilitators in meeting an adequate intake of dairy and seafood in pre-conception and during pregnancy and lactation.
6. Opinions on the best way to deliver dietary recommendations which are understandable and practical, regarding iodine nutrition.

As part of the interview process, participants were given coloured photos of different foods (dairy products, milk, salt, red meat, sushi, vegetables, fish and seafood) and were asked to name the sources of iodine. They were also provided with pictures of iodine-rich food portions (a glass of milk, milk in drinks, a portion of cheese, a pot of yoghurt, portions of fish), to estimate a combination that would cover their requirement for iodine in pregnancy.

The interview topic guide was pre-tested for clarity and comprehension in a group of women that did not take part in the main study. Validity and reliability were secured in the study during the design of the topic guide, the interviews process, and analysis, by following Yardley's [29] principles for assessment of qualitative research (i.e., sensitivity to context, commitment and rigour, transparency and coherence, impact and importance). In every step of the study, the authors followed the criteria of quality assessment, from the level of design to the level of data presentation.

Interviews were completed after reaching saturation in the upcoming themes. Interviews stopped when a lack of novel contributions was evident; the data collected were transcribed verbatim. Transcripts were reviewed by two researchers; after agreement that data saturation was reached, study recruitment closed.

2.5. Data Analysis and Statistics

All quantitative data from the socio-demographics and FFQ questionnaires were entered in an SPSS database. Descriptive statistics were calculated. Parametric data were described as mean and standard deviation and non-parametric as median and interquartile range (IQR). The FFQ data were analysed according to Combet and Lean [26]. The statistical software SPSS version 21.0 (IBM Corporation, New York, NY, USA) was used.

All interviews were audio-recorded, transcribed verbatim, and analysed with thematic analysis by following the four stages of the analysis: familiarisation with transcripts and data, generation of initial codes, searching for themes, and reviewing themes. NVivo version 11 (QSR International, Doncaster, Australia) was used in the analysis.

3. Results

3.1. Participants' Characteristics and Awareness of Iodine Importance

Only women meeting all inclusion criteria were recruited to the study. A total of 54 women were recruited to the study, of which six failed to complete the interviews and the short questionnaire, resulting in 48 women taking part. At the time of their participation, 38% were pregnant, 35% were breastfeeding, 10% were planning to start a family or were actively trying to conceive, and 17% had a baby or a toddler (younger than two years old) but were not breastfeeding. A minority were following a vegetarian diet (n = 4, 8%), and 17% were obese. All participants' characteristics are shown in Table 1. Out of the 48 interviews, 40 were phone and eight face-to-face interviews, with an average duration of 10:46 min (range 06:33–18:06 min).

Table 1. Participants' characteristics.

Demographic Data	Mean	SD
Maternal Age (years) n = 48	30.8	4.3
Pregnant n = 18	31.6	3.5
Breastfeeding/with baby n = 25	31.0	4.7
Planning a pregnancy n = 5	27.2	3.0
Child Age (weeks) n = 23	39.7	24.5
	Median	**IQR**
Maternal BMI (kg/m²) [1]	24	21–29
% WHO iodine recommendation achieved		
Increased demands (250 µg/day) (n = 35)	81	56–122
Basic demands (150 µg/day) (n = 13)	99	57–134
Total daily iodine intake (µg/day)		
Increased demands (n = 35)	203	140–304
Basic demands (n = 13)	148	85–202
	n	**%**
Ethnicity		
White Scottish	16	33
Other White British	26	54
Other ethnic groups	6	13
Residence		
Scotland	27	56
England, Wales, Northern Ireland	21	44
Education		
School level	3	6
College level	6	13
Undergraduate degree	24	50
Postgraduate degree	14	29
Parity		
0 (or expecting first)	15	31
1	27	56
2 or more	6	13
Use of supplements—all (n = 29/48)		
Iodised	17	35 [2]
Non-iodised	12	25
Increased demands (n = 24/35)		
Iodised	16	67 [3]
Non-iodised	8	33
Basic demands (n = 5/13)		
Iodised	1	20 [4]
Non-iodised	4	80
Smokers	1	2
Aware about iodine [5]	11	23
Low iodine confidence (1–3 points) [6]	34	72

[1] For pregnant women, the BMI (body mass index) has been calculated based on the pre-pregnancy weight reported by the participants; [2] Proportion of women taking iodised/non-iodised supplements out of the total sample; [3] Proportion of women taking iodised/non-iodised supplements out of the women with increased demands; [4] Proportion of women taking iodised/non-iodised supplements out of the women with basic demands; [5] Iodine awareness was defined as positive when the answer to the question "When it comes to healthy eating in pregnancy and lactation, have you heard of, or were you informed about iodine" was "yes"; [6] Iodine confidence referred to confidence on how to achieve an adequate iodine intake in pregnancy and lactation and was measured with a 7-point Likert scale (1: very low confidence −7: very high confidence). SD: standard deviation, IQR: interquartile range, WHO: World Health Organization.

Participants' awareness of iodine was poor. Only 23% (n = 11) had heard about iodine, lower than for other nutrients: folic acid 100% (n = 48), iron 92% (n = 44), calcium 85% (n = 41), vitamin D 75% (n = 36), and vitamin A 63% (n = 30). Only 25% (n = 12) reported awareness of the role of iodine in the development of the unborn baby. Confidence on how to achieve adequate iodine intake during pregnancy was low (score 1, 2, or 3 in a 7-point Likert scale) in 72% (n = 34) of the participants (mode = 1).

3.2. Iodine Intake

Out of the 48 participants, 73% (n = 35) had increased daily iodine demands according to WHO/UNICEF/ICCIDD and EFSA as they were pregnant or breastfeeding. Table 2 shows the median iodine intakes in those with basic or increased demands and the contributions of a range of food sources, as well as the proportion of the WHO/UNICEF/ICCIDD recommended intake achieved in each group, through diet and supplements.

Table 2. Iodine and iodine rich foods intake in participants with increased demands (250 µg/day, pregnant and breastfeeding) and normal adult demands (150 µg/day).

	Increased Demands (n = 35)		Basic Demands (n = 13)	
	Median	IQR	Median	IQR
Milk (g/day)	200	100–500	113	11–270
Other dairy (g/day) [1]	119	86–192	106	80–233
Fish (g/day)	39	9–65	43	0–101
Total daily iodine from dairy (µg/day)	120	90–185	121	62–146
Total daily iodine from milk (µg/day)	54	27–136	31	3–73
Total daily iodine from fish (µg/day)	21	8–31	29	0–53
% daily iodine from dairy	83	75–97	77	68–99
% daily iodine from milk	45	23–54	24	5–47
% daily iodine from fish	16	3–24	22	0–32
Total daily iodine from food (µg/day)	152	120–199	148	85–202
Total daily iodine with supplements (µg/day)—whole sample	203	140–304	148	85–202
Total daily iodine with supplements (µg/day) only in those taking supplement	299 [2]	215–233	550 [3]	550–550
% WHO recommendation achieved	81	56–122	99	57–134

[1] Other dairy includes all dairy products listed in the FFQ (food frequency questionnaire) excluding milk (i.e., cheese (hard and soft), yoghurts, milk/cream-based puddings, cheese-based dishes); [2] n = 16; [3] n = 1.

Dietary change in pregnancy varied among participants, with up to 16% reporting to decrease at least one type of dairy product, 22% reporting to cut-out a type of fish or seafood product, while 40% and 16% reported increasing dairy or fish/seafood, respectively.

3.3. Qualitative Results

Five main themes emerged from the analysis of the 48 interviews, summarised in Figure 1 with associated subthemes and their inter-relationships. The first theme included views about information received during the periods of preconception and pregnancy and focused on sources, content, and form of information, as well as perceived problems related to this information and attitudes of participants towards this advice. The second theme focused on the level of participants' iodine knowledge as a nutrient and the recommendations for pregnancy. The third theme was around the exploration of the acceptance of iodine sources and any barriers related to their intake. The fourth theme included views on preferred ways of dietary information delivery in the perinatal period of life. In parallel, the emotional dimension of receiving nutritional guidance in pregnancy emerged throughout the interviews.

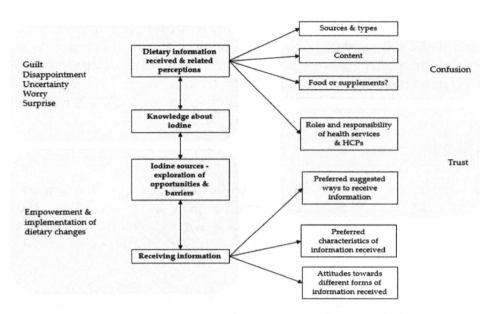

Figure 1.   Themes and main subthemes of the analysis and their relationships.   HCPs: healthcare professionals.

3.3.1. Dietary Information Received and Related Perceptions

Sources and Form of Received Dietary Information

There were differences in the type of informational support that participants had received in pregnancy nutrition, by case and between UK regions. Most had received written guidance (leaflets/booklets) from community midwives, mainly during the first antenatal care appointment (IT39: *"It was really only some leaflets that I was given by the midwife. I don't think she actually talked to me through or anything, it was just literature she handed over."*). Those living in Scotland mentioned the "Ready Steady Baby" as a source of information about pregnancy nutrition either as a book, a website, or an application. No similar resource was mentioned by participants from other geographical areas.

Verbal information was seldom commented on (IT14: *"My midwife on my first appointment asked whether I was aware (about dietary guidelines for pregnancy), I said I was generally aware but then she gave me general points."*). Short discussions with the midwives regarding nutrition were less frequent and mainly included a brief summary of the written information, mostly after participants' personal enquiry (IT05: *"It was I who brought it up with my midwife on one of the first visits. I had a couple of questions about how cheese and various things like that and it was me that actually brought it up with her. She didn't bring it up with me and really she answered a couple of questions but then told me to refer to this folder I've been given."*). Apart from the community midwives, who were mostly providing nutrition-related advice, general practitioners were also mentioned in providing verbal guidance, as well as friends and family. A quarter of the participants said that no one has spoken to them about nutrition in pregnancy. Participants interested in learning more about nutrition, including those that have received some form of information, did personal research, either online or using books.

Nutrition Information Content

Pregnancy nutrition-related information fell under three themes: eating a healthy balanced diet, avoiding certain foods, and taking folic acid and/or other multivitamin supplements. Most participants could not remember or list specific received nutrition information, and when they could, it was mainly about (i) avoiding uncooked and unpasteurised foods, alcohol, caffeine; and (ii) taking supplements. Lack of information regarding diet during lactation was also reported.

Around half of the participants highlighted how the information received during pregnancy was mainly related to the foods and other things to avoid (e.g., smoking, alcohol, raw fish and meat, vitamin

A, certain types of cheese) rather than foods to increase or maintain in their diet (IT21: *"It was more about what you couldn't eat though than what you should eat. It was more about avoiding things like caffeine and certain types of food rather than what was the best to eat."*). A group of the participants who reported having received information on what should be eaten during pregnancy believed that messages regarding foods to avoid were the most powerful.

Multiparous participants reported having received less information in subsequent pregnancies compared to their first one, as prior knowledge was assumed (IT42: *"I think I didn't receive a lot this time round, because this is my second pregnancy I think they kind of assumed I that I knew it from before."*).

Foods or Supplements?

A minor theme focused on multivitamins and folic acid with little information or knowledge on the foods that contain the required micronutrients (IT15: *"When I was told in the beginning from my midwife you shouldn't have too much vitamin A, nothing was really explained why and I am still not really clear what foods vitamin A is in, how I should avoid vitamin A."*). Many participants reported knowing that they should be taking supplements during pregnancy (mainly folic acid, vitamin D, or a multivitamin), having received this advice from their midwife, without information about food sources of the nutrient. A suggestion made was that iodine should be included in pregnancy supplements to cover needs, especially for those who do not know how to eat a balanced diet. Worryingly, some participants taking multivitamins felt confident that the needs are covered, justifying not paying attention to their diet (IT42: *"Since I became pregnant I've just been taking a multivitamin designed for pregnancy, so I am hoping that kind of covers most things."*). Only one participant reported that she forgot her supplements and was not taking them regularly, so found food recommendations easier to implement.

Role and Responsibility of Health Services and Healthcare Professionals

Participants usually referred to the health services (including the midwife, the general practitioner, the obstetrician, the health services literature, tools and services) for guidance during pregnancy. There was a high expectation that the health services would provide all the required dietary information during the first (booking) appointment or an earlier appointment, through verbal discussions, leaflets, booklets and referrals to online sources, websites, and applications. Most participants received this at their first antenatal care appointment with the community midwife (around eight to twelve weeks of pregnancy). Midwives were recognised to have experience in the field of pregnancy nutrition and were usually the first port of call when pregnant women were unsure about their diet (IT37: *"I trust very much what the midwife has to say in terms of my nutrition regarding my pregnancy, because they are quite experienced in that field."*). However, expectations were not always met, as described below (see Section 3.3.5 "Trust").

3.3.2. Knowledge about Iodine

Iodine was an unknown nutrient for most participants, with a minority linking it to infant brain development (through personal interest, reading or research, and seldom through their community midwife). Knowledge of the relation between iodine nutrition and the thyroid hormones was limited, without any deeper specific knowledge of its importance in pregnancy.

Most participants admitted not knowing the dietary sources of iodine and attempted to guess the correct iodine-rich foods from a selection of foods depicted. Most answers were chosen randomly and were often incorrect. Only a minority identified the iodine-rich foods being dairy and seafood products.

Participants were also asked to estimate the food combination that would cover requirements for iodine in pregnancy, using pictures with portions of iodine-rich foods (a glass of milk, milk in drinks such as tea, chocolate or coffee, a portion of cheese, a pot of yoghurt, a portion of white fish, and a portion of salmon). Most food combinations proposed would not have provided a sufficient iodine intake for pregnancy and lactation. The exercise triggered surprise and hesitation in the participants (evident through their expressions, pauses, and frequent change of answers).

3.3.3. Iodine Sources—Opportunities and Barriers

Attitudes towards dairy products were generally positive as half of the participants reported finding it quite easy to include or increase dairy in the diet in substantial amounts if necessary. Milk was believed to alleviate heartburn symptoms and was often craved during pregnancy (IT25: *"Milk, I probably, I had quite a lot of milk when I was pregnant, a lot of it was because of heartburn but I would say I could drink a lot of milk."*). In cases of dislike, participants still tried to increase dairy consumption via yogurts and/ or cheese (IT36: *"I do not drink milk but I do take a lot of cheese and yoghurts."*). The main barriers towards dairy consumption included taste (mainly of milk), lactose intolerance or other health conditions believed to be associated with dairy products (such as eczema), morning sickness in the first months of pregnancy, and perceptions about the unhealthfulness of cheese in products (fat, processed foods) (IT33: *"I think with cheese I try not to each too much because I think it is quite fat ... "*).

Fish and seafood consumption was perceived as harder to increase or maintain during pregnancy. Less than a fifth reported finding this easy and the barriers were further explored. For most, the main barrier was a general dislike of fish and seafood products. During pregnancy, this was exacerbated by heartburn, morning sickness, and change in taste and smell. Another major cause of fish exclusion was partners' and familial preferences, as well as lack of cooking skills and low knowledge (IT30: *"Well, I don't eat a lot of fish probably because my husband doesn't enjoy it and I don't like to cook more than one meal at once."*; IT09: *"People probably don't have as much knowledge on how to cook fish."*). However, even for participants with a high intention to consume fish and seafood, confusion regarding the recommendations, compounded by the worry of eating the wrong fish species, prevented the consumption of any fish and seafood type. Cost implications, low availability, and a habit of not buying or eating these products were also regularly described barriers (IT42: *"We are not in a habit of eating a lot of fish and that's one of the things we often say to ourselves we should have a little bit more of..."*). Vegetarians did not generally intend to change habits by including fish in their diet during pregnancy.

3.3.4. Receiving Dietary Information

Receiving Dietary Information—Attitudes towards Different Formats

The majority of views around verbal information were positive, with only a couple of participants stating not finding a discussion helpful regarding something important about pregnancy (IT48: *"If I was to go to the doctors and ask for advice there I don't think that would be as beneficial because (...) I feel it would be quite overwhelming (...) so if the midwife mentioned something to me I would remember but wouldn't really know too much about it so I would have to go and look into it for myself"*). During discussions with midwives, the participants recalled the opportunity to ask questions and get more in-depth knowledge regarding the importance of the advice received, even when the discussion was short. Discussion with an expert was proposed as more useful if accompanied by a leaflet, booklet, or another visual source to refer to later, as a reminder and prompt. However, it was agreed by most that such discussions rarely happen, with leaflets usually given without going through them verbally (IT05: *"So for me, the best thing for me would have been if the midwife had given me a brief overview and then maybe given me a leaflet or a web, specific web address to take away that I could then look into more depth afterwards"*).

A common theme that emerged was also around the written information received, especially leaflets and booklets. Leaflets were read by many participants, but too many were received during pregnancy and subsequently lost, thrown out, or misplaced when required (IT48: *"I was also given information in leaflet form but during pregnancy the amount of leaflets you get is unbelievable so you don't really pay attention, well I don't really pay attention to a lot of the hand out stuff I was given."*). However, participants self-characterised as "old school" written information in the form of bright, colourful leaflets with pictures that catch the attention, mainly given from the midwife or combined with verbal advice, a good and practical way of receiving information about pregnancy, diet, and specific nutrients. The information expected to appear on leaflets should be "clear", "specific", "comprehensive", and "straight forward". Leaflets were perceived as useful to remind participants about a key piece of information, more practical, smaller, and easier to read compared to books. If the leaflets were not brightly designed, participants mentioned forgetting them or not reading them (IT22: *"Basically kind of brightly designed or whatever, I would definitely pay attention to."*).

Most participants (who were often highly educated) referred to the internet as a source of information in pregnancy. Participants admitted using simple "Google" searches to obtain information about nutrition and pregnancy, and combining information from several online sources, including several websites, BabyCentre (BabyCentre® L.L.C., San Francisco, CA, USA) and healthcare services websites, fora, social media and weekly emails with leaflets, booklets, and verbal advice. However, the use of social media and other online sources is not always reliable, and often prompted by excitement about the new pregnancy and the intention to do everything right (IT05: *"These days obviously everybody goes straight on the internet, and that's what was one of the first things that I did, but the problem I think with that is that you google various phrases and it's more luck than judgement which websites you come up on"*; IT02: *"Well the first thing I do is look on the internet, but then you cannot really rely on that."*). Participants preferred the internet when looking for information, but recognised that a reliable source, complete with all the required information and presented by an expert, is needed (IT30: *"I like to look online and read things of a reliable source. I might use the NHS website or something similar rather than a forum. But you need to know to look, that's the problem."*). The combination with other sources (leaflets, discussions) was also perceived as an effective way of getting information, as well as the weekly emails that healthcare services or other reliable sources send to pregnant women (IT37: *"The emails from the NHS, once you are registered for your pregnancy are really good because you get an email like once a week or something like that (. . .) they are really helpful."*).

Mobile applications were considered an interactive way of dealing with nutritional requirements and increasing knowledge and awareness about specific dietary needs. For many participants, an application on a smartphone would be useful, easy, and innovative if they needed to get informed about a nutrient (e.g., iodine) and try to increase it in their diet. As technology is progressing and smartphones and tablets are becoming mainstream, especially in young women, participants suggested mobile applications during pregnancy and lactation to meet an information gap related to healthy eating, supplements reminder, fitness tips, and information about fetus development. Participants proposed that if the information relating to the importance of a nutrient was integrated with one of these mobile applications, or if a new specific mobile application could be developed, that would be useful, easy, and practical, especially if endorsed by the doctor or the midwife (IT25: *"You can get apps now for everything, so maybe an app that you could give out like different ideas on how you can get that nutrient you need in the right amount, maybe like meal ideas or something like that."*; IT05: *"The best thing for me would have been if the midwife had given me a brief overview and then maybe given me a leaflet or a web, specific web address to take away that I could then look into more depth afterwards."*). Tracking dietary intake by adding or ticking a checklist of foods commonly consumed daily via a mobile application was highlighted, with a view to tailor advice on dietary needs, including directions on what to consume to increase intake of a specific nutrient. A minority disagreed with the use of mobile applications, which they found overwhelming and burdensome (search, download, usage), preferring information from a booklet, a leaflet, or a conversation with their midwife instead (IT08: *"I found the most useful just conversation really I suppose rather than apps and research cause that's how I think you can get a bit overwhelming for pregnant mums and for first time pregnant mums."*).

Receiving Dietary Information—Preferred Formats and Stakeholders' Suggestions

Half of the participants interviewed stated that the information should be easier, quicker, clearer, more practical, basic, straight forward, and easy to remember and understand. They expressed the view that if the information was presented in a more visual, bright, and colourful way, including pictures or easy infographics, charts, and associations of nutrients with foods and portion sizes, it would stand to attention and be more likely to be remembered.

While understanding which nutrients are important in pregnancy, a gap was identified regarding portion size and the quantity of food required to obtain the correct amount of a nutrient (IT42: *"I think having something visual that kind of shows you clearly what, like what the portions equate to is really helpful"*). While some participants were confident about the nutrients of importance in pregnancy, they were unable to translate dietary requirements to a balanced meal. There was specific uncertainty on where to get nutrients from the diet, which and how much food, and the impact of different cooking methods.

Participants were asked what they consider the best way to convey or receive information about a specific nutrient. A clear majority believed that the healthcare services were best placed to deliver this advice. The midwife, general practitioner, other healthcare professionals (health visitors, nurses, and pharmacists), dieticians, and nutritionists were in most cases considered as the best sources of nutrition information. A face-to-face discussion, early in pregnancy or at the first booking appointment, or even in an antenatal class, was often suggested. Many participants proposed that a combination of this discussion alongside written and/or online information (a leaflet, a website) would be ideal—providing the choice to return to that information later for reference. The healthcare services website and emails were also suggested, as well as the internet in general (other websites, Google search, social media, fora).

For practical advice on how to increase iodine intake, some participants reported that advice from their midwife or doctor, potentially in combination with a reference to a website, a leaflet, or a booklet, would be sufficient. For others, knowledge of key nutritional focus points was also enough—with the future health of their child being an incentive to take the required steps to initiate change. Many other ideas were discussed, including iodised supplements use; iodised salt consumption; a tick sheet or a pin board with reminders for main foods, portions, and importance of iodine; internet websites; recipes or meal plans online and in books; fridge magnets and small reference cards; supermarket magazines; advertisements; food packaging information; and the use of a mobile application with relevant information. Understanding the portion sizes and the iodine content of the foods was considered important to manage an increased need in iodine during pregnancy.

When thinking innovatively, participants proposed different tools that could be designed to deliver information regarding iodine, nutrition, and pregnancy. Approximately half of the participants preferred a mobile application for their smartphone or tablet, accessible at all times, to track dietary intake and get reminders when to adapt their diet. Mobile application tailored meal plans were also suggested, as well as improved knowledge on portion sizes, recommended intakes, and needs; a comparator was mobile applications focusing on weight management. Visual prompts were identified as important for those with low literacy. Others preferred an easy, pictorial-based, and quick to refer to tool. Recipes, meal plans ideas, pictorial-based bright leaflets, and association of foods and portions with nutritional requirements were described as desirable ways of delivering information. Other proposals included TV programmes and advertisements, public health campaigns, weekly healthcare services emails, and infographics. A minority still supported a one-to-one discussion with their midwife or doctor and a referral to a reliable website, booklet, or leaflet, as sufficient sources of information.

3.3.5. Emotional Dimensions of Receiving Dietary Advice and Information

Confusion

Confusion about the information received was often observed. Participants reported finding different pregnancy recommendations between the UK and other countries, getting different advice between different UK areas, and receiving conflicting information from different healthcare professionals (IT09: *"And then a different midwife had a completely different attitude."*). The lack of a single reference place with comprehensive information about all nutrients was also reported (IT26: *"They should tell you exactly what you need to have, you need to have a leaflet or like a website … It should be clearer, now it is not clear at all."*). Some recommendations were perceived as difficult to understand

and implement in terms of know-how (e.g., vitamin A content of foods, recognising unpasteurised products), and overwhelming in the context of all other dietary recommendations available.

Empowerment—Implementation of Dietary Changes

Analysis highlighted a theme of clear commitment to change behaviour if prompted or made aware (IT06: *"If I knew how important it was, I would increase it."*). Almost half of the participants highlighted the fact that if they had the knowledge, the information, and the awareness about the importance of a factor during their pregnancy (in this case mainly referring to increasing their iodine intake), they would make a conscious effort to change their behaviour or practice. The intention was already high, even from the period of preconception, as participants believed that those at that stage of life want the best for their baby and themselves. Proactivity was also evident in many cases, as nutrition was a topic often brought up by participants to their midwives. Participants asked questions and ended-up looking online for advice when they did not get the level of advice they required or expected. All participants reported having read or considered the information given to them, with the majority stating that they adjusted their diet (with a minority not changing habits through belief of already achieving a balanced diet). To feel confident of meeting all nutrients' recommended intake, multivitamin supplements were frequently adopted.

Trust

A trustful source of information was very important for most participants. A clear theme of trust emerged towards the health services and the healthcare professionals. The health services were very often mentioned during the interviews and were considered as the norm for the provision of trustful dietary and pregnancy advice. The most trustful and suitable advisors were "an expert", "the midwife", and "the general practitioner/ doctor", as well as the staff running antenatal classes (IT47: *"I think probably is verbally so that we could ask questions rather than just written information, and maybe not necessarily one to one but along with those pre-antenatal type classes."*). However, although initial attitudes expressed towards the health services were high expectations and trust, they were followed by disappointment regarding the actual amount of advice received. Similar feelings arose towards the general practitioner surgeries that did not provide nutrition information, which had been an expectation from several participants.

The internet and smartphone applications were considered useful sources of information, but the issue of source reliability emerged. As a result, the healthcare services website or websites proposed by experts were the online sources that participants trusted most. Moreover, the health services application and the BabyCentre application (BabyCentre® L.L.C., San Francisco, CA, USA) were widely used as reliable sources.

Negative Feelings

Pregnancy is a stage of life when the fetus totally depends on its mother for the supply of nutrients—a fact appreciated by most participants. For this reason, participants were usually positive in making dietary and lifestyle changes (as mentioned above in *"Empowerment—implementation of dietary changes"*), but at the same time, this responsibility triggered negative feelings. Apart from the disappointment mentioned above, uncertainty regarding the dietary recommendations was expressed. This triggered, in some cases, worry and lack of confidence on adequate adherence to guidance (example of fish recommendations, as mentioned in Section 3.3.3.)

Towards the end of the interview, the importance of iodine for fetal development, and the richest dietary sources of iodine, were presented to the participants, alongside an indicative food combination selected to achieve the pregnancy daily recommended iodine intake. Some participants expressed surprise and disappointment at that point, and questioned why iodine had not been mentioned to them in peri-natal care. Worry and stress were also apparent through tone of voice and expressions, when participants realised the importance of iodine and were unsure whether needs had been covered

(IT27: *"There is not enough guidance. As I say I felt I am quite surprised, even a little bit disappointed I didn't know how important iodine, how important the role is it plays in the fetal development."*). In a couple of cases, participants reported feeling overwhelmed and under pressure to follow the pregnancy recommendations, resulting in guilt for not "getting everything right" (IT08: *"That put a lot of pressure and a lot of guilt on me, but the second time round I decided to be a bit more relaxed and trust my body a bit more."*).

4. Discussion

4.1. Main Findings

ID is a global public health concern, with the latest ICCIDD data highlighting the general populations in as many as 20 countries, and the pregnant populations of as many as 39 countries being mildly to severely deficient [30]. Correcting ID is especially important in high risk groups, such as pregnant women and their infants. To achieve this, it is essential to understand the underlying causes of ID and the understanding of iodine nutrition by the populations concerned [22].

We explored the lack of iodine awareness and knowledge in pregnancy and the dietary and nutrition information received in and around pregnancy, to identify potential ways to improve information delivery at that stage of life. After an in-depth discussion with stakeholders, around the themes of dietary advice received in pregnancy, preferred ways of information delivery, and the knowledge and awareness of iodine nutrition, we identified gaps related to dietary advice in pregnancy and the way it is provided. Our results agree and strengthen previous findings that awareness and knowledge are low amongst pregnant women [8], even though more pregnant women achieved the WHO recommended iodine intake [2] in this sample compared to previous results (81% in this study vs. 46% in 1st trimester/40% in second and third trimesters previously [8]). Dietary guidance during pregnancy was described as confusing, focusing mostly on foods to avoid, supplements, and selected nutrients of interest (not iodine), and was not always perceived as sufficient or helpful enough to trigger effective dietary changes. Participants highlighted the need for clearer recommendations, with a clearer focus on foods and portion sizes, but also emphasised their trust in the health services.

4.2. Barriers to Iodine Sufficiency

Until recently, the UK was thought to be iodine replete; however, the inadequate iodine status of the British population was highlighted in a multi-centre survey of school girls [7]. The reasons behind the re-emergence of iodine insufficiency are multifaceted and need to be explored systematically.

Most countries have implemented mandatory salt iodisation in table and food industry salt [31]. In the UK, the regulatory and legislative framework means that salt iodisation is voluntary. Iodised salt availability is low [32], and mandatory iodine fortification is still perceived to conflict with the public health message for salt reduction and chronic diseases [33]. In our study, a single participant used iodised salt and 60% reported rarely or never using salt at the table—meaning that voluntary fortification is not likely to effectively address iodine insufficiency through the consumption of table salt alone, since most sodium is consumed through ready-meals and processed foods. Universal salt iodisation has been successful in correcting ID in population level worldwide. However, studies in Italy [34], Turkey [35], and Tasmania [36] showed that ID in pregnant women persisted after the application of universal salt iodisation and awareness and knowledge of the female population regarding iodine's role and sources remained poor after salt fortification [37]. Iodine reference intake for pregnancy has not been reviewed by the UK Department of Health since 1991, and remains similar to those of non-pregnant adults—a possible contributor to the lack of awareness. Iodine is also often lacking from pregnancy supplements and dietary guidance does not specifically cover the importance of iodine or its dietary sources.

Pregnant women depend on community midwives during antenatal care. The health services are the main providers of dietary and lifestyle advice in pregnancy, in agreement with previous findings from Australia [38]. Consequently, dietary guidance starts around the 10th week of pregnancy, possibly too late for addressing the impact of any iodine insufficiency on fetal neurodevelopment, as the myelination process is complete in the first trimester. Our results highlight the role and importance of the health services in the provision of dietary information around pregnancy. Two contrasting feelings—one of trust, the other of disappointment, were apparent in respect to the relationship with the healthcare professionals and the delivery of information on nutrition and iodine. Awareness and knowledge regarding iodine nutrition in pregnancy have been previously found to be low amongst healthcare professionals in the UK [39] and other countries [23,40–43], and may partially contribute toward the shift from trust to disappointment. The lack of nutrition education that midwives receive is an important area to tackle [44,45], while recognising the stresses and burdens experienced by this group of healthcare professionals, especially the restricted time to cover several complex aspects of pregnancy care and related advice.

As healthcare professionals lack nutritional knowledge, the iodine and nutrition information pregnant women receive is limited, fostering poor knowledge and awareness [8]. We highlighted divergent experiences of receiving dietary guidance in pregnancy (depth and breadth), with variations between healthcare teams, geographical areas, and parity, but also personal interest of the pregnant women, previous pregnancy experience, and educational background. Our findings confirm our previous results, showing that although information on pregnancy guidelines comes from several sources, confusion and uncertainty prevail, under the need of a reference source of reliable information. The way dietary guidance was delivered during pregnancy, and the level of depth covered, also varies between geographical areas in the UK, with inconsistencies amongst antenatal care teams, and is largely influenced by the personal interest of the pregnant women, their previous experience of pregnancy, and their educational background. As a result, our study highlights a clear need for a trustful, more comprehensive source of dietary advice in pregnancy for women to follow without feeling confused by different conflicting or unclear guidelines.

An important aspect in the landscape of strategies to address iodine insufficiency is the availability and choice of iodine-rich foods (dairy products, fish and seafood, including seaweed, iodised salt) and the potential barriers to their consumption. Since the 1970s, the demand for milk and milk products has decreased steadily [46], but barriers to their consumption are often overlooked. In an area without known ID (Sabadell, Catalonia, Spain), the iodine status of 600 pregnant women was found to be inadequate, based on their UIC (104 µg/L). The FFQ results associated milk and supplements intake with a 41% and 78% lower risk, respectively, of having UIC levels below 150 µg/L [47]. In this study, we highlight the organoleptic and behavioural dimensions linked to milk and other dairy products avoidance, including taste and smell, and, less often, adherence to a strict vegetarian or vegan diet, or its association with health-related issues (perceived or diagnose lactose intolerance). Other studies which have explored drivers of dairy food choices also identified family members' taste preferences and needs, cost and health benefits [48–50], but also gender, age, and socioeconomic status [51]. Choice behaviours regarding milk and dairy products in the context of iodine nutrition are compounded by environmental factors: milk iodine concentration is lower in the spring and summer and in organic milk products [52,53]; therefore, seasonality and milk type should be taken into consideration when making recommendations and measuring intake [54], as milk remains the main source of iodine in the UK [10].

Attitudes were generally more negative towards fish and seafood products. Main barriers included general dislike due to taste and smell, followed by family's preferences, lack of cooking skills, cost, and availability, in agreement with previous results [55]. However, an important barrier for fish and seafood consumption in pregnancy lay in the confusion in the dietary recommendations in pregnancy, namely restricting the intake of certain fish species due to heavy metals, toxins, and bacterial risk. In extreme cases, this confusion and perception of a risk led to total avoidance of fish, despite two portions of fish per week (one of which oil-rich) being advised [56]. This is consistent with the findings of Bloomingdale et al. in Boston, who found that women would rather exclude fish intake in pregnancy than risk harming themselves or their infant's health [57].

Even though dietary information received during pregnancy is plenty, the way this information is delivered is a key factor in facilitating their implementation (including memorisation, understanding, behaviour change). Clear information, with more focus on portion sizes and foods rather than nutrients, are some of the main characteristics desired by participants. With 90% of people aged 16–24 and 87% of those aged 25–34 owning a smartphone in the UK in 2015 [58], technologically-based information delivery should be reinforced. However, the use of technology can alienate minorities (e.g., women of low socioeconomic status, low education, homeless, socially deprived, urban migrant groups) and care should be taken to avoid exclusion of those groups from accessing information, since they are often the groups needing advice the most [59]. Although technology usage, broadly, and internet access is increasing, the quality of information available online is often questionable, and quality control is needed [60]. The BabyCentre (BabyCentre® L.L.C., San Francisco, CA, USA) website and application, for example, belong to the Johnson & Johnson group, a commercial entity, which participants still trusted despite the lack of affiliation to the health services. Overall, health information technology can be effective for preventive health and increasing adherence to guidelines, but cost-effectiveness data are limited and inconclusive [61].

4.3. Strengths and Limitations

The choice of qualitative design helped in the deep investigation of the topic of iodine nutrition in pregnancy and perceptions on the way dietary guidance is delivered in the perinatal period of life. This deep understanding of the reasons why iodine insufficiency is present in those life stages is needed to effectively address this public health issue.

Iodine intake was quantified with our previously validated iodine specific FFQ for women of childbearing age [26], as a suitable way to classify participants based on their habitual intake of micronutrients, giving us the opportunity to know whether the perceptions of the study population would represent women with a range of different levels of intake.

Recruitment mainly took place online, to reach a population across the UK. As a result, women residing in England, Scotland, Wales, and Northern Ireland were recruited, increasing the sample's representativeness. The study population is highly educated, with less than 30% of the participants not having a Bachelor's degree or higher. This is however in agreement with the national statistics, as the level of education improves with the years and is higher in females of that age (childbearing age) compared to males. The 16 to 24 year old individuals Not in Education, Employment, or Training in 2014–2015 have decreased by three points since 2010–2011, accounting for only 15.3% in females of that age [62]. Comparing the study population with the British population, the education level is higher but worryingly, even in that educated young population which could also be biased in terms of interest in pregnancy nutrition, the lack of awareness regarding iodine nutrition in pregnancy remains low.

Our sample also did not include a high percentage of obese women (17% versus 26% in the UK [63]) or smokers (1% versus 14.1% of women in the UK [64]), and had no drug or alcohol dependent women, but included 13% of non-British women. In more vulnerable groups, it is possible that dietary advice would be supplanted by focus on areas deemed more pressing—such as tobacco or alcohol dependencies. This is a dimension not explored in this study.

Lastly, information about iodine was already in the information sheet participants had received, and the question regarding the sources of iodine was asked both in the questionnaire they filled in and during the interviews. As a result, their answers were potentially influenced by these factors.

5. Conclusions

The lack of iodine fortification in the UK provides an unusual, highly appropriate, ecological terrain to study the impact of a simple food or education-based intervention to tackle iodine insufficiency and its endocrine and neurodevelopmental consequences. The approach used in this study assumed that evaluating needs and expectations of stakeholders (mothers and women planning a pregnancy or breastfeeding) would enhance the design of suitable and impactful dietary recommendations and information packages, ultimately to improve iodine sufficiency.

Iodine nutrition is important during pregnancy and lactation, but awareness and knowledge is low amongst women of childbearing age, even with high educational attainment, and among healthcare professionals in the UK.

Dietary guidance received in pregnancy is not clear, leading to confusion over recommendations. There is a need to focus on specific foods and portion sizes, rather than nutrients, supplements, and specific recommendations that are not tethered to a balanced diet and the associated know-how, that many assume is in place (such as cooking skills and knowledge of foods). Future work should incorporate users' input to design and implement tailored health promotion approaches. In Scotland, a nutrition education intervention in pregnancy was found to be acceptable in 16–18 year old pregnant women; however, with limited effectiveness in term of changing dietary habits [65]. There is scope to build on such an intervention to improve iodine status in pregnancy. However, it is likely that, to tackle iodine insufficiency in and around pregnancy, a multi-sprung approach will be required, tackling several different angles of the problem [22]. Mobile health tools open an existing range of opportunities for personalised health, which, combined with regulatory steps, conventional dietary advice through health care professionals, and targeted awareness campaigns, would form a comprehensive approach to the public health challenge iodine has become.

Acknowledgments: M.B. received a Ph.D. scholarship from Glasgow Children's Hospital Charity (Grant Number: YRSS-2014-05).

Author Contributions: E.C. and M.B. conceived and designed the study. M.B. recruited participants, completed the interviews, and analysed the data, as part of a Ph.D. programme under the supervision of E.C. and M.E.J.L. E.C. and M.B. reviewed the transcripts. All authors contributed to the preparation of the manuscript, for which M.B. wrote the first draft.

Abbreviations

The following abbreviations are used in this manuscript:

EFSA	European Food Safety Authority
FFQ	Food frequency questionnaire
HCP	Healthcare professional
ICCIDD	International Council for the Control of Iodine Deficiency Disorders
ID	Iodine deficiency
IQ	Intelligence quotient
IQR	Interquartile range
UIC	Urinary Iodine Concentration
UK	United Kingdom
UNICEF	United Nations Children's Fund
WHO	World Health Organisation

References

1. World Health Organisation. *Urinary Iodine Concentrations for Determining Iodine Status in Populations;* World Health Organisation: Geneva, Switzerland, 2013.

2. World Health Organisation; United Nations Children's Fund; International Council for the Control of Iodine Deficiency Disorders. *Assessment of Iodine Deficiency Disorders and Monitoring Their Elimination. A Guide for Programme Managers;* World Health Organisation: Geneva, Switzerland, 2007.

3.   Bath, S.C.; Steer, C.D.; Golding, J.; Emmett, P.; Rayman, M.P. Effect of inadequate iodine status in UK pregnant women on cognitive outcomes in their children: Results from the Avon Longitudinal Study of Parents and Children (ALSPAC). *Lancet* **2013**, *382*, 331–337. [CrossRef]

4.   Bath, S.C.; Rayman, M.P. A review of the iodine status of UK pregnant women and its implications for the offspring. *Environ. Geochem. Health* **2015**, *37*, 619–629. [CrossRef] [PubMed]

5.   Lampropoulou, M.; Lean, M.; Combet, E. Iodine status of women of childbearing age in Scotland. In Proceedings of the Translational Nutrition: Integrating Research, Practice and Policy, London, UK, 16–19 July 2012.

6.   Kibirige, M.S.; Hutchison, S.; Owen, C.J.; Delves, H.T. Prevalence of maternal dietary iodine insufficiency in the north east of England: Implications for the fetus. *Arch. Dis. Child. Fetal Neonatal Ed.* **2004**, *89*, F436–F439. [CrossRef] [PubMed]

7.   Vanderpump, M.P.; Lazarus, J.H.; Smyth, P.P.; Laurberg, P.; Holder, R.L.; Boelaert, K.; Franklyn, J.A. Iodine status of UK schoolgirls: A cross-sectional survey. *Lancet* **2011**, *377*, 2007–2012. [CrossRef]

8.   Combet, E.; Bouga, M.; Pan, B.; Lean, M.E.J.; Christopher, C.O. Iodine and pregnancy—A UK cross-sectional survey of dietary intake, knowledge and awareness. *Br. J. Nutr.* **2015**, *114*, 108–117. [CrossRef] [PubMed]

9.   Zimmermann, M.B. Iodine and iodine deficiency disorders. In *Present Knowledge in Nutrition*; Wiley-Blackwell: Hoboken, NJ, USA, 2012; pp. 554–567.

10.   Bates, B.; Cox, L.; Nicholson, S.; Page, P.; Prentice, A.; Steer, T.; Swan, G. *National Diet and Nutrition Survey. Results from Years 5–6 (Combined) of the Rolling Programme (2012/13–2013/14)*; Public Health England: London, UK, 2016.

11.   Rasmussen, L.B.; Ovesen, L.; Bulow, I.; Jorgensen, T.; Knudsen, N.; Laurberg, P.; Pertild, H. Dietary iodine intake and urinary iodine excretion in a Danish population: Effect of geography, supplements and food choice. *Br. J. Nutr.* **2002**, *87*, 61–69. [CrossRef] [PubMed]

12.   Remer, T.; Neubert, A.; Manz, F. Increased risk of iodine deficiency with vegetarian nutrition. *Br. J. Nutr.* **1999**, *81*, 45–49. [CrossRef] [PubMed]

13.   Combet, E. Iodine Status, Thyroid Function, and Vegetarianism. In *Vegetarian and Plant-Based Diets in Health and Disease Prevention*; Elsevier: Amsterdam, The Netherlands, 2017; pp. 769–790.

14.   Krajčovičová-Kudláčková, M.; Bučková, K.; Klimeš, I.; Šeboková, E. Iodine Deficiency in Vegetarians and Vegans. *Ann. Nutr. Metab.* **2003**, *47*, 183–185. [CrossRef] [PubMed]

15.   Leung, A.M.; Lamar, A.; He, X.; Braverman, L.E.; Pearce, E.N. Iodine status and thyroid function of Boston-area vegetarians and vegans. *J. Clin. Endocrinol. Metab.* **2011**, *96*, E1303–E1307. [CrossRef] [PubMed]

16.   Bougma, K.; Aboud, F.E.; Harding, K.B.; Marquis, G.S. Iodine and mental development of children 5 years old and under: A systematic review and meta-analysis. *Nutrients* **2013**, *5*, 1384–1416. [CrossRef] [PubMed]

17.   Abel, M.; Ystrom, E.; Caspersen, I.; Meltzer, H.; Aase, H.; Torheim, L.; Askeland, R.; Reichborn-Kjennerud, T.; Brantsæter, A. Maternal Iodine Intake and Offspring Attention-Deficit/Hyperactivity Disorder: Results from a Large Prospective Cohort Study. *Nutrients* **2017**, *9*, 1239. [CrossRef] [PubMed]

18.   Monahan, M.; Boelaert, K.; Jolly, K.; Chan, S.; Barton, P.; Roberts, T.E. Costs and benefits of iodine supplementation for pregnant women in a mildly to moderately iodine-deficient population: A modelling analysis. *Lancet Diabetes Endocrinol.* **2015**, *3*, 715–722. [CrossRef]

19.   Zhou, S.J.; Skeaff, S.A.; Ryan, P.; Doyle, L.W.; Anderson, P.J.; Kornman, L.; McPhee, A.J.; Yelland, L.N.; Makrides, M. The effect of iodine supplementation in pregnancy on early childhood neurodevelopment and clinical outcomes: Results of an aborted randomised placebo-controlled trial. *Trials* **2015**, *16*, 563. [CrossRef] [PubMed]

20.   He, F.J.; Ma, Y.; Feng, X.; Zhang, W.; Lin, L.; Guo, X.; Zhang, J.; Niu, W.; Wu, Y.; MacGregor, G.A. Effect of salt reduction on iodine status assessed by 24 hour urinary iodine excretion in children and their families in northern China: A substudy of a cluster randomised controlled trial. *BMJ Open* **2016**, *6*, e011168. [CrossRef] [PubMed]

21.   The Lancet Diabetes Endocrinology. Iodine deficiency in the UK: Grabbing the low-hanging fruit. *Lancet Diabetes Endocrinol.* **2016**, *4*, 469.

22.   Bouga, M.; Lean, M.E.J.; Combet, E. Contemporary challenges to iodine status and nutrition—The role of foods, dietary recommendations, fortification and supplementation. *Proc. Nutr. Soc.* **2018**, in press.

23. Lucas, C.J.; Charlton, K.E.; Brown, L.; Brock, E.; Cummins, L. Antenatal shared care: Are pregnant women being adequately informed about iodine and nutritional supplementation? *Aust. N. Z. J. Obstet. Gynaecol.* **2014**, *54*, 515–521. [CrossRef] [PubMed]

24. O'Kane, S.M.; Pourshahidi, L.K.; Farren, K.M.; Mulhern, M.S.; Strain, J.J.; Yeates, A.J. Iodine knowledge is positively associated with dietary iodine intake among women of childbearing age in the UK and Ireland. *Br. J. Nutr.* **2016**, *116*, 1728–1735. [CrossRef] [PubMed]

25. Rosenstock, I. *The Health Belief Model: Explaining Health Behavior through Expectancies*; Jossey-Bass: San Francisco, CA, USA, 1990; pp. 39–62.

26. Combet, E.; Lean, M.E.J. Validation of a short food frequency questionnaire specific for iodine in UK females of childbearing age. *J. Hum. Nutr. Diet.* **2014**, *27*, 599–605. [CrossRef] [PubMed]

27. Ritchie, J.; Lewis, J.; McNaughton Nicholls, C.; Ormston, R. *Qualitative Research Practice*; SAGE: London, UK, 2014.

28. Braun, V.; Clarke, V. *Successful Qualitative Research: A Practical Guide for Beginners*; SAGE: London, UK, 2013.

29. Yardley, L. Dilemmas in qualitative health research. *Psychol. Health* **2000**, *15*, 215–228. [CrossRef]

30. IDD Newsletter. *Global Iodine Scorecard 2017*; IDD Newsletter: Indianapolis, IN, USA, 2017.

31. World Health Organisation. *Fortification of Food—Grade Salt with Iodine for the Prevention and Control of Iodine Deficiency Disorders*; World Health Organisation: Geneva, Switzerland, 2014.

32. Bath, S.C.; Button, S.; Rayman, M.P. Availability of iodised table salt in the UK—Is it likely to influence population iodine intake? *Public Health Nutr.* **2014**, *17*, 450–454. [CrossRef] [PubMed]

33. Charlton, K.; Webster, J.; Kowal, P. To legislate or not to legislate? A comparison of the UK and South African approaches to the development and implementation of salt reduction programs. *Nutrients* **2014**, *6*, 3672–3695. [CrossRef] [PubMed]

34. Marchioni, E.; Fumarola, A.; Calvanese, A.; Piccirilli, F.; Tommasi, V.; Cugini, P.; Ulisse, S.; Rossi Fanelli, F.; D'Armiento, M. Iodine deficiency in pregnant women residing in an area with adequate iodine intake. *Nutrition* **2008**, *24*, 458–461. [CrossRef] [PubMed]

35. Kut, A.; Gursoy, A.; Senbayram, S.; Bayraktar, N.; Budakoglu, I.İ.; Akgun, H.S. Iodine intake is still inadequate among pregnant women eight years after mandatory iodination of salt in Turkey. *J. Endocrinol. Investig.* **2010**, *33*, 461–464. [CrossRef] [PubMed]

36. Burgess, J.R.; Seal, J.A.; Stilwell, G.M.; Reynolds, P.J.; Taylor, E.R.; Parameswaran, V. A case for universal salt iodisation to correct iodine deficiency in pregnancy: Another salutary lesson from Tasmania. *Med. J. Aust.* **2007**, *186*, 574–576. [PubMed]

37. Charlton, K.; Yeatman, H.; Lucas, C.; Axford, S.; Gemming, L.; Houweling, F.; Goodfellow, A.; Ma, G. Poor Knowledge and Practices Related to Iodine Nutrition during pregnancy and Lactation in Australian Women: Pre- and Post-Iodine fortification. *Nutrients* **2012**, *4*, 1317–1327. [CrossRef] [PubMed]

38. Charlton, K.E.; Gemming, L.; Yeatman, H.; Ma, G. Suboptimal iodine status of Australian pregnant women reflects poor knowledge and practices related to iodine nutrition. *Nutrition* **2010**, *26*, 963–968. [CrossRef] [PubMed]

39. Williamson, C.; Lean, M.E.; Combet, E. Dietary iodine: Awareness, knowledge and current practice among midwives. In Proceedings of the Translational Nutrition: Integrating Research, Practice and Policy, London, UK, 16–19 July 2012.

40. De Leo, S.; Pearce, E.N.; Braverman, L.E. Iodine Supplementation in Women during Preconception, Pregnancy, and Lactation: Current Clinical Practice by U.S. Obstetricians and Midwives. *Thyroid* **2016**, *27*, 434–439. [CrossRef] [PubMed]

41. Guess, K.; Malek, L.; Anderson, A.; Makrides, M.; Zhou, S.J. Knowledge and practices regarding iodine supplementation: A national survey of healthcare providers. *Women Birth* **2017**, *30*, e56–e60. [CrossRef] [PubMed]

42. Kut, A.; Kalli, H.; Anil, C.; Mousa, U.; Gursoy, A. Knowledge, attitudes and behaviors of physicians towards thyroid disorders and iodine requirements in pregnancy. *J. Endocrinol. Investig.* **2015**, *38*, 1057–1064. [CrossRef] [PubMed]

43. Nithiananthan, V.; Carroll, R.; Krebs, J. Iodine supplementation in pregnancy and breastfeeding: A New Zealand survey of user awareness. *N. Z. Med. J.* **2013**, *126*, 94–97. [PubMed]

44. Moore, H.; Adamson, A.J.; Gill, T.; Waine, C. Nutrition and the health care agenda: A primary care perspective. *Fam. Pract.* **2000**, *17*, 197–202. [CrossRef] [PubMed]

45.   Arrish, J.; Yeatman, H.; Williamson, M. Midwives and nutrition education during pregnancy: A literature review. *Women Birth* **2014**, *27*, 2–8. [CrossRef] [PubMed]

46.   Revoredo-Giha, C. Understanding consumers' trends on the purchases of dairy products. In *Improving Health Attributes of Dairy Chains Workshop*; Scotland's Rural College: Edinburgh, UK, 2013.

47.   Alvarez-Pedrerol, M.; Ribas-Fitó, N.; García-Esteban, R.; Rodriguez, À.; Soriano, D.; Guxens, M.; Mendez, M.; Sunyer, J. Iodine sources and iodine levels in pregnant women from an area without known iodine deficiency. *Clin. Endocrinol.* **2010**, *72*, 81–86. [CrossRef] [PubMed]

48.   Hammond, G.K.; Chapman, G.E. Decision-making in the dairy aisle: Maximizing taste, health, cost and family considerations. *Can. J. Diet. Pract. Res.* **2008**, *69*, 66–70. [CrossRef] [PubMed]

49.   Richardson-Harman, N.J.; Stevens, R.; Walker, S.; Gamble, J.; Miller, M.; Wong, M.; McPherson, A. Mapping consumer perceptions of creaminess and liking for liquid dairy products. *Food Qual. Prefer.* **2000**, *11*, 239–246. [CrossRef]

50.   Hagy, L.F.; Brochetti, D.; Duncan, S.E. Focus groups identified women's perceptions of dairy foods. *J. Women Aging* **2000**, *12*, 99–115. [CrossRef] [PubMed]

51.   Ares, G.; Gambaro, A. Influence of gender, age and motives underlying food choice on perceived healthiness and willingness to try functional foods. *Appetite* **2007**, *49*, 148–158. [CrossRef] [PubMed]

52.   Payling, L.M.; Juniper, D.T.; Drake, C.; Rymer, C.; Givens, D.I. Effect of milk type and processing on iodine concentration of organic and conventional winter milk at retail: Implications for nutrition. *Food Chem.* **2015**, *178*, 327–330. [CrossRef] [PubMed]

53.   Bath, S.C.; Button, S.; Rayman, M.P. Iodine concentration of organic and conventional milk: Implications for iodine intake. *Br. J. Nutr.* **2012**, *107*, 935–940. [CrossRef] [PubMed]

54.   Bath, S.C.; Button, S.; Rayman, M.P. Does farm-management system affect milk-iodine concentration? Comparison study of organic and conventional milk. In Proceedings of the 70th Anniversary: From Plough through Practice to Policy, London, UK, 4–6 July 2011.

55.   Verbeke, W.; Vackier, I. Individual determinants of fish consumption: Application of the theory of planned behaviour. *Appetite* **2005**, *44*, 67–82. [CrossRef] [PubMed]

56.   Public Health England. *The Eatwell Guide*; Public Health England: London, UK, 2016.

57.   Bloomingdale, A.; Guthrie, L.B.; Price, S.; Wright, R.O.; Platek, D.; Haines, J.; Oken, E. A qualitative study of fish consumption during pregnancy. *Am. J. Clin. Nutr.* **2010**, *92*, 1234–1240. [CrossRef] [PubMed]

58.   Statista. Smartphone Ownership Penetration in the United Kingdom (UK) in 2012–2015, by Age. Available online: http://www.statista.com/statistics/271851/smartphone-owners-in-the-united-kingdom-uk-by-age/ (accessed on 16 May 2017).

59.   Adams, O. *Falling through the Net: Defining the Digital Divide*; A Report on the Telecommunications and Information Technology Gap in America: US Department of Commerce; National Telecommunications and Information Administration (NTIA): Washington, DC, USA, 2000. Available online: http://www.ntia.doc.gov/ntiahome/fttn99/contents.html (accessed on 30 January 2018).

60.   Eysenbach, G. Consumer health informatics. *Br. Med. J.* **2000**, *320*, 1713–1716. [CrossRef]

61.   Chaudhry, B.; Wang, J.; Wu, S.; Maglione, M.; Mojica, W.; Roth, E.; Morton, S.C.; Shekelle, P.G. Systematic review: Impact of health information technology on quality, efficiency, and costs of medical care. *Ann. Intern. Med.* **2006**, *144*, 742–752. [CrossRef] [PubMed]

62.   Department for Education. *Education and Training Statistics for the United Kingdom*; Department for Education: London, UK, 2015.

63.   NHS Digital. *Statistics on Obesity, Physical Activity and Diet—England 2017 Report*; NHS Didital: Leeds, UK, 2017.

64.   Office for National Statistics; Public Health England. *Statistical Bulletin: Adult Smoking Habits in the UK: 2016*; Office for National Statistics: South Wales, UK, 2017.

65.   Symon, A.G.; Wrieden, W.L. A qualitative study of pregnant teenagers' perceptions of the acceptability of a nutritional education intervention. *Midwifery* **2003**, *19*, 140–147. [CrossRef]

6

Iodine Status in Schoolchildren and Pregnant Women of Lazio, a Central Region of Italy

Enke Baldini [1], Camilla Virili [2], Eleonora D'Armiento [3], Marco Centanni [2] and Salvatore Ulisse [1,*]

[1]   Department of Surgical Sciences, "Sapienza" University of Rome, 00161 Rome, Italy
[2]   Department of Medico-Surgical Sciences and Biotechnologies, "Sapienza" University of Rome, 04100 Latina, Italy
[3]   Department of Internal Medicine and Medical Specialties, "Sapienza" University of Rome, 00161 Rome, Italy
*   Correspondence: salvatore.ulisse@uniroma1.it

Abstract: The inhabitants of Lazio, similarly to those of other Italian regions, have been historically exposed to the detrimental effects of an inadequate intake of iodine. The latter is a micronutrient essential for the biosynthesis of thyroid hormones (TH). Iodine deficiency is responsible for a number of adverse effects on human health known as iodine deficiency disorders (IDD), the most common of which worldwide are goiter and hypothyroidism. In order to reduce IDD, a national salt iodination program was started in Italy in 2005. In this article we reviewed the available data regarding iodine intake in the Lazio population before and after the introduction of the national salt iodination program, in order to evaluate its efficacy and the eventual problem(s) limiting its success. On the whole, the information acquired indicates that, following the introduction of the program, the dietary iodine intake in the Lazio population is improved. There is, however, still much work ahead to ameliorate the iodine prophylaxis in this region. In fact, although a generally adequate iodine intake in school-age children has been observed, there are still areas where a mild iodine insufficiency is present. Moreover, two independent epidemiological surveys on pregnant women evidenced a low urinary iodine concentration with respect to the reference range conceived by the World Health Organization. These findings demonstrate the need for greater attention to the iodine prophylaxis by health care providers (i.e., obstetricians, gynecologists, pediatricians, etc.), and the implementation of effective advertising campaigns aimed at increasing the knowledge and awareness of the favorable effects of iodine supplementation on population health.

Keywords: iodine deficiency; schoolchildren; pregnancy; iodine prophylaxis; iodine deficiency disorders; goiter; hypothyroidism

1. Introduction

Iodine is an indispensable micronutrient required by the thyroid gland for the appropriate synthesis of the thyroid hormones (TH), i.e., triiodothyronine (T_3) and its prohormone thyroxine (T_4) [1]. By modulating key cellular processes (i.e., proliferation, differentiation, apoptosis, and metabolism), TH affect multiple body tasks from the early stages of prenatal life, when maternal thyroxinemia plays a fundamental role in neural growth and differentiation, to adulthood, in which they regulate metabolism, thermogenesis, feeding, memory/learning abilities, and cardiovascular and reproductive functions [2–5]. To guarantee an appropriate TH biosynthesis, the daily dietary iodine intake recommended by the World Health Organization (WHO), the United Nations Children's Emergency Fund (UNICEF), and the International Council for the Control of Iodine Deficiency Disorders (ICCIDD) is 90 µg for preschool children (0 to 59 months), 120 µg for schoolchildren (6 to 12 years), 150 µg for adolescents (above 12 years) and adults, 250 µg for pregnant and lactating women [6]. Failure to meet these requirements is held responsible for a number of adverse effects on human health known as iodine deficiency disorders

(IDD) [7]. These affect almost 1.9 billion people worldwide and constitute a major public health issue in different countries, including Italy [6,8,9]. IDD may occur at all ages, from the early stages of fetal life to adulthood. Of particular relevance are the detrimental effects of an insufficient maternal intake of iodine on development and maturation of the fetal brain, which represents a foremost preventable cause of mental defects [10]. Further adverse effects include abortion, stillbirth, impairment of cognitive functions, delayed growth and puberty, hypothyroidism, goiter, and infertility [11–17].

The epidemiological criteria established by the WHO to evaluate the prevalence and severity of iodine deficiency in a specific population refer to the median urinary iodine concentration (UIC) in morning spot urine samples, along with the presence of goiter [6]. Assuming a daily diuresis of 1.5 liters, a given land area is considered iodine sufficient when the median UIC of the population is comprised between 100 and 199 µg/L, and goiter prevalence in school-age children (≥6 years) is below 5% [6]. In pregnant women, median UIC should be comprised between 150 and 250 µg/L to guarantee normal fetal development. Reported in Table 1 are the WHO reference values of UIC for classifying the iodine status in a population.

Table 1. Median urinary iodine concentrations (UIC) and iodine status in school-age children and pregnant women according to the World Health Organization (see reference [6]).

School-Age Children		Pregnant Women	
UIC (µg/L)	Iodine Status	UIC (µg/L)	Iodine Status
<20	Severe iodine deficiency	<150	Insufficient
20–49	Moderate iodine deficiency	150–249	Adequate
50–99	Mild iodine deficiency	250–499	Above requirements
100–199	Adequate iodine nutrition	≥500	Excessive
200–299	More than adequate		
≥300	Excessive		

In the attempt to establish an efficient iodine prophylaxis and to eradicate IDD, the law n.55/2005, introducing a national salt iodination program (30 mg of potassium iodate per kilogram of salt), was promulgated in 2005 in Italy [9]. The rules laid down by this law make the sale of iodized salt compulsory and favor the silent prophylaxis. Specifically, the sale points of salt for direct consumption have to expose iodine enriched salt while ensuring the availability of non-iodized salt, which is provided only upon specific request of the consumer. In the public catering sector, such as bars and restaurants, and in workplace or community canteens, iodine-enriched salt should also be available to consumers. Furthermore, the law recommends the use of iodized salt in the food industries as an ingredient in preparation and food storage [9].

In the present manuscript, we will review the available information on iodine status in Lazio (a region of central Italy) before and after the introduction of the Italian law n.55/2005, along with the encountered problems hampering the actuation of the national iodine prophylaxis program. All papers analyzed have been obtained from PubMed. Additional data are from the National Observatory for the Monitoring of Iodoprophylaxis in Italy (OSNAMI) of the Italian National Institute of Health.

2. Iodine Status in the Lazio Region before the Introduction of the National Iodine Prophylaxis Program

The Italian population, including the inhabitants of Lazio, has historically been exposed to the negative effects of iodine food shortages [9,18–20].

In the seventies of the last century, epidemiological studies carried out in about 5700 school-age children (6–13 years old) of southern Lazio documented the presence of iodine deficiency [21]. Reported mean UIC values varied from 22 µg per gram of creatinine (µg/g Cr) to 40 µg/g Cr, consistent with an iodine deficiency of moderate degree, as shown in Figure 1 and Table 1. In these children the prevalence of goiter, evaluated by palpation, varied from 6.9% to 11.7%, as shown in Figure 1. In a subsequent case study, performed in 1998 in the city of Rome, UIC and goiter prevalence were investigated in 1040 school-age children (6–14 years old) [22]. A median UIC value of 92 μg/L (mean UIC value of 98 μg/L), consistent with a mild iodine deficiency, as shown in Table 1, was still observed, as shown in Figure 1. On the other hand, goiter prevalence determined by ultrasound was 4.7% [22]. Hence, before the introduction of the nationwide iodine prophylaxis program, the data collected indicated a condition of mild to moderate iodine deficiency of children residing in Lazio. To the best of our knowledge, no studies were performed on iodine status in pregnant women before 2005.

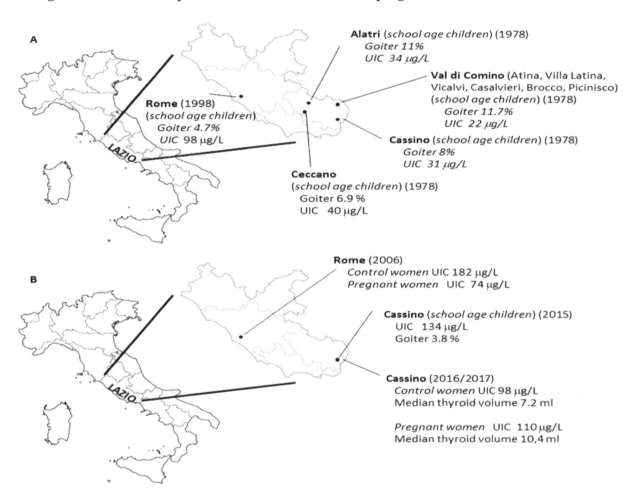

Figure 1. Urinary iodine concentrations (UIC) and goiter prevalence in the inhabitants of Lazio before (**A**) and after (**B**) the introduction of the national salt iodination program.

3. Iodine Status in the Lazio Region after the Introduction of the National Iodine Prophylaxis Program

Following the introduction of the iodine prophylaxis program, three independent studies were performed in order to assess iodine status in both school-age children and pregnant women [23–25].

A first observational study was realized in 2006 in the city of Rome to evaluate iodine intake in pregnant women compared to non-pregnant age-matched ones [23]. The study enrolled 51 clinically healthy pregnant women in their first gestational trimester, and 100 clinically healthy non-pregnant women [23]. The median UIC value observed in control women was 182 μg/L, suggestive of an adequate iodine intake, as shown in Figure 1. However, pregnant women showed poor iodine consumption, attested by a median UIC value of 74 μg/L. In particular, the UIC was found below the normal range only in 4% of control women but in 92% of pregnant women. These observations pointed out that, despite the iodine sufficiency recognized in control women, the majority of pregnant women and their fetuses were exposed to detrimental consequences of iodine deficiency.

After that, a new survey was performed in 2015 in the city of Cassino, located in the south of Lazio, whose residents were previously found to have a moderate iodine deficiency, as shown in Figure 1B [24]. In this study, UIC and thyroid volume measured by ultrasonography were evaluated in 234 school-age children (13–14 years old). At the same time an inquiry was conducted to estimate the percentage of iodized salt sold in the preceding year by the major local retailers. The latter showed only 42% of all salt sold in 2014 in this city was iodized. Despite that, a median UIC of 134 µg/L was observed in the school children under examination, suggesting an adequate iodine intake. This result was also corroborated by the low prevalence of goiter, encountered only in 3.8% of subjects. However, when children were grouped based on the regular consumption of iodized salt or milk or both, those referring no consumption of either iodized salt or milk had a median UIC value (96.4 µg/L), compatible with a mild iodine deficiency. On the other hand, optimal median UIC values were found in school children regularly taking either iodized salt (132.1 µg/L) or milk (131 µg/L) or both (147.9 µg/L). Such evidence strengthens the importance of eating iodized salt and iodine-rich food to achieve the right amount of iodine in the body for thyroid function [24].

A further study was aimed to analyze iodine intake in pregnant women from the same area of Cassino [25]. Study participants were enrolled in the period from January 2016 to April 2017, for a total of 96 pregnant women and 79 age-matched non-pregnant women. In the control group, median UIC was nearby 98 µg/L, consistent with a mild iodine deficiency, while pregnant women had a median UIC of about 110 µg/L, below the lower value (150 µg/L) recommended by the WHO for categorizing iodine adequacy in a pregnant population. In agreement with this finding, a significantly increased thyroid volume was recorded in pregnant women compared to non-pregnant ones, as shown in Figure 1 [25]. In this study the effects of iodized salt and/or milk consumption on UIC levels of both control and pregnant women, considered as a whole, were also examined. The analysis showed an increasing trend of UIC from women not using either iodized salt or milk (median UIC 79.8 µg/L) compared to those using iodized salt (median UIC 94 µg/L) or milk (median UIC 112 µg/L) or both (median UIC 118 µg/L) [25]. Thus, once again the data obtained highlight the need to implement the national salt iodination program, as well as the importance of inserting initiatives targeted at control of iodine prophylaxis and prevention of IDD in regional health plans. It has to be mentioned, however, that the aforementioned studies rely on a limited number of subjects analyzed and should be corroborated on larger case studies.

4. Encountered Problems Hampering the Actuation of the National Iodine Prophylaxis Program

As reported above, the available epidemiological data demonstrated that, following the introduction of the national salt iodination program, the iodine intake in the inhabitants of Lazio is somewhat improved. However, prevention measures are still needed to fully avoid the risks of IDD in this region. In particular, there are three main lines of action that should be pursued.

The first is devising strategies to increment the amount of iodized salt sold by retailers. In fact, due to the lack of penalties related to non-compliance with the law n.55/2005, vendors are not discouraged from exhibiting non-iodized salt on store shelves, and they sell both iodized salt and or even just non-iodized salt [24]. This, at least in part, may explain the low percentage of iodized salt sold (42%) in the city of Cassino, and why 45% of the school children and 50% of women of child-bearing age do not use iodized salt. Moreover, the latest data provided by OSNAMI indicated that the percentage of iodized salt used in collective catering is still very low (about 24%), and that used by the food industry is even lower (3–8%) [26]. Thus, it is of great importance to encourage this manufacturing sector to make more extensive use of iodized salt.

The second line of intervention should be to adequately inform the population on the beneficial effects on human health deriving from the consumption of iodized salt. This task could be accomplished by creating effective advertising campaigns able to reach every single citizen. In this context, an initiative of the Ministry of Health is taking place that aims to provide all students with comprehensive information about the beneficial effects of the use of iodized salt through meetings with medical staff organized by individual schools [27].

Finally, greater attention by the major health care providers of the National Health System is highly desirable, especially obstetricians, gynecologists, and pediatricians. Different surveys, in fact, noticed that obstetricians and midwives do not recommend iodine supplementation either to women planning pregnancy or during pregnancy or lactation [28,29]. To this regard, a position statement on the use of iodized salt in adulthood and children was signed by the Italian Ministry of Health, the National Institute of Health, the Italian Society of Endocrinology, the Italian Thyroid Association, the Medical Association of Endocrinologists, the Italian Society of Pediatric Endocrinology and Diabetology, the Italian Society of Pediatrics, the Italian Society of Gynecology and Obstetrics, the Italian Association of Consultative Gynecologists, the Italian Society of Human Nutrition, the Italian Society of Nutraceuticals, the Italian Association of Dietetics and Clinical Nutrition, the Italian Society for the Study of Food Behavior Disorders, the Italian Federation of Nutrition, and the National Federation of General Practitioners [30]. The joint implementation of all these actions should provide a consistent contribution toward the eradication of iodine deficiency in Italy.

5. Conclusions

The available epidemiological data indicate that, following the introduction of the national salt iodination program, the iodine intake of the inhabitants of Lazio has only partially improved. In fact, although a generally adequate iodine intake in school-age children has been observed, pregnant women still show an iodine deficiency. Thus, it is necessary to encourage compliance with the law in order to reach optimal iodine nutrition and to completely eradicate the IDD in this region. The situation recorded in Lazio corroborates the recent Krakow Declaration on Iodine reporting an increased concern about the fading commitment of policymakers to address iodine deficiency in Europe and the poor attention of policymakers, opinion leaders, and the public toward the resolution of IDD [31]. Thus, it has become of primary importance to join forces with policymakers, public health officials, and scientists to guarantee that existing European strategies to prevent IDD are fulfilled and implemented.

Author Contributions: All authors participated in the review design, contributed to the first draft and manuscript revisions, and approved the final version.

References

1. Citterio, C.E.; Targovnik, H.M.; Arvan, P. The role of thyroglobulin in thyroid hormonogenesis. *Nat. Rev. Endocrinol.* **2019**. [CrossRef] [PubMed]
2. Cheng, S.Y.; Leonard, J.L.; Davis, P.J. Molecular aspects of thyroid hormone actions. *Endocr. Rev.* **2010**, *31*, 139–170. [CrossRef] [PubMed]
3. Bernal, J. Thyroid hormone receptors in brain development and function. *Nat. Clin. Pract. Endocrinol. Metab.* **2007**, *3*, 249–259. [CrossRef] [PubMed]
4. Angelousi, A.; Kassi, E.; Nasiri-Ansari, N.; Weickert, M.O.; Randeva, H.; Kaltsas, G. Clock genes alterations and endocrine disorders. *Eur. J. Clin. Investig.* **2018**, *48*, e12927. [CrossRef] [PubMed]
5. Krassas, G.E.; Poppe, K.; Glinoer, D. Thyroid function and human reproductive health. *Endocr. Rev.* **2010**, *31*, 702–755. [CrossRef] [PubMed]
6. World Health Organization; International Council for the Control of Iodine Deficiency Disorders; United Nations Children's Fund (WHO/ICCIDD/UNICEF). *Assessment of the Iodine Deficiency Disorders and Monitoring Their Elimination*, 3rd ed.; World Health Organization: Geneva, Switzerland, 2007; Available online: https://apps.who.int/iris/bitstream/handle/10665/43781/9789241595827_eng.pdf?sequence=1 (accessed on 4 June 2019).
7. Hetzel, B.S. Iodine deficiency disorders (IDD) and their eradication. *Lancet* **1983**, *2*, 1126–1129. [CrossRef]

8.   Vanderpump, M.P.J. The epidemiology of thyroid disease. *Br. Med. Bull.* **2011**, *99*, 39–51. [CrossRef] [PubMed]

9.   Olivieri., A.; Di Cosmo, C.; De Angelis, S.; Da Cas, R.; Stacchini, P.; Pastorelli, A.; Vitti, P.; Regional Observatories for Goiter Prevention. The way forward in Italy for iodine. *Minerva Med.* **2017**, *108*, 159–168. [PubMed]

10.   Delange, F. Iodine deficiency as a cause of brain damage. *Postgrad. Med. J.* **2001**, *77*, 217–220. [CrossRef] [PubMed]

11.   Salazar, P.; Cisternas, P.; Martinez, M.; Inestrosa, N.C. Hypothyroidism and Cognitive Disorders during Development and Adulthood: Implications in the Central Nervous System. *Mol. Neurobiol.* **2019**, *56*, 2952–2963. [CrossRef]

12.   Walsh, V.; Brown, J.V.E.; McGuire, W. Iodine supplementation for the prevention of mortality and adverse neurodevelopmental outcomes in preterm infants. *Cochrane Database Syst. Rev.* **2019**, *2*, CD005253. [CrossRef]

13.   Farebrother, J.; Naude, C.E.; Nicol, L.; Sang, Z.; Yang, Z.; Jooste, P.L.; Andersson, M.; Zimmermann, M.B. Effects of Iodized Salt and Iodine Supplements on Prenatal and Postnatal Growth: A Systematic Review. *Adv. Nutr.* **2018**, *9*, 219–237. [CrossRef] [PubMed]

14.   Eastman, C.J.; Zimmermann, M.B. The Iodine Deficiency Disorders. In *Endotext [Internet]*; Feingold, K.R., Anawalt, B., Boyce, A., Chrousos, G., Dungan, K., Grossman, A., Hershman, J.M., Kaltsas, G., Koch, C., Kopp, P., et al., Eds.; MDText.com, Inc.: South Dartmouth, MA, USA, 2018. Available online: https://www.ncbi.nlm.nih.gov/books/NBK285556/ (accessed on 4 June 2019).

15.   Dunn, J.T.; Delange, F. Damaged reproduction: The most important consequence of iodine deficiency. *J. Clin. Endocrinol. Metab.* **2001**, *86*, 2360–2363. [CrossRef]

16.   Ferri, N.; Ulisse, S.; Aghini-Lombardi, F.; Graziano, F.M.; Di Mattia, T.; Russo, F.P.; Arizzi, M.; Baldini, E.; Trimboli, P.; Attanasio, D.; et al. Iodine supplementation restores fertility of sheep exposed to iodine deficiency. *J. Endocrinol. Investig.* **2003**, *26*, 1081–1087. [CrossRef] [PubMed]

17.   Baldini, E.; Sorrenti, S.; Catania, A.; Tartaglia, F.; Pironi, D.; Vergine, M.; Monti, M.; Filippini, A.; Ulisse, S. Nodular thyroid disease with aging. In *Aging: Exploring a Complex Phenomenon*; Shamin, A., Ed.; Taylor and Francis/CRC Press: Abingdon, UK, 2018; pp. 95–118.

18.   Aghini-Lombardi, F.; Antonangeli, L.; Vitti, P.; Pinchera, A. Status of iodine nutrition in Italy. In *Iodine Deficiency in Europe*; Delange, F., Dunn, J.T., Glinoer, D., Eds.; Plenum Press: New York, NY, USA, 1993; pp. 403–408.

19.   Vitti, P.; Rago, T.; Aghini-Lombardi, F.; Pinchera, A. Iodine deficiency disorders in Europe. *Public Health Nutr.* **2001**, *4*, 529–535. [CrossRef] [PubMed]

20.   Andersson, M.; de Benoist, B.; Darton-Hill, I.; Delange, F. *Iodine Deficiency in Europe: A Continuing Public Health Problem*; WHO Press: Geneva, Switzerland, 2007; Available online: https://www.who.int/nutrition/publications/VMNIS_Iodine_deficiency_in_Europe.pdf (accessed on 5 June 2019).

21.   Baschieri, L.; Costa, A.; Basile, A. L'endemia. In *Il Gozzo*; Fegiz, G., Ed.; Edizioni Luigi Pozzo: Rome, Italy, 1978; pp. 399–427.

22.   Panunzi, C.; Manca Bitti, M.L.; Di Paolo, A.; Fabbrini, R.; Valle, D.; Spadoni, G.L.; Del Duca, E.; Guglielmi, R.; Valente, M.; Finocchi, A.; et al. Goiter prevalence and urinary excretion of iodine in a sample of school age children in the city of Rome. *Ann. Ist. Super. Sanità* **1998**, *34*, 409–412. [PubMed]

23.   Marchioni, E.; Fumarola, A.; Calvanese, A.; Piccirilli, F.; Tommasi, V.; Cugini, P.; Ulisse, S.; Rossi Fanelli, F.; D'Armiento, M. Iodine deficiency in pregnant women residing in an area with adequate iodine intake. *Nutrition* **2008**, *24*, 458–461. [CrossRef]

24.   Coccaro, C.; Tuccilli, C.; Prinzi, N.; D'Armiento, E.; Pepe, M.; Del Maestro, F.; Cacciola, G.; Forlini, B.; Verdolotti, S.; Bononi, M.; et al. Consumption of iodized salt may not represent a reliable indicator of iodine adequacy: Evidence from a cross-sectional study on schoolchildren living in an urban area of central Italy. *Nutrition* **2016**, *32*, 662–666. [CrossRef]

25.   Tuccilli, C.; Baldini, E.; Truppa, E.; D'Auria, B.; De Quattro, D.; Cacciola, G.; Aceti, T.; Cirillo, G.; Faiola, A.; Indigeno, P.; et al. Iodine deficiency in pregnancy: Still a health issue for the women of Cassino city, Italy. *Nutrition* **2018**, *50*, 60–65. [CrossRef]

26.   OSNAMI, Osservatorio Nazionale per il Monitoraggio della Iodoprofilassi in Italia. Istituto Superiore di Sanità. Available online: http://old.iss.it/binary/osna/cont/dati_vendita.pdf (accessed on 4 June 2019).

27.   OSNAMI, Osservatorio Nazionale per il Monitoraggio della Iodoprofilassi in Italia. Istituto Superiore di Sanità. Available online: http://old.iss.it/osnami/index.php?lang=1&anno=2019&tipo=27 (accessed on 9 July 2019).

28.   De Leo, S.; Pearce, E.N.; Braverman, L.E. Iodine supplementation in women during preconception, pregnancy, and lactation: Current clinical practice by U.S. obstetricians and midwives. *Thyroid* **2017**, *27*, 434–439. [CrossRef]

29.   Malek, L.; Umberger, W.; Makrides, M.; Zhou, S.J. Poor adherence to folic acid and iodine supplement recommendations in preconception and pregnancy: A cross-sectional analysis. *Aust. N. Z. J. Public Health* **2016**, *40*, 424–429. [CrossRef] [PubMed]

30.   Ministero della Salute. Available online: http://www.salute.gov.it/imgs/C_17_pubblicazioni_2593_allegato.pdf (accessed on 4 June 2019).

31.   The EUthyroid Consortium. The Krakow Declaration on Iodine. Available online: https://www.iodinedeclaration.eu/wp-content/uploads/2018/04/Krakow-Declaration-2018_03_29.pdf (accessed on 9 July 2019).

7

Interference on Iodine Uptake and Human Thyroid Function by Perchlorate-Contaminated Water and Food

Giuseppe Lisco [1], Anna De Tullio [2], Vito Angelo Giagulli [2,3], Giovanni De Pergola [4] and Vincenzo Triggiani [2,*]

[1]   ASL Brindisi, Unit of Endocrinology, Metabolism & Clinical Nutrition, Hospital "A. Perrino", Strada per Mesagne 7, 72100 Brindisi, Puglia, Italy; g.lisco84@gmail.com
[2]   Interdisciplinary Department of Medicine—Section of Internal Medicine, Geriatrics, Endocrinology and Rare Diseases, University of Bari "Aldo Moro", School of Medicine, Policlinico, Piazza Giulio Cesare 11, 70124 Bari, Puglia, Italy; annadetullio16@gmail.com (A.D.T.); vitogiagulli58@gmail.com (V.A.G.)
[3]   Clinic of Endocrinology and Metabolic Disease, Conversano Hospital, Via Edmondo de Amicis 36, 70014 Conversano, Bari, Puglia, Italy
[4]   Department of Biomedical Sciences and Human Oncology, Section of Internal Medicine and Clinical Oncology, University of Bari Aldo Moro, Piazza Giulio Cesare 11, 70124 Bari, Puglia, Italy; gdepergola@libero.it
*   Correspondence: vincenzotriggiani@uniba.it

Abstract: Background: Perchlorate-induced natrium-iodide symporter (NIS) interference is a well-recognized thyroid disrupting mechanism. It is unclear, however, whether a chronic low-dose exposure to perchlorate delivered by food and drinks may cause thyroid dysfunction in the long term. Thus, the aim of this review was to overview and summarize literature results in order to clarify this issue. Methods: Authors searched PubMed/MEDLINE, Scopus, Web of Science, institutional websites and Google until April 2020 for relevant information about the fundamental mechanism of the thyroid NIS interference induced by orally consumed perchlorate compounds and its clinical consequences. Results: Food and drinking water should be considered relevant sources of perchlorate. Despite some controversies, cross-sectional studies demonstrated that perchlorate exposure affects thyroid hormone synthesis in infants, adolescents and adults, particularly in the case of underlying thyroid diseases and iodine insufficiency. An exaggerated exposure to perchlorate during pregnancy leads to a worse neurocognitive and behavioral development outcome in infants, regardless of maternal thyroid hormone levels. Discussion and conclusion: The effects of a chronic low-dose perchlorate exposure on thyroid homeostasis remain still unclear, leading to concerns especially for highly sensitive patients. Specific studies are needed to clarify this issue, aiming to better define strategies of detection and prevention.

Keywords: perchlorate; Natrium/Iodide symporter; iodine; endocrine disruptors; review; drinking and Food; Hypothyroidism

1. Introduction

Endocrine disrupting chemicals (EDCs) have been defined as a group of compounds or a mixture of natural or man-housed exogenous chemicals which interfere with the hormonal network, or induce endocrine cell damage [1]. Interference may be attributable to several mechanisms such as receptor agonism or antagonism, modulation of receptor expression, modification of signal transduction, hormone synthesis or incretion, plasmatic distribution and clearance [2]. Moreover, epigenetic effects have been hypothesized for EDCs and concerns about a possible "transmission" of EDCs across the generations is a topic of debate [3,4]. To date, a wide range of environmental chemicals have been identified as being involved in the pathogenesis of thyroid diseases [5,6] and several chemicals or common pollutants may act as thyroid disruptors [7–9]. Perfluorooctanoic acid [10], a chemical largely employed for the manufacturing of waxes, cosmetics, carpets, cleaning or waterproof products, and bisphenols [11], hugely used as plasticizers, were found to increase the prevalence of thyroid diseases in exposed patients [12], including thyroid autoimmunity [13]. Moreover, legacy pesticides were experimentally shown to affect thyroid function [14] and, despite some controversy, they may also induce hypothyroidism, thyroid autoimmunity, thyroid volume enlargement or nodules in humans [15]. The bactericide triclosan was mostly found in personal hygiene products (oral care, shampoos, hand sanitizers, soaps), and was proven to increase the risk of thyroid diseases, too [16]. Thyroid disruption includes different pathways, and may be due to either interference or synergism among different EDCs [17]. The leading mechanisms of thyroid interference by pollutant agents have been explored, and frequently include the inhibition of thyroperoxidase activity, competitive natrium-iodide symporter (NIS) inhibition, impairment of binding protein transport and peripheral deiodinase activity, enhancement of liver catabolism [18]. Since food and drinks are also a relevant source of thyroid disruptors, a lifelong human exposure to these chemicals could induce potentially harmful consequences on thyroidal homeostasis. Given this consideration, this review aims to specifically focalize on NIS interference by specific agents, mainly perchlorate compounds, which are commonly found in food and drinks.

2. Materials and Methods

The authors summarized iodine metabolism and its importance in thyroid homeostasis and hormonal synthesis. Furthermore, the authors searched PubMed/MEDLINE, Scopus, Web of Science, institutional websites and Google for relevant information about the fundamental mechanism of NIS interference induced by perchlorate compounds orally assumed and the consequences on thyroidal health status associated with chronic exposure to these chemicals.

3. Results

3.1. Overview on Iodine Metabolism in Healthy Humans

The primary source of iodine (I) is represented by natural food (seafood, milk, eggs, vegetables, legumes, fruits), fortified food (salt) and mineral waters. I is basically available in two forms, organic and inorganic (iodide); the latter form is absorbed at the level of stomach and duodenum [19] through a specific natrium-iodide symporter (NIS) which regulates iodine homeostasis in human body [20]. After gastrointestinal absorption, I enters the circulation, undergoing to a large distribution into the plasma, red blood cell cytoplasm and extracellular fluid, and is finally intercepted by tissues [21]. A wide range of tissues express the NIS, including salivary glands, breast, and thyroid [22]. Nevertheless, thyroid represents the most important reservoir of the ion considering that, in a healthy human body, the gland normally stores up to 80% of the entire iodine pool (15–20 mg). The NIS is a 13-domain transmembrane protein which mediates transmembrane I and sodium (1 to 2 ratio) transport at the level of thyrocyte's basolateral membrane [23,24]. Transmembrane sodium gradient is generated by the sodium-potassium ATPase pump which indirectly provides energy for an almost continuous intrathyroidal I uptake (secondary active transport). Given this thyroid avidity, I concentration in thyrocytes is 30 to 60 times higher than its plasmatic levels [25]. As a mean, thyroid secretes 80 μg a day of I in the form of both levothyroxine and triiodothyronine [26]. Due to peripheral metabolism of thyroid hormones, I circulates in bloodstream finally undergoing to both renal and hepato-biliary clearance and thyroidal re-uptake, as well. An intrathyroidal I recycling has also been described [27]. Thyroidal uptake considerably fluctuates according to I intake, and ranges from 10% to over 80% of the entire amount of ingested I. Contrariwise, urinary I excretion is inversely correlated with thyroid uptake, and in the case of adequate I intake, more than 90% of the ion is cleared by the kidneys with urine [28]. Urinary I concentration is thus a reliable biomarker of I intake, and is a useful tool for screening patients suspected for I deficiency [25]. Both the thyroid hormone synthesis and urinary I excretion increase during pregnancy [29], while 126 to 269 μg of I could be excreted with each liter of breast milk in lactating women [30]. Iodine intake is generally recommended at 150 μg per day for adults in order to ensure the daily iodine recycle [31]. Thus, the recommended dose of iodine intake raises at 200 - 250 μg per day during pregnancy and lactation for sustaining an increased requirement [32]. I is an essential micronutrient for thyroid hormones synthesis [33,34]. Afterward the transition into thyrocyte cytoplasm, I moves towards the apical surface of thyrocyte's plasmatic membrane into the follicular lumen. This transport is mediated by a ionic carrier belonging to the SLC26A family, otherwise known as pendrin [35], and is also expressed at the level of the inner ear, kidney and bowel. Specifically, pendrin is essential for favoring the efflux of iodine into follicular space in exchange of chloride (1 to 1 ratio) and a defective synthesis or function of this carrier is responsible for a the so called Pendred's syndrome [36]. Once into follicular lumen, I undergoes oxidation by thyroperoxidase, thus becoming promptly available for thyroglobulin's organification. Thyroid I content is the most important regulator of thyroid hormone synthesis. Indeed, I overload reduces the expression of NIS, decreases both the thyroid peroxidase and deiodinases activities, and finally leads to a transient impairment of thyroid hormone synthesis [37]. In predisposed patients, iodine excess increases oxidative stress, and may induce or exacerbate thyroid autoimmunity and hypothyroidism (Wolff–Chaikoff effect) [38]. Finally, I overload may exacerbate a latent hyperthyroidism in patient with single thyroid nodule or multinodular goiter [39].

3.2. Perchlorate Compounds and Iodine Interference

The evidence that high doses of perchlorate (ClO_4^-) anion decreased thyroid hormone synthesis has been known since the 1950s [40], and given this peculiarity, it has been used to effectively treat hyperthyroidism such as in Graves' disease and amiodarone-induced hyperthyroidism [41]. Specifically, ClO_4^- competes with I at the level of the NIS (Figure A1), the former having a 30-fold higher affinity for the symporter when compared to the latter [42]. A dose-response sigmoid curve has been reported for describing NIS sensitivity to ClO_4^- inhibition in different species and the half maximal inhibiting concentration in humans was found at 1.566 μM [43]. To confirm these experimental results, an orally delivered acute exposure to up to 520 μg/kg of body weight (bw) induced a significant increase in serum thyroid stimulating hormone (TSH) levels, with a relevant decline in serum-free levothyroxine concentrations [44]. On the other hand, it is thought that a chronic low-dose exposure to ClO_4^-, normally observed as the consequence of food and drink intake, could impair thyroid function by reducing iodine uptake particularly in predisposed individuals, such as those with an underlying iodine deficiency [45,46].

3.3. Perchlorate Compounds in Food and Water

ClO_4^- may naturally occur in the atmosphere from spontaneous photogenic reaction between chloride and ozone, or arises from man-made products such as oxidizers, fertilizers, explosives, propellants, fireworks, airbag inflators spread into environment. In addition, ClO_4^- can be also produced from the degradation of the common water disinfectant hypochlorite [47]. Perchlorate compounds occur in different form, such as metal perchlorate, ammonium and alkali metal forms, organic and inorganic forms and salts. Antarctic ice represents the most important sediment of ClO_4^- in the planet, with different concentrations depending on drilling areas [48]. The Atacama desert (Chile, South America) is another important natural source of geogenic ClO_4^-, and elevated concentrations of its compounds have been found in soil (290 to 2565 μg/Kg) and surface waters (744 to 1480 μg/L) [49]. Other relevant sources of natural ClO_4^- have been discovered in Alaska, Puerto Rico, New Mexico, Texas, California (United States of America, USA), and Bolivia (South America). Anthropogenic ClO_4^- compounds have been found in soil, sea and rainwater, surface and groundwaters, indoor and outdoor dust, ice and snow [50]. Given data from ice drilling analyses, anthropogenic ClO_4^- started to accumulate in Arctic ice from the 1980s [51]. In Devon Island (Canada, North America), ClO_4^- compounds were found in ice and snow at variable concentrations ranging from 1 to 18 ng/L [52]. A great variability in rainwater ClO_4^- levels was observed due to differences in analyzed geographical sites and seasonality. In fact, ClO_4^- concentration ranges from 0.02 to 1.6 μg/L in Texas (USA) [53], 0.02 to 6.9 μg/L in India (Asia) [54], and 0.35 to 27.3 ng/mL in China (Asia) [55]. Moreover, Munster et al. evaluated the levels ClO_4^- in total deposition from November 2005 to July 2007 in Long Island (New York State), relieving a mean concertation of 0.21 μg/L and with a maximum level of 2.81 μg/L recorded after fireworks displays occurred during the Independence day celebration [56]. Another observation reported different levels of ClO_4^- in wet deposition only, ranging from <5 to 105 ng/L (mean 14 ng/L) with higher concentrations recorded in spring and summer than winter [57]. Soil usually does not retain ClO_4^- and more than 90% is confined in the aqueous phase [58] where ClO_4^- spreads and persists due to its high solubility and resistance to photolysis and anaerobic bacterial biodegradation [59]. Fruits and vegetables represent a relevant food source of ClO_4^-, particularly because of the widespread use of perchlorate-based fertilizers [60]. In particular, leafy vegetables, spinach, salad plants, raspberries, apricots, asparagus, cantaloupes, and tomatoes accumulate ClO_4^- as a consequence of farming techniques [61]. The mean concentration of perchlorate in tested food appears variable and the highest levels have been found in Guatemalan cantaloupes (156 μg/Kg), spinach (133 μg/Kg), Chilean green grapes (45.5 μg/Kg) and Romaine lettuce (29 μg/Kg) [62]. Vega et al. reported variable concentration of ClO_4^- in Chilean drinking waters which ranged from 4 to 120 μg/L [63]. Conversely, lower levels of ClO_4^- in drinking water have been observed in the USA [64] and Europe, including Italy (0.5–75 μg/L) [65].

3.4. Chronic Esposure to Perchlorate Compounds by Food and Drinking Water

The 2018 "Italian Institute for Food and Agriculture Market Services" ranking reported the USA as the most valuable country in exporting fruits and vegetables, followed by Mexico and Chile. Given the volume of exports, Spain (4th) and Italy (7th) are responsible for the 42% of the entire European market of fruits and vegetables, ahead of Poland, France and Greece [66]. Chile has a remarkable export economy [67], and usually exports several thousands of millions of kilograms of fruits a year worldwide [68]. Specifically, the European Union is Chile's third-largest trade partner in the world, after China and the USA, and currently imports 19% of the Chilean global export of vegetable products [69]. Cherries and table grapes, followed by apples, Chilean blueberries and plums are the most exported vegetable products to Europe. Vegetables from Chile are notoriously rich in ClO_4^- and the excessive consumption of these products could have chronically negative consequences on thyroid homeostasis. Indeed, ClO_4^- food exposure is essentially driven by vegetables and fruits and widely ranged according to geographical area as well as seasonality [70]. To confirm this assumption, ClO_4^- was detected in a wide range of vegetable samples, ranging from 21 to 162 μg/kg [71]. Vegetables consumption in Italy seems to slightly but continuously increase over time and some of the most consumed vegetable products, such as spinach, leaf vegetables and spices were found to be a relevant source of ClO_4^- [72]. Normal consumption of these vegetables does not usually lead to exceeding the maximal total daily dose according to the European Food Safety Authority 2014 (0.3 μg/Kg of bw). However, a higher daily consumption of these products led to a relevant exceeding of the maximal tolerated dose by 32% in adults, 61% in children and 56% in infant [72]. In addition, tea and herbal infusions could represent another relevant source of ClO_4^-, oscillating from 630 to 730 μg/Kg for dark tea; 80 to 430 μg/Kg for black tea; and 250 to 500 μg/Kg for green tea [73]. Therefore, the consumption of the aforementioned products should be moderate and intermittent for avoiding a consistent ClO_4^- overload. Indeed, acute exposure to high or very high levels of ClO_4^- normally is not enough for overcoming thyroidal compensation and ability to maintain normal serum concentration of thyroid hormones in healthy individuals [64]. Chronic consumption of ClO_4^- in adults has been estimated as high as 0.07 to 0.34 μg/Kg of body weight per day in Europe [70], and 0.2 to 0.4 μg/Kg of body weight per day in the USA [74]. Despite ClO_4^- consumption being generally below the level of recommended reference dose in adults [75], it may become critical, especially in some categories, such as children, high sensitive patients, cigarette smokers, iodine deficient people, and pregnant and breast feeding women as well [76–78]. Indeed, the inhibition of I uptake and any potential downstream effects induced by ClO_4^- are strictly dependent on the exposure to other environmental NIS inhibitors, such as thiocyanates and nitrates, and iodine intake itself [79]. These potential confounders should therefore be considered in future studies and calculations for risk assessment [80]. Finally, breast milk and infant formulas are the most significant sources of ClO_4^- for newborns and infants [81–83]. Compared with adults, infants and children exhibited a greater ClO_4^- exposure per Kg of bw per day [75,84], particularly breastfed children (0.22 µg/Kg of bw/day) respective to those fed by cow milk-based formula (0.1 µg/Kg of bw/day) or soy-based formula (0.027 µg/Kg of bw/day) [85]. Food intake more than drinking water is considered the main source of ClO_4^- for children [81] and adults [86], since ClO_4^- exposure from drinking water alone is not able to suppress thyroid function [87]. Nevertheless, this assumption is controversial considering that other results suggest opposite conclusions [70,74].

3.5. Perchlorate Compounds Toxicity

From this point of view, concerns have been supposed in case of ClO_4^- exposure during fetal and infantile life [88,89]. The placental NIS ensures maternal-to-fetal transition of I [90], therefore allowing fetal uptake of ClO_4^- and other goitrogen chemicals, too. Blount et al. specifically analyzed the perinatal exposure to goitrogen chemicals in 150 mothers from New Jersey (USA), showing that the placental barrier was more permeable to I respective to goitrogens and maternal urinary ClO_4^- concentrations were directly correlated with ClO_4^- concentration in amniotic fluid, thus resulting an useful tool for assessing fetal exposure [91]. As observed in a Chinese population, ClO_4^- was detected in infant's urine (22.4 ng/mL) and cord blood serum (3.2 ng/mL) at a concentration about 22 times greater compared to that reported by Blount (0.14 µg/L) [92]. This finding is difficult to explain, but could be attributable to different environmental exposures or dissimilarities in assay or both. Several studies analyzed the impact of a mild-to-moderate exposure to ClO_4^- in early pregnancy on both maternal thyroid function and several neonatal outcomes. In a cross-sectional trial in Athens (Greece), 139 first-trimester pregnant women with mild iodine deficiency were chronically exposed to dietary sources of ClO_4^- as suggested by median levels of urinary ClO_4^- concentration at around 4 µg/L. The authors specifically found that ClO_4^- urinary concentration, possibly associated with a moderate iodine deficiency, was inversely related with plasmatic levels of triiodothyronine and thyroxin in this cluster of patients [93]. A cross-sectional study in 200 first-trimester Thai pregnant women (<14 weeks of gestation age) confirmed a chronic low-level environmental exposure to ClO_4^- compounds (and thiocyanates) and this exposure was positively associated with serum TSH concentration and negatively related with serum levothyroxine levels [94]. Data from San Diego (South California) reported a mean urinary ClO_4^- concentration of 8.5 µg/L in first-trimester pregnant women, and the higher the level of ClO_4^-, the higher the level of TSH and the lower those of total thyroxine and free thyroxine [95]. Pearce et al. analyzed the effects of environmental exposure to ClO_4^- in a cohort of 1600 first-trimester pregnant women, with mild-to-moderate iodine deficiency, who had been enrolled in the Controlled Antenatal Thyroid Screening Study (CATS) from Cardiff (Wales) and Turin (Italy). The results of this observation displayed a low-level environment exposure to ClO_4^- in all participants but no thyroidal impairment due to this contamination was noted [96]. These findings were also confirmed in first-trimester pregnant women from Los Angeles (California) and Cordoba (Argentina) in whom a low concentration of urinary ClO_4^- were detected (mean of 7.8 and 13.5 µg/L, respectively) but no correlation with ClO_4^- exposure and thyroid function was demonstrated [97]. A cross-sectional association between urinary ClO_4^-, thiocyanate and nitrate concentration and thyroid function was also assessed in healthy pregnant women living in New York City (New York State). The results confirm that a co-occurrent exposure to ClO_4^-, thiocyanate and nitrate may possibly impair thyroid homeostasis leading to hypothyroidism and ClO_4^- specifically displayed the largest weight in driving this outcome [98]. Taylor et al. evaluated the relationship between maternal ClO_4^- exposure and neurocognitive development in first-trimester pregnant women with hypothyroidism or hypothyroxinemia and mild iodine deficiency. The results display that maternal urinary ClO_4^- concentration in the highest 10% of the population were associated with an higher risk of offspring's verbal intellective quotient impairment [odds ratio 3.14 (1.38–7.13), p 0.006] and levothyroxine replacement did not improve the outcome [99]. In addition, a high risk of mild reduction in the verbal intellective quotient in 3-year-old children who were prenatally exposed to ClO_4^- was observed irrespective of their mother's thyroid function during pregnancy [100]. Furthermore, maternal ClO_4^- concentration was found to positively correlate with male infant bodyweight, especially in preterm [101].

Several observations assessed the relationship between maternal perchlorate exposure and neonatal or infant thyroid homeostasis with controversial results according to the different clinical end-points used for the assessment of euthyroidism [102–104]. ClO_4^- may affect children growth as reported by Mervish et al., who observed that girls with higher ClO_4^- exposure displayed lower body mass index and waist circumference than controls [105]. In addition, the results of a cross-sectional study in 3151 participants (12–80 years old) displayed for each logarithmic unit increased exposure to both ClO_4^- and thiocyanate, the level of free thyroxine decreased by 8% in adolescent girls and 9% in adolescent boys, respectively [106].

3.6. Overview on Other Halogenate Compounds

Other halogenated compounds may interfere with I uptake as similarly observed for ClO_4^-, including bromine and brominated compounds [107] and fluoride and fluorinated compounds [108]. Bromine compounds naturally occur in marine and terrestrial plants, but industrial compounds account for 80% of bromine production [109]. In particular, bromine compounds are essentially found in phytochemical, pharmaceutics, pesticides, dyes, and photographic and water treatment chemicals [109]. Bromine has been found at higher concentrations in seawater (65 to 80 mg/L) compared to natural waters (in mean 0.5 mg/L) and groundwaters (1 to several mg/L) [110]. In addition, potassium bromate is an inexpensive oxidizing agent used as dough improver in the baking industry [111]. Specifically, it leads to the formation of disulfide bonds between gluten proteins, ameliorating bread's proprieties, such as swelling and volume [112]. Chronic exposure to potassium bromate was associated with toxic effects and carcinogenicity in animal models [113–115]. However, no data are currently available to also confirm toxicity and carcinogenicity in humans, thus the International Agency for Research on Cancer classified potassium bromate in group 2B (possibly carcinogen to humans) [116]. Given these considerations, potassium bromate has been precautionarily banned from several countries, such as those in Europe, the United Kingdom, Canada, Nigeria, China, South Korea, and several countries in South America, but it is still considered safe in the United States. Indeed, according to the Food and Drug Administration, no sufficient evidence of potassium bromate adverse effects has been collected in humans thus allowing the use of additives in the bread baking industry not exceeding 75 parts per million [117]. For this reason, bromate levels should be constantly and reliably monitored in bread whether potassium bromate has been used as an additive in flour processing [112]. In one observational study in Nanchang (China), bromine was detected in all 131 whole blood samples, thus suggesting a higher prevalence of contamination among people [84]. The daily intake of bromide ranged from 2 to 8 mg in the USA and 9 mg in Europe (the Netherlands) [110]. Regulatory agencies defined limits of concentration bromide in drinking-waters at 6 mg/L for adults and 2 mg/L for children and acceptable daily intake currently ranges from 0 to 1 mg/Kg of bw [110]. Human exposure to brominated compounds usually occurs by food intake and consistently increases over time, resulting particularly higher in Occidental countries [118]. Breast milk as well as hair and adipose tissue may accumulate these chemicals, thus resulting as reservoirs for further persistence of brominated compounds in the human body [118]. Bromide may interfere with thyroid homeostasis, particularly competing with I uptake and I clearance [119,120] however, human toxicity data demonstrated that polybrominated compounds may interfere with gonadal function and sexual steroids' metabolism [118]. Fluoride and fluorinated compounds has been found in different rock-forming minerals, fertilizers, pesticides, and propellants, and has also been found in drinking water generally at acceptable levels according to regulatory agencies (<1.5 mg/L or <4 mg/L) [121] and groundwater [122]. Considering that a low dose of fluoride increases overall oral health, several countries add it to their public water supply at 0.7 to 1.5 mg/L [118]. In Italy, public waters are naturally rich in fluoride (1 mg/L), thus making fluoride addition in public supply unnecessary [123]. However, fluoride concentration in public waters differs among regions, and is particularly higher in Lazio, where an excessive consumption of public drinking-water may lead to a fluoride overexposure [123]. Concerns over fluoride overexposure through drinking water have been raised in several countries [124], in which the levels of fluoride intake exceed safety limits, leading to a relevant increase in the prevalence of both dental and skeletal fluorosis [125]. Fluoride has been found to block I uptake by two fundamental mechanisms: inhibition of sodium-potassium ATPase and a cytokine-mediated reduction in NIS gene expression [126]. Indeed, fluoride exposure in early stages of life, mostly for preventing dental caries, is believed to be linked with an higher risk of future development of several diseases, including hypothyroidism and impaired intellective quotient [127]. Moreover, the exposure to fluoride concentration at 100 ppm (mg/L) in experimental conditions were associated with apoptosis, organelle damage and oxidative stress resulting in neurodegeneration, endocrine dysfunction and diabetes mellitus [128]. Due to anthropogenic and industrial activities, a great number of pollutant entry in water systems leading to possible concerns for wildlife and human health. Defluoridation of water may contribute in reducing the level of fluoride contamination in water and different physicochemical and electrochemical methods have been used for this purpose [129]. Among these, biosorption should be considered an easily available, recyclable and inexpensive tool [129].

4. Discussion

I sufficiency and euthyroidism are essential for preventing negative neurodevelopmental [130] outcomes and processing disorders [131], thus I deficiency or interference should be hazardous particularly during pregnancy and earlier stages of life given the particularly vulnerable thyroid function in this developmental phase. Conventionally, I deficiency has been defined as a 24-h urinary excretion <100 µg/L [132]. Given this criteria, more than 2 billion people worldwide are at high risk of iodine insufficiency and at least half of European citizens exhibit a mild to moderate I deficiency [133]. Italy has been historically defined as being endemic for I deficiency, particularly in the northern mountainous regions. Strategies of implementation of iodine intake have been allowed by law since 1972 through the use, on a voluntary basis, of fortified salt with an I content of 15 µg/Kg, subsequently augmented to 30 µg/kg (law 55/2005). Supplementation provided a slow but progressive improvement of iodine status over time but did not completely eradicate the risk [134,135] and the prevalence of mild-to-moderate I deficiency remains a current matter [136], especially in pregnancy and lactation [137]. Of note, patients with I deficiency should be considered as highly susceptible for developing I interference by food intake. ClO_4^- has a short half-life (up to 8 h) due to a quick renal clearance [138], thus its accumulation in human body is clearly due to chronic exposure to drinks and food [139,140]. ClO_4^- exposure may be harmful for thyroid homeostasis, especially in childhood and pregnancy. Two trials were performed to assess short term effects of a ClO_4^- acute exposure (2 weeks) to either 0.5 or 3 mg daily, showing no effect on thyroid function [141,142]. However, 2 weeks of ClO_4^- exposure at higher doses (10 to 30 mg per day) resulted in significantly reduced iodine uptake, potentially affecting thyroid hormone synthesis [143,144]. The results of these studies should be interpreted with caution, particularly considering that short-term exposure is usually insufficient to affect thyroid secretion of levothyroxine. Moreover, to achieve these levels of exposure, it could be necessary to have an extremely high daily consumption of ClO_4^- for a limited period of time which is normally not reproducible in real life (i.e., 2 litres of drinking water at ClO_4^- content as high as 200 µg/L). On the other hand, studies which assessed the effect of a chronic ClO_4^- exposure (i.e., occupational) on thyroid hormone synthesis reported inclusive or equivocal results, despite I uptake being usually impaired in almost all participants [145–147]. Given these findings, it was difficult to make an unequivocal conclusion. The National Research Council of the National Academics sustained that, in healthy individuals, I uptake would be reduced by at least 75% for months in order to significantly impair thyroid hormone synthesis [47]. Thus, a sustained exposure to 0.5 mg/Kg of bw/day of ClO_4^- would be most likely to induce a significant decline in I uptake consequentlyaffecting thyroid hormone synthesis [47]. However, the US Environmental Protection Agency adopted a recommended reference dose for ClO_4^- at 0.7 µg/kg of bw/day [141]. This conservative decision was based upon a non-observed effect level found by Greer et al. in 2002 (7 µg/Kg of bw/day) divided for an uncertainty factor of 10 attributable to intra-human variability intended to calculate an acceptable daily intake [144]. The Office of Environmental Health Hazards Assessment developed a public health target for ClO_4^- in drinking water of 6 µg/L in 2002 to 1 µg/L in 2012 [148]. In 2011, the Joint Food and Agriculture Organization—World Health Organization recognized a maximum tolerable daily intake of 10 µg/kg of body weight [149]. In Europe (France and Germany), the acceptable level of exposure to ClO_4^- was set at 0.7 µg/kg of bw with a tolerable concentration in drinking water of 15 µg/L, successively reduced to 4 µg/L [47]. Furthermore, the European Food Safety Authority in 2014 predisposed the maximum tolerable daily dose of 0.3 µg/Kg of bw/day [70]. Water and soil contaminations have become a concern due to detrimental consequences for both wildlife and human health. Efficient methods for reducing the levels of ClO_4^- in fruits and vegetables represent useful tools to decrease the levels of exposure. Considering that the contamination of fruits and vegetables should reflect ClO_4^- concentration in soil, water for irrigation and fertilizers, several processes found application in this field [150]. As an example, ion exchangers, which replace ClO_4^- with other resident anions, such as bicarbonate, sulfate and nitrate, are one of the most used methods for removing ClO_4^- from water and may be considered as a tool for dropping ClO_4^- levels throughout soil watering [151]. Biological degradation by perchlorate-reductase producer bacteria [152] or plants [150] could be counted as another useful method for reducing ClO_4^- in water and soil, respectively. Photocatalytic reduction of aqueous oxyanions converts toxic anions (such as ClO_4^- or bromate) into harmless and less and/or not toxic ions in contaminated waters [153]. However, several limitations have been described for this method, which include high costs of technologies, sunlight harvesting capability and generation of dangerous radical substances [153]. Physical methods include reverse osmosis coupled with nanofiltration membrane systems [154], or a less expensive semipermeable membrane system coupled with electrodialysis [155]. Moreover, iron-media adsorbent have been used for removing ClO_4^- and other anions in aqueous solutions [156]. In particular, granular ferric hydroxide was found to induce a rapid uptake of ClO_4^- in water, considering that its maximum absorption and equilibrium were achieved in 30 and 60 min, respectively at 25 °C with optimal pH at 3–7 [157]. ClO_4^- contamination of soil and water is strictly related to geogenic ClO_4^- naturally occurred in the atmosphere and subsequently precipitated. However, fertilizes may be considered a source of ClO_4^- accumulated in food chain [158]. Among fertilizers, higher levels of ClO_4^- were detected in nitrogenous fertilizers (32.6 mg/Kg) compared to natrium-phosphorus-potassium (12.6 mg/Kg), non-nitrogen (10.2 mg/Kg) and phosphates (11.5 mg/Kg) fertilizers [159]. Thus, the type and the amount of fertilizer may influence the source of entry for ClO_4^- in crops. Additionally, agronomic practices of fertilization may also contribute in this risk. As an example, fertigation is an innovative and less expensive methods of fertilization which allows for less water being wasted, better distribution of fertilizers and superior micronutrient assimilation by crops, but given these principles, it may be easier to foster more significant accumulations of ClO_4- in fruits and vegetables [60].

5. Conclusions

In conclusion, acute exposure to ClO_4^- by food and drink should not be a harmful concern for thyroid homeostasis in healthy individuals. Generally, chronic exposure to ClO_4^- by eating and drinking does not exceed the safety reference levels. However, lifelong effects of a low-dose exposure to ClO_4^- are currently unknown and concerns remain, especially for highly susceptible individuals such as pregnant and breastfeeding women, infants and children, cigarette smokers and high vegetable consumers, such as vegans. These clusters of patients should be advised about this worry, and encouraged to limit daily consumption of rich in perchlorate vegetables, as well as to implement I intake.

On the other hand, producers should be encouraged to use specific culture systems, fertilizers (as an example nitrate-free) as well as technologies for reducing the level of ClO_4^- in soil and irrigation waters in order to prevent an unnecessary ClO_4^- enrichment of crops. For this purpose, economic sustainment should be considered particularly for small and medium-size companies in order to reduce management costs.

Finally, further and specific long-term studies are probably needed to better explore this issue, aiming to clarify whether monitoring of perchlorate exposure over time, especially in individuals at risk, could be of interest for endocrinologists for better defining strategies of detection and prevention in exposed patients.

Author Contributions: V.T. conceived the review. V.T., G.L. and A.D.T. provided database search. G.L. and A.D.T. drafted the manuscript. All the authors (V.T., G.L., A.D.T., V.A.G., G.D.P.) read, gave feedback, and approved the final manuscript. All authors have read and agreed to the published version of the manuscript.

Appendix A

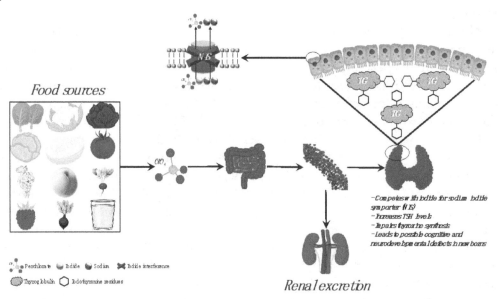

Figure A1. Simplified representation of perchlorate metabolism, distribution and iodide interference (specifically at the level of thyroid gland).

References

1. Thomas Zoeller, R.; Brown, T.R.; Doan, L.L.; Gore, A.C.; Skakkebaek, N.E.; Soto, A.M.; Woodruff, T.J.; Vom Saal, F.S. Endocrine-disrupting chemicals and public health protection: A statement of principles from the Endocrine Society. *Endocrinology* **2012**, *153*, 4097–4110. [CrossRef]
2. La Merrill, M.A.; Vandenberg, L.N.; Smith, M.T.; Goodson, W.; Browne, P.; Patisaul, H.B.; Guyton, K.Z.; Kortenkamp, A.; Cogliano, V.J.; Woodruff, T.J.; et al. Consensus on the key characteristics of endocrine-disrupting chemicals as a basis for hazard identification. *Nat. Rev. Endocrinol.* **2020**, *16*, 45–57. [CrossRef]

3. Langer, P.; Kočan, A.; Tajtáková, M.; Koška, J.; Rádiková, Ž.; Kšinantová, L.; Imrich, R.; Hučková, M.; Drobná, B.; Gašperíková, D.; et al. Increased thyroid volume, prevalence of thyroid antibodies and impaired fasting glucose in young adults from organochlorine cocktail polluted area: Outcome of transgenerational transmission? *Chemosphere* **2008**, *73*, 1145–1150. [CrossRef]

4. Street, M.E.; Angelini, S.; Bernasconi, S.; Burgio, E.; Cassio, A.; Catellani, C.; Cirillo, F.; Deodati, A.; Fabbrizi, E.; Fanos, V.; et al. Current knowledge on endocrine disrupting chemicals (EDCs) from animal biology to humans, from pregnancy to adulthood: Highlights from a national italian meeting. *Int. J. Mol. Sci.* **2018**, *19*, 1647. [CrossRef] [PubMed]

5. Ferrari, S.M.; Fallahi, P.; Antonelli, A.; Benvenga, S. Environmental issues in thyroid diseases. *Front. Endocrinol.* **2017**, *8*, 50. [CrossRef]

6. Yilmaz, B.; Terekeci, H.; Sandal, S.; Kelestimur, F. Endocrine disrupting chemicals: Exposure, effects on human health, mechanism of action, models for testing and strategies for prevention. *Rev. Endocr. Metab. Disord.* **2019**, *21*, 127–147. [CrossRef]

7. Boas, M.; Feldt-Rasmussen, U.; Main, K.M. Thyroid effects of endocrine disrupting chemicals. *Mol. Cell. Endocrinol.* **2012**, *355*, 240–248. [CrossRef] [PubMed]

8. Calsolaro, V.; Pasqualetti, G.; Niccolai, F.; Caraccio, N.; Monzani, F. Thyroid disrupting chemicals. *Int. J. Mol. Sci.* **2017**, *18*, 2583. [CrossRef] [PubMed]

9. Mughal, B.B.; Fini, J.B.; Demeneix, B.A. Thyroid-disrupting chemicals and brain development: An update. *Endocr. Connect.* **2018**, *7*, R160–R186. [CrossRef] [PubMed]

10. Melzer, D.; Rice, N.; Depledge, M.H.; Henley, W.E.; Galloway, T.S. Association between serum perfluorooctanoic acid (PFOA) and thyroid disease in the U.S. National Health and Nutrition Examination Survey. *Environ. Health Perspect.* **2010**, *118*, 686–692. [CrossRef]

11. MacKay, H.; Abizaid, A. A plurality of molecular targets: The receptor ecosystem for bisphenol-A (BPA). *Horm. Behav.* **2018**, *101*, 59–67. [CrossRef] [PubMed]

12. Wang, N.; Zhou, Y.; Fu, C.; Wang, H.; Huang, P.; Wang, B.; Su, M.; Jiang, F.; Fang, H.; Zhao, Q.; et al. Influence of Bisphenol A on Thyroid Volume and Structure Independent of Iodine in School Children. *PLoS ONE* **2015**, *10*, e0141248. [CrossRef]

13. Li, L.; Ying, Y.; Zhang, C.; Wang, W.; Li, Y.; Feng, Y.; Liang, J.; Song, H.; Wang, Y. Bisphenol A exposure and risk of thyroid nodules in Chinese women: A case-control study. *Environ. Int.* **2019**, *126*, 321–328. [CrossRef] [PubMed]

14. Leemans, M.; Couderq, S.; Demeneix, B.; Fini, J.B. Pesticides With Potential Thyroid Hormone-Disrupting Effects: A Review of Recent Data. *Front. Endocrinol.* **2019**, *10*, 743. [CrossRef] [PubMed]

15. Campos, É.; Freire, C. Exposure to non-persistent pesticides and thyroid function: A systematic review of epidemiological evidence. *Int. J. Hyg. Environ. Health* **2016**, *219*, 481–497. [CrossRef] [PubMed]

16. Witorsch, R.J. Critical analysis of endocrine disruptive activity of triclosan and its relevance to human exposure through the use of personal care products. *Crit. Rev. Toxicol.* **2014**, *44*, 535–555. [CrossRef] [PubMed]

17. Demeneix, B.A. Evidence for Prenatal Exposure to Thyroid Disruptors and Adverse Effects on Brain Development. *Eur. Thyroid J.* **2019**, *8*, 283–292. [CrossRef]

18. Pearce, E.N.; Braverman, L.E. Environmental pollutants and the thyroid. *Best Pract. Res. Clin. Endocrinol. Metab.* **2009**, *23*, 801–813. [CrossRef]

19. Pironi, L.; Guidetti, M.; Agostini, F. Iodine status in intestinal failure in adults. *Curr. Opin. Clin. Nutr. Metab. Care* **2015**, *18*, 582–587. [CrossRef] [PubMed]

20. Nicola, J.P.; Carrasco, N.; Masini-Repiso, A.M. Dietary I– Absorption: Expression and Regulation of the Na+/I– Symporter in the Intestine. *Vitam. Horm.* **2015**, *98*, 1–31.

21. Cavalieri, R.R. Iodine metabolism and thyroid physiology: Current concepts. *Thyroid* **1997**, *7*, 177–181. [CrossRef] [PubMed]

22. Ravera, S.; Reyna-Neyra, A.; Ferrandino, G.; Amzel, L.M.; Carrasco, N. The Sodium/Iodide Symporter (NIS): Molecular Physiology and Preclinical and Clinical Applications. *Annu. Rev. Physiol.* **2017**, *79*, 261–289. [CrossRef] [PubMed]

23. Dai, G.; Levy, O.; Carrasco, N. Cloning and characterization of the thyroid iodide transporter. *Nature* **1996**, *379*, 458–460. [CrossRef] [PubMed]

24. Carrasco, N. Iodide transport in the thyroid gland. *BBA Rev. Biomembr.* **1993**, *1154*, 65–82. [CrossRef]

25. Milanesi, A.; Brent, G.A. Iodine and Thyroid Hormone Synthesis, Metabolism, and Action. *Mol. Genet. Nutr. Asp. Major Trace Miner.* **2017**, 143–150.

26. Lee, S.Y.; Chang, D.L.F.; He, X.; Pearce, E.N.; Braverman, L.E.; Leung, A.M. Urinary iodine excretion and serum thyroid function in adults after iodinated contrast administration. *Thyroid* **2015**, *25*, 471–477. [CrossRef]

27. Dunn, J.T.; Dunn, A.D. Update on intrathyroidal iodine metabolism. *Thyroid* **2001**, *11*, 407–414. [CrossRef]

28. Rohner, F.; Zimmermann, M.; Jooste, P.; Pandav, C.; Caldwell, K.; Raghavan, R.; Raiten, D.J. Biomarkers of Nutrition for Development—Iodine Review. *J. Nutr.* **2014**, *144*, 1322S–1342S. [CrossRef]

29. Glinoer, D. The regulation of thyroid function in pregnancy: Pathways of endocrine adaptation from physiology to pathology. *Endocr. Rev.* **1997**, *18*, 404–433. [CrossRef]

30. Osei, J.; Andersson, M.; van der Reijden, O.; Dold, S.; Smuts, C.M.; Baumgartner, J. Breast-milk iodine concentrations, iodine status, and thyroid function of breastfed infants aged 2–4 months and their mothers residing in a south african township. *JCRPE J. Clin. Res. Pediatr. Endocrinol.* **2016**, *8*, 381–391. [CrossRef]

31. Guideline: Fortification of Food-Grade Salt with Iodine for the Prevention and Control of Iodine Deficiency Disorders. Available online: https://www.who.int/publications-detail/9789241507929 (accessed on 3 June 2020).

32. De Groot, L.; Abalovich, M.; Alexander, E.K.; Amino, N.; Barbour, L.; Cobin, R.H.; Eastman, C.J.; Lazarus, J.H.; Luton, D.; Mandel, S.J.; et al. Management of thyroid dysfunction during pregnancy and postpartum: An endocrine society clinical practice guideline. *J. Clin. Endocrinol. Metab.* **2012**, *97*, 2543–2565. [CrossRef] [PubMed]

33. Triggiani, V.; Tafaro, E.; Giagulli, V.; Sabba, C.; Resta, F.; Licchelli, B.; Guastamacchia, E. Role of Iodine, Selenium and Other Micronutrients in Thyroid Function and Disorders. *Endocr. Metab. Immune Disord. Drug Targets* **2009**, *9*, 277–294. [CrossRef] [PubMed]

34. Guastamacchia, E.; Giagulli, V.; Licchelli, B.; Triggiani, V. Selenium and Iodine in Autoimmune Thyroiditis. *Endocr. Metab. Immune Disord. Targets* **2015**, *15*, 288–292. [CrossRef] [PubMed]

35. Bizhanova, A.; Kopp, P. Minireview: The sodium-iodide symporter NIS and pendrin in iodide homeostasis of the thyroid. *Endocrinology* **2009**, *150*, 1084–1090. [CrossRef] [PubMed]

36. Wémeau, J.L.; Kopp, P. Pendred syndrome. *Best Pract. Res. Clin. Endocrinol. Metab.* **2017**, *31*, 213–224. [CrossRef]

37. Leung, A.M.; Braverman, L.E. Consequences of excess iodine. *Nat. Rev. Endocrinol.* **2014**, *10*, 136–142. [CrossRef]

38. Sundick, R.S.; Bagchi, N.; Brown, T.R. The role of iodine in thyroid autoimmunity: From chickens to humans: A review. *Autoimmunity* **1992**, *13*, 61–68. [CrossRef]

39. Katagiri, R.; Yuan, X.; Kobayashi, S.; Sasaki, S. Effect of excess iodine intake on thyroid diseases in different populations: A systematic review and meta-analyses including observational studies. *PLoS ONE* **2017**, *12*, e0173722. [CrossRef]

40. Stanbury, J.B.; Wyngaarden, J.B. Effect of perchlorate on the human thyroid gland. *Metabolism* **1952**, *1*, 533–539.

41. Leung, A.M.; Pearce, E.N.; Braverman, L.E. Perchlorate, iodine and the thyroid. *Best Pract. Res. Clin. Endocrinol. Metab.* **2010**, *24*, 133–141. [CrossRef]

42. Tonacchera, M.; Pinchera, A.; Dimida, A.; Ferrarini, E.; Agretti, P.; Vitti, P.; Santini, F.; Crump, K.; Gibbs, J. Relative potencies and additivity of perchlorate, thiocyanate, nitrate, and iodide on the inhibition of radioactive iodide uptake by the human sodium iodide symporter. *Thyroid* **2004**, *14*, 1012–1019. [CrossRef] [PubMed]

43. Concilio, S.C.; Zhekova, H.R.; Noskov, S.Y.; Russell, S.J. Inter-species variation in monovalent anion substrate selectivity and inhibitor sensitivity in the sodium iodide symporter (NIS). *PLoS ONE* **2020**, *15*, e0229085. [CrossRef] [PubMed]

44. Chen, H.X.; Ding, M.H.; Li, Y.G.; Liu, Q.; Peng, K.L. Dose-Response Relationship between Orally Administered Ammonium Perchlorate and Urine Perchlorate Concentrations in Rats: Possible Biomarker to Quantify Environmental Ammonium Perchlorate Exposure on Thyroid Homeostasis. *Arch. Environ. Occup. Health* **2015**, *70*, 286–290. [CrossRef] [PubMed]

45. Hershman, J.M. Perchlorate and thyroid function: What are the environmental issues? *Thyroid* **2005**, *15*, 427–431. [CrossRef]

46. Suh, M.; Abraham, L.; Hixon, J.G.; Proctor, D.M. The effects of perchlorate, nitrate, and thiocyanate on free thyroxine for potentially sensitive subpopulations o. The 2001–2002 and 2007–2008 National Health and Nutrition Examination Surveys. *J. Expo. Sci. Environ. Epidemiol.* **2014**, *24*, 579–587. [CrossRef]

47. EFSA Panel on Contaminants in the Food Chain (CONTAM). Scientific Opinion on the risks to public health related to the presence of perchlorate in food, in particular fruits and vegetables. *EFSA J.* **2014**, *12*, 3869. [CrossRef]

48. Kounaves, S.P.; Stroble, S.T.; Anderson, R.M.; Moore, Q.; Catling, D.C.; Douglas, S.; Mckay, C.P.; Ming, D.W.; Smith, P.H.; Tamppari, L.K.; et al. Discovery of natural Perchlorate in the Antarctic Dry Valleys and its global implications. *Environ. Sci. Technol.* **2010**, *44*, 2360–2364. [CrossRef]

49. Calderón, R.; Palma, P.; Parker, D.; Molina, M.; Godoy, F.A.; Escudey, M. Perchlorate levels in soil and waters from the Atacama Desert. *Arch. Environ. Contam. Toxicol.* **2014**, *66*, 155–161. [CrossRef]

50. Kumarathilaka, P.; Oze, C.; Indraratne, S.P.; Vithanage, M. Perchlorate as an emerging contaminant in soil, water and food. *Chemosphere* **2016**, *150*, 667–677. [CrossRef]

51. Furdui, V.I.; Zheng, J.; Furdui, A. Anthropogenic Perchlorate Increases since 1980 in the Canadian High Arctic. *Environ. Sci. Technol.* **2018**, *52*, 972–981. [CrossRef]

52. Furdui, V.I.; Tomassini, F. Trends and sources of perchlorate in Arctic snow. *Environ. Sci. Technol.* **2010**, *44*, 588–592. [CrossRef] [PubMed]

53. Dasgupta, P.K.; Martinelango, P.K.; Jackson, W.A.; Anderson, T.A.; Tian, K.; Tock, R.W.; Rajagopalan, S. The origin of naturally occurring perchlorate: The role of atmospheric processes. *Environ. Sci. Technol.* **2005**, *39*, 1569–1575. [CrossRef]

54. Kannan, K.; Praamsma, M.L.; Oldi, J.F.; Kunisue, T.; Sinha, R.K. Occurrence of perchlorate in drinking water, groundwater, surface water and human saliva from India. *Chemosphere* **2009**, *76*, 22–26. [CrossRef]

55. Qin, X.; Zhang, T.; Gan, Z.; Sun, H. Spatial distribution of perchlorate, iodide and thiocyanate in the aquatic environment of Tianjin, China: Environmental source analysis. *Chemosphere* **2014**, *111*, 201–208. [CrossRef] [PubMed]

56. Munster, J.; Hanson, G.N.; Jackson, W.A.; Rajagopalan, S. The fallout from fireworks: Perchlorate in total deposition. *Water Air Soil Pollut.* **2009**, *198*, 149–153. [CrossRef]

57. Rajagopalan, S.; Anderson, T.; Cox, S.; Harvey, G.; Cheng, Q.; Jackson, W.A. Perchlorate in Wet Deposition Across North America. *Environ. Sci. Technol.* **2009**, *43*, 616–622. [CrossRef] [PubMed]

58. Urbansky, E.T.; Brown, S.K. Perchlorate retention and mobility in soils. *J. Environ. Monit.* **2003**, *5*, 455–462. [CrossRef]

59. Dugan, N.R.; Williams, D.J.; Meyer, M.; Schneider, R.R.; Speth, T.F.; Metz, D.H. The impact of temperature on the performance of anaerobic biological treatment of perchlorate in drinking water. *Water Res.* **2009**, *43*, 1867–1878. [CrossRef]

60. Calderón, R.; Palma, P.; Eltit, K.; Arancibia-Miranda, N.; Silva-Moreno, E.; Yu, W. Field study on the uptake, accumulation and risk assessment of perchlorate in a soil-chard/spinach system: Impact of agronomic practices and fertilization. *Sci. Total Environ.* **2020**, *719*, 137411. [CrossRef]

61. Calderón, R.; Godoy, F.; Escudey, M.; Palma, P. A review of perchlorate (ClO4−) occurrence in fruits and vegetables. *Environ. Monit. Assess.* **2017**, *189*, 82. [CrossRef]

62. Wang, Z.; Forsyth, D.; Lau, B.P.Y.; Pelletier, L.; Bronson, R.; Gaertner, D. Estimated dietary exposure of canadians to perchlorate through the consumption of fruits and vegetables available in Ottawa markets. *J. Agric. Food Chem.* **2009**, *57*, 9250–9255. [CrossRef] [PubMed]

63. Vega, M.; Nerenberg, R.; Vargas, I.T. Perchlorate contamination in Chile: Legacy, challenges, and potential solutions. *Environ. Res.* **2018**, *164*, 316–326. [CrossRef]

64. Steinmaus, C.M. Perchlorate in Water Supplies: Sources, Exposures, and Health Effects. *Curr. Environ. Health Rep.* **2016**, *3*, 136–143. [CrossRef] [PubMed]

65. Iannece, P.; Motta, O.; Tedesco, R.; Carotenuto, M.; Proto, A. Determination of Perchlorate in Bottled Water from Italy. *Water* **2013**, *5*, 767–779. [CrossRef]

66. Agrarmarkt Informations-Gesellschaft MbH. European Statistics Handbook—FRUIT LOGISTICA 2019. Available online: www.AMI-informiert.de (accessed on 2 March 2020).

67. OEC. Chile (CHL) Exports, Imports, and Trade Partners. Available online: https://oec.world/en/profile/country/chl/ (accessed on 11 May 2020).

68. Chilean Table Grape Exports to Europe Increase by 36%. Available online: https://www.freshplaza.com/article/9196058/chilean-table-grape-exports-to-europe-increase-by-36/ (accessed on 11 May 2020).

69. Chile—Trade—European Commission. Available online: https://ec.europa.eu/trade/policy/countries-and-regions/countries/chile/ (accessed on 11 May 2020).

70. Arcella, D.; Binaglia, M.; Vernazza, F. Dietary exposure assessment to perchlorate in the European population. *EFSA J.* **2017**, *15*, e05043.

71. Dong, H.; Xiao, K.; Xian, Y.; Wu, Y.; Zhu, L. A novel approach for simultaneous analysis of perchlorate (ClO4−) and bromate (BrO3−) in fruits and vegetables using modified QuEChERS combined with ultrahigh performance liquid chromatography-tandem mass spectrometry. *Food Chem.* **2019**, *270*, 196–203. [CrossRef]

72. Vejdovszky, K.; Grossgut, R.; Unterluggauer, H.; Inreiter, N.; Steinwider, J. Risk assessment of dietary exposure to perchlorate for the Austrian population. *Food Addit. Contam. Part A Chem. Anal. Control. Expo. Risk Assess.* **2018**, *35*, 623–631. [CrossRef]

73. Liu, Y.; Sun, H.; Zhou, L.; Luo, F.; Zhang, X.; Chen, Z. Quantitative determination and contamination pattern of perchlorate in tea by ultra performance liquid chromatography and tandem mass spectrometry. *Food Chem.* **2019**, *274*, 180–186. [CrossRef]

74. Huber, D.R.; Blount, B.C.; Mage, D.T.; Letkiewicz, F.J.; Kumar, A.; Allen, R.H. Estimating perchlorate exposure from food and tap water based on US biomonitoring and occurrence data. *J. Expo. Sci. Environ. Epidemiol.* **2011**, *21*, 395–407. [CrossRef]

75. Blount, B.C.; Valentin-Blasini, L.; Osterloh, J.D.; Mauldin, J.P.; Pirkle, J.L. Perchlorate exposure of the US population, 2001–2002. *J. Expo. Sci. Environ. Epidemiol.* **2007**, *17*, 400–407. [CrossRef]

76. Zoeller, T.R. Environmental chemicals targeting thyroid. *Hormones* **2010**, *9*, 28–40. [CrossRef]

77. Vandenberg, L.N.; Colborn, T.; Hayes, T.B.; Heindel, J.J.; Jacobs, D.R.; Lee, D.H.; Shioda, T.; Soto, A.M.; vom Saal, F.S.; Welshons, W.V.; et al. Hormones and endocrine-disrupting chemicals: Low-dose effects and nonmonotonic dose responses. *Endocr. Rev.* **2012**, *33*, 378–455. [CrossRef] [PubMed]

78. Lee, S.Y.; McCarthy, A.M.; Stohl, H.; Ibrahim, S.; Jeong, C.; Braverman, L.E.; Ma, W.; He, X.; Mestman, J.H.; Schuller, K.E.; et al. Urinary Iodine, Perchlorate, and Thiocyanate Concentrations in U.S. Lactating Women. *Thyroid* **2017**, *27*, 1574–1581. [CrossRef] [PubMed]

79. Leung, A.M.; LaMar, A.; He, X.; Braverman, L.E.; Pearce, E.N. Iodine status and thyroid function of Boston-area vegetarians and vegans. *J. Clin. Endocrinol. Metab.* **2011**, *96*, E1303–E1307. [CrossRef] [PubMed]

80. De Groef, B.; Decallonne, B.R.; Van der Geyten, S.; Darras, V.M.; Bouillon, R. Perchlorate versus other environmental sodium/iodide symporter inhibitors: Potential thyroid-related health effects. *Eur. J. Endocrinol.* **2006**, *155*, 17–25. [CrossRef]

81. Téllez, R.T.; Chacón, P.M.; Abarca, C.R.; Blount, B.C.; Van Landingham, C.B.; Crump, K.S.; Gibbs, J.P. Long-term environmental exposure to perchlorate through drinking water and thyroid function during pregnancy and the neonatal period. *Thyroid* **2005**, *15*, 963–975. [CrossRef]

82. Maffini, M.V.; Trasande, L.; Neltner, T.G. Perchlorate and Diet: Human Exposures, Risks, and Mitigation Strategies. *Curr. Environ. Health Rep.* **2016**, *3*, 107–117. [CrossRef]

83. Borjan, M.; Marcella, S.; Blount, B.; Greenberg, M.; Zhang, J.; Murphy, E.; Valentin-Blasini, L.; Robson, M. Perchlorate exposure in lactating women in an urban community in New Jersey. *Sci. Total Environ.* **2011**, *409*, 460–464. [CrossRef]

84. Zhang, T.; Wu, Q.; Sun, H.W.; Rao, J.; Kannan, K. Perchlorate and iodide in whole blood samples from infants, children, and adults in Nanchang, China. *Environ. Sci. Technol.* **2010**, *44*, 6947–6953. [CrossRef]

85. Valentín-Blasini, L.; Blount, B.C.; Otero-Santos, S.; Cao, Y.; Bernbaum, J.C.; Rogan, W.J. Perchlorate exposure and dose estimates in infants. *Environ. Sci. Technol.* **2011**, *45*, 4127–4132. [CrossRef]

86. Lau, F.K.; Decastro, B.R.; Mills-Herring, L.; Tao, L.; Valentin-Blasini, L.; Alwis, K.U.; Blount, B.C. Urinary perchlorate as a measure of dietary and drinking water exposure in a representative sample of the United States population 2001–2008. *J. Expo. Sci. Environ. Epidemiol.* **2013**, *23*, 207–214. [CrossRef]

87. Crump, C.; Michaud, P.; Téllez, R.; Reyes, C.; Gonzalez, G.; Montgomery, E.L.; Crump, K.S.; Lobo, G.; Becerra, C.; Gibbs, J.P. Does perchlorate in drinking water affect thyroid function in newborns or school-age children? *J. Occup. Environ. Med.* **2000**, *42*, 603–612. [CrossRef] [PubMed]

88. Levie, D.; Korevaar, T.I.M.; Bath, S.C.; Murcia, M.; Dineva, M.; Llop, S.; Espada, M.; van Herwaarden, A.E.; de Rijke, Y.B.; Ibarluzea, J.M.; et al. Association of Maternal Iodine Status With Child IQ: A Meta-Analysis of Individual Participant Data. *J. Clin. Endocrinol. Metab.* **2019**, *104*, 5957–5967. [CrossRef] [PubMed]

89. Knight, B.A.; Shields, B.M.; He, X.; Pearce, E.N.; Braverman, L.E.; Sturley, R.; Vaidya, B. Effect of perchlorate and thiocyanate exposure on thyroid function of pregnant women from South-West England: A cohort study. *Thyroid Res.* **2018**, *11*, 9. [CrossRef] [PubMed]

90. Mitchell, A.M.; Manley, S.W.; Morris, J.C.; Powell, K.A.; Bergert, E.R.; Mortimer, R.H. Sodium iodide symporter (NIS) gene expression in human placenta. *Placenta* **2001**, *22*, 256–258. [CrossRef] [PubMed]

91. Blount, B.C.; Rich, D.Q.; Valentin-Blasini, L.; Lashley, S.; Ananth, C.V.; Murphy, E.; Smulian, J.C.; Spain, B.J.; Barr, D.; Ledoux, T.; et al. Perinatal exposure to perchlorate, thiocyanate, and nitrate in New Jersey mothers and newborns. *Environ. Sci. Technol.* **2009**, *43*, 7543–7549. [CrossRef]

92. Zhang, T.; Ma, Y.; Wang, D.; Li, R.; Chen, X.; Mo, W.; Qin, X.; Sun, H.; Kannan, K. Placental transfer of and infantile exposure to perchlorate. *Chemosphere* **2016**, *144*, 948–954. [CrossRef]

93. Pearce, E.N.; Alexiou, M.; Koukkou, E.; Braverman, L.E.; He, X.; Ilias, I.; Alevizaki, M.; Markou, K.B. Perchlorate and thiocyanate exposure and thyroid function in first-trimester pregnant women from Greece. *Clin. Endocrinol.* **2012**, *77*, 471–474. [CrossRef]

94. Charatcharoenwitthaya, N.; Ongphiphadhanakul, B.; Pearce, E.N.; Somprasit, C.; Chanthasenanont, A.; He, X.; Chailurkit, L.; Braverman, L.E. The association between perchlorate and thiocyanate exposure and thyroid function in first-trimester pregnant Thai women. *J. Clin. Endocrinol. Metab.* **2014**, *99*, 2365–2371. [CrossRef]

95. Steinmaus, C.; Pearl, M.; Kharrazi, M.; Blount, B.C.; Miller, M.D.; Pearce, E.N.; Valentin-Blasini, L.; DeLorenze, G.; Hoofnagle, A.N.; Liaw, J. Thyroid hormones and moderate exposure to perchlorate during pregnancy in women in southern California. *Environ. Health Perspect.* **2016**, *124*, 861–867. [CrossRef]

96. Pearce, E.N.; Lazarus, J.H.; Smyth, P.P.A.; He, X.; Dall'Amico, D.; Parkes, A.B.; Burns, R.; Smith, D.F.; Maina, A.; Bestwick, J.P.; et al. Perchlorate and thiocyanate exposure and thyroid function in first-trimester pregnant women. *J. Clin. Endocrinol. Metab.* **2010**, *95*, 3207–3215. [CrossRef] [PubMed]

97. Pearce, E.N.; Spencer, C.A.; Mestman, J.H.; Lee, R.H.; Bergoglio, L.M.; Mereshian, P.; He, X.; Leung, A.M.; Braverman, L.E. Effect of environmental perchlorate on thyroid function in pregnant women from Córdoba, Argentina, and Los Angeles, California. *Endocr. Pract.* **2011**, *17*, 412–417. [CrossRef] [PubMed]

98. Horton, M.K.; Blount, B.C.; Valentin-Blasini, L.; Wapner, R.; Whyatt, R.; Gennings, C.; Factor-Litvak, P. CO-occurring exposure to perchlorate, nitrate and thiocyanate alters thyroid function in healthy pregnant women. *Environ. Res.* **2015**, *143*, 1–9. [CrossRef] [PubMed]

99. Taylor, P.N.; Okosieme, O.E.; Murphy, R.; Hales, C.; Chiusano, E.; Maina, A.; Joomun, M.; Bestwick, J.P.; Smyth, P.; Paradice, R.; et al. Maternal perchlorate levels in women with borderline thyroid function during pregnancy and the cognitive development of their offspring: Data from the controlled antenatal thyroid study. *J. Clin. Endocrinol. Metab.* **2014**, *99*, 4291–4298. [CrossRef]

100. Brent, G.A. Perchlorate exposure in pregnancy and cognitive outcomes in children: It's not your mother's thyroid. *J. Clin. Endocrinol. Metab.* **2014**, *99*, 4066–4068. [CrossRef]

101. Rubin, R.; Pearl, M.; Kharrazi, M.; Blount, B.C.; Miller, M.D.; Pearce, E.N.; Valentin-Blasini, L.; DeLorenze, G.; Liaw, J.; Hoofnagle, A.N.; et al. Maternal perchlorate exposure in pregnancy and altered birth outcomes. *Environ. Res.* **2017**, *158*, 72–81. [CrossRef]

102. Buffler, P.A.; Kelsh, M.A.; Lau, E.C.; Edinboro, C.H.; Barnard, J.C.; Rutherford, G.W.; Daaboul, J.J.; Palmer, L.; Lorey, F.W. Thyroid function and perchlorate in drinking water: An evaluation among California newborns, 1998. *Environ. Health Perspect.* **2006**, *114*, 798–804. [CrossRef]

103. Amitai, Y.; Winston, G.; Sack, J.; Wasser, J.; Lewis, M.; Blount, B.C.; Valentin-Blasini, L.; Fisher, N.; Israeli, A.; Leventhal, A. Gestational exposure to high perchlorate concentrations in drinking water and neonatal thyroxine levels. *Thyroid* **2007**, *17*, 843–850. [CrossRef]

104. Steinmaus, C.; Miller, M.D.; Smith, A.H. Perchlorate in drinking water during pregnancy and neonatal thyroid hormone levels in California. *J. Occup. Environ. Med.* **2010**, *52*, 1217–1224. [CrossRef]

105. Mervish, N.A.; Pajak, A.; Teitelbaum, S.L.; Pinney, S.M.; Windham, G.C.; Kushi, L.H.; Biro, F.M.; Valentin-Blasini, L.; Blount, B.C.; Wolff, M.S. Thyroid antagonists (perchlorate, thiocyanate, and nitrate) and childhood growth in a longitudinal study of U.S. girls. *Environ. Health Perspect.* **2016**, *124*, 542–549. [CrossRef]

106. McMullen, J.; Ghassabian, A.; Kohn, B.; Trasande, L. Identifying subpopulations vulnerable to the thyroid-blocking effectsof perchlorateandthiocyanate. *J. Clin. Endocrinol. Metab.* **2017**, *102*, 2637–2645. [CrossRef] [PubMed]

107. Van Sande, J.; Massart, C.; Beauwens, R.; Schoutens, A.; Costagliola, S.; Dumont, J.E.; Wolff, J. Anion selectivity by the sodium iodide symporter. *Endocrinology* **2003**, *144*, 247–252. [CrossRef] [PubMed]

108. Jianjie, C.; Wenjuan, X.; Jinling, C.; Jie, S.; Ruhui, J.; Meiyan, L. Fluoride caused thyroid endocrine disruption in male zebrafish (Danio rerio). *Aquat. Toxicol.* **2016**, *171*, 48–58. [CrossRef] [PubMed]

109. Yoffe, D.; Frim, R.; Ukeles, S.D.; Dagani, M.J.; Barda, H.J.; Benya, T.J.; Sanders, D.C. Bromine Compounds. In *Ullmann's Encyclopedia of Industrial Chemistry*; Wiley-VCH Verlag GmbH & Co. KGaA: Weinheim, Germany, 2013; pp. 1–31.

110. Bromine as a Drinking-Water Disinfectant Alternative Drinking-Water Disinfectants: Bromine. 2018. Available online: http://apps.who.int/bookorders (accessed on 27 May 2020).

111. Thewlis, B.H. The fate of potassium bromate when used as a breadmaking improver. *J. Sci. Food Agric.* **1974**, *25*, 1471–1475. [CrossRef]

112. Shanmugavel, V.; Komala Santhi, K.; Kurup, A.H.; Kalakandan, S.; Anandharaj, A.; Rawson, A. Potassium bromate: Effects on bread components, health, environment and method of analysis: A review. *Food Chem.* **2020**, *311*, 125964. [CrossRef] [PubMed]

113. Mitsumori, K.; Maita, K.; Kosaka, T.; Miyaoka, T.; Shirasu, Y. Two-year oral chronic toxicity and carcinogenicity study in rats of diets fumigated with methyl bromide. *Food Chem. Toxicol.* **1990**, *28*, 109–119. [CrossRef]

114. Kurokawa, Y.; Maekawa, A.; Takahashi, M.; Hayashi, Y. Toxicity and carcinogenicity of potassium bromate—A new renal carcinogen. *Environ. Health Perspect.* **1990**, *87*, 309–335.

115. Umemura, T.; Sai, K.; Takagi, A.; Hasegawa, R.; Kurokawa, Y. A possible role for cell proliferation in potassium bromate (KBrO3) carcinogenesis. *J. Cancer Res. Clin. Oncol.* **1993**, *119*, 463–469. [CrossRef]

116. Last eval.: Potassium Bromate (IARC Summary & Evaluation, Volume 73, 1999). Available online: http://www.inchem.org/documents/iarc/vol73/73-17.html (accessed on 31 May 2020).

117. FDA CFR—Code of Federal Regulations Title 21. Available online: https://www.accessdata.fda.gov/scripts/cdrh/cfdocs/cfcfr/CFRSearch.cfm?fr=172.730 (accessed on 31 May 2020).

118. Wu, Z.; He, C.; Han, W.; Song, J.; Li, H.; Zhang, Y.; Jing, X.; Wu, W. Exposure pathways, levels and toxicity of polybrominated diphenyl ethers in humans: A review. *Environ. Res.* **2020**, *187*, 109531. [CrossRef]

119. Pavelka, S. Metabolism of Bromide and Its Interference With the Metabolism of Iodine. *Physiol. Res.* **2004**, *53* (Suppl. 1), S81–S90.

120. Block, J. Nineteenth-Century Homeopathic Materia Medica Texts Predict Source Materials Whose Physiological Actions Influence Thyroid Activity. *Homeopathy* **2019**, *108*, 214–222. [CrossRef] [PubMed]

121. Yadav, K.K.; Gupta, N.; Kumar, V.; Khan, S.A.; Kumar, A. A review of emerging adsorbents and current demand for defluoridation of water: Bright future in water sustainability. *Environ. Int.* **2018**, *111*, 80–108. [CrossRef] [PubMed]

122. Kurwadkar, S. Occurrence and distribution of organic and inorganic pollutants in groundwater. *Water Environ. Res.* **2019**, *91*, 1001–1008. [CrossRef] [PubMed]

123. La Fluorazione Delle Acque in Italia. Available online: https://www.epicentro.iss.it/cavo_orale/nota (accessed on 27 May 2020).

124. WHO. Water-Related Diseases. Available online: https://www.who.int/water_sanitation_health/diseases-risks/diseases/fluorosis/en/ (accessed on 31 May 2020).

125. Srivastava, S.; Flora, S.J.S. Fluoride in Drinking Water and Skeletal Fluorosis: A Review of the Global Impact. *Curr. Environ. Health Rep.* **2020**, *7*. [CrossRef]

126. Waugh, D.T. Fluoride exposure induces inhibition of sodium/iodide symporter (NIS) contributing to impaired iodine absorption and iodine deficiency: Molecular mechanisms of inhibition and implications for public health. *Int. J. Environ. Res. Public Health* **2019**, *16*, 1086. [CrossRef]

127. Nakamoto, T.; Ralph Rawls, H. Fluoride exposure in early life as the possible root cause of disease in later life. *J. Clin. Pediatr. Dent.* **2018**, *42*, 325–330. [CrossRef]

128. Johnston, N.R.; Strobel, S.A. Principles of fluoride toxicity and the cellular response: A review. *Arch. Toxicol.* **2020**, *94*, 1051–1069. [CrossRef]

129. Hegde, R.M.; Rego, R.M.; Potla, K.M.; Kurkuri, M.D.; Kigga, M. Bio-inspired materials for defluoridation of water: A review. *Chemosphere* **2020**, *253*. [CrossRef]

130. Leung, A.K.C.; Leung, A.A.C. Evaluation and management of the child with hypothyroidism. *World J. Pediatr.* **2019**, *15*, 124–134. [CrossRef]

131. Hay, I.; Hynes, K.L.; Burgess, J.R. Mild-to-moderate gestational iodine deficiency processing disorder. *Nutrients* **2019**, *11*, 19674. [CrossRef]

132. Urinary Iodine Concentrations for Determining Iodine Status in Populations. Available online: https://apps.who.int/iris/bitstream/handle/10665/85972/WHO_NMH_NHD_EPG_13.1_eng.pdf?ua=1 (accessed on 3 June 2020).

133. Zimmermann, M.B. Iodine deficiency. *Endocr. Rev.* **2009**, *30*, 376–408. [CrossRef] [PubMed]

134. Baldini, E.; Virili, C.; D'Armiento, E.; Centanni, M.; Ulisse, S. Iodine status in schoolchildren and pregnant women of lazio, a central region of Italy. *Nutrients* **2019**, *11*, 1674. [CrossRef] [PubMed]

135. Giordano, C.; Barone, I.; Marsico, S.; Bruno, R.; Bonofiglio, D.; Catalano, S.; Andò, S. Endemic goiter and iodine prophylaxis in calabria, a region of southern Italy: Past and present. *Nutrients* **2019**, *11*, 2428. [CrossRef]

136. Zimmermann, M.B.; Andersson, M. Assessment of iodine nutrition in populations: Past, present, and future. *Nutr. Rev.* **2012**. [CrossRef] [PubMed]

137. Li, M.; Eastman, C.J. NATURE REVIEWS | ENDOCRINOLOGY The changing epidemiology of iodine deficiency. *Nat. Publ. Gr.* **2012**. [CrossRef]

138. Soldin, O.P.; Braverman, L.E.; Lamm, S.H. Perchlorate Clinical Pharmacology and Human Health: A Review. *Ther. Drug Monit.* **2001**, *23*, 316. [CrossRef]

139. Murray, C.W.; Egan, S.K.; Kim, H.; Beru, N.; Bolger, P.M. US food and drug administration's total diet study: Dietary intake of perchlorate and iodine. *J. Expo. Sci. Environ. Epidemiol.* **2008**, *18*, 571–580. [CrossRef]

140. Mantovani, A. Endocrine disrupters and the safety of food chains. *Horm. Res. Paediatr.* **2016**, *86*, 279–288. [CrossRef]

141. Council, N.R. Health Implications of Perchlorate Ingestion. 2005. Available online: https://books.google.com/books?hl=it&lr=&id=05F0iOqvwgAC&oi=fnd&pg=PR1&ots=1byRT87Mff&sig=Kf3cQjhexKXGQ24WspdAKos7iNM (accessed on 10 May 2020).

142. Lawrence, J.; Lamm, S.; Braverman, L.E. Low dose perchlorate (3 mg daily) and thyroid function. *Thyroid* **2001**, *11*, 295. [CrossRef] [PubMed]

143. Lawrence, J.E.; Lamm, S.H.; Pino, S.; Richman, K.; Braverman, L.E. The effect of short-term low-dose perchlorate on various aspects of thyroid function. *Thyroid* **2000**, *10*, 659–663. [CrossRef]

144. Greer, M.A.; Goodman, G.; Pleus, R.C.; Greer, S.E. Health effects perchlorate contamination: The dose response for inhibition of thyroidal radioiodine uptake in humans. *Environ. Health Perspect.* **2002**, *110*, 927–937. [CrossRef] [PubMed]

145. Gibbs, J.P.; Ahmad, R.; Crump, K.S.; Houck, D.P.; Leveille, T.S.; Findley, J.E.; Francis, M. Evaluation of a population with occupational exposure to airborne ammonium perchlorate for possible acute or chronic effects on thyroid function. *J. Occup. Environ. Med.* **1998**, *40*, 1072–1082. [CrossRef] [PubMed]

146. Lamm, S.H.; Braverman, L.E.; Li, F.X.; Richman, K.; Pino, S.; Howearth, G. Thyroid health status of ammonium perchlorate workers: A cross-sectional occupational health study. *J. Occup. Environ. Med.* **1999**, *41*, 248–260. [CrossRef] [PubMed]

147. Braverman, L.E.; He, X.; Pino, S.; Cross, M.; Magnani, B.; Lamm, S.H.; Kruse, M.B.; Engel, A.; Crump, K.S.; Gibbs, J.P. The Effect of Perchlorate, Thiocyanate, and Nitrate on Thyroid Function in Workers Exposed to Perchlorate Long-Term. *J. Clin. Endocrinol. Metab.* **2005**, *90*, 700–706. [CrossRef] [PubMed]

148. Alexeeff, G.V.; Rodriquez, M.; Brown Governor, E.G., Jr. Office of Environmental Health Hazard Assessment OEHHA Adopts Updated Public Health Goal for Perchlorate. 2015. Available online: www.oehha.ca.gov (accessed on 10 May 2020).

149. WHO|JECFA. Evaluations of the Joint FAO/WHO Expert Committee on Food Additives (JECFA). Available online: https://apps.who.int/food-additives-contaminants-jecfa-database/chemical.aspx?chemID=5885 (accessed on 11 May 2020).

150. Srinivasan, A.; Viraraghavan, T. Perchlorate: Health effects and technologies for its removal from water resources. *Int. J. Environ. Res. Public Health* **2009**, *6*, 1418–1442. [CrossRef]

151. Batista, J.R.; McGarvey, F.X.; Vieira, A.R. The Removal of Perchlorate from Waters Using Ion-Exchange Resins. In *Perchlorate in the Environment*; Springer: Boston, MA, USA, 2000; pp. 135–145.

152. Xu, J.; Song, Y.; Min, B.; Steinberg, L.; Logan, B.E. Microbial degradation of perchlorate: Principles and applications. *Environ. Eng. Sci.* **2003**, *20*, 405–422. [CrossRef]

153. Zhao, X.; Zhang, G.; Zhang, Z. TiO2-based catalysts for photocatalytic reduction of aqueous oxyanions: State-of-the-art and future prospects. *Environ. Int.* **2020**, *136*. [CrossRef]

154. Han, J.; Kong, C.; Heo, J.; Yoon, Y.; Lee, H.; Her, N. Removal of perchlorate using reverse osmosis and nanofiltration membranes. *Environ. Eng. Res.* **2012**, *17*, 185–190. [CrossRef]

155. Roquebert, V.; Booth, S.; Cushing, R.S.; Crozes, G.; Hansen, E. Electrodialysis reversal (EDR) and ion exchange as polishing treatment for perchlorate treatment. *Desalination* **2000**, *131*, 285–291. [CrossRef]

156. Kumar, E.; Bhatnagar, A.; Hogland, W.; Marques, M.; Sillanpää, M. Interaction of inorganic anions with iron-mineral adsorbents in aqueous media—A review. *Adv. Colloid Interface Sci.* **2014**, *203*, 11–21. [CrossRef]

157. Kumar, E.; Bhatnagar, A.; Ji, M.; Jung, W.; Lee, S.H.; Kim, S.J.; Lee, G.; Song, H.; Choi, J.Y.; Yang, J.S.; et al. Defluoridation from aqueous solutions by granular ferric hydroxide (GFH). *Water Res.* **2009**, *43*, 490–498. [CrossRef] [PubMed]

158. Susarla, S.; Collette, T.W.; Garrison, A.W.; Wolfe, N.L.; Mccutcheon, S.C. Perchlorate identification in fertilizers. *Environ. Sci. Technol.* **1999**, *33*, 3469–3472. [CrossRef]

159. Calderon, R.; Rajendiran, K.; Kim, U.J.; Palma, P.; Arancibia-Miranda, N.; Silva-Moreno, E.; Corradini, F. Sources and fates of perchlorate in soils in Chile: A case study of perchlorate dynamics in soil-crop systems using lettuce (Lactuca sativa) fields. *Environ. Pollut.* **2020**, *264*. [CrossRef] [PubMed]

Stable Iodine Nutrition During Two Decades of Continuous Universal Salt Iodisation in Sri Lanka

Renuka Jayatissa [1],*, Jonathan Gorstein [2], Onyebuchi E. Okosieme [3], John H. Lazarus [3] and Lakdasa D. Premawardhana [3]

[1]   Department of Nutrition, Medical Research Institute, Danister De Silva Mawatha, Colombo 8, Sri Lanka
[2]   University of Washington, Department of Global Health, Seattle, WA 98195, USA; jgorstein@ign.org
[3]   Centre for Endocrine and Diabetes Sciences and Thyroid Research Group, C2 Link Corridor, University Hospital of Wales, Heath Park, Cardiff CF14 4XN, UK; Okosiemeoe@cardiff.ac.uk (O.E.O.); Lazarus@cardiff.ac.uk (J.H.L.); PremawadhanaLD@cardiff.ac.uk (L.D.P.)
*   Correspondence: renukajayatissa@ymail.com

Abstract: Universal salt iodisation (USI) was introduced in Sri Lanka in 1995. Since then, four national iodine surveys have assessed the iodine nutrition status of the population. We retrospectively reviewed median urine iodine concentration (mUIC) and goitre prevalence in 16,910 schoolchildren (6–12 years) in all nine provinces of Sri Lanka, the mUIC of pregnant women, drinking-water iodine level, and the percentage of households consuming adequately (15 mg/kg) iodised salt (household salt iodine, HHIS). The mUIC of schoolchildren increased from 145.3 µg/L (interquartile range (IQR) = 84.6–240.4) in 2000 to 232.5 µg/L (IQR = 159.3–315.8) in 2016, but stayed within recommended levels. Some regional variability in mUIC was observed (178.8 and 297.3 µg/L in 2016). There was positive association between mUIC in schoolchildren and water iodine concentration. Goitre prevalence to palpation was a significantly reduced from 18.6% to 2.1% (p < 0.05). In pregnant women, median UIC increased in each trimester (102.3 (61.7–147.1); 217.5 (115.6–313.0); 273.1 (228.9–337.6) µg/L (p = 0.000)). We conclude that the introduction and maintenance of a continuous and consistent USI programme has been a success in Sri Lanka. In order to sustain the programme, it is important to retain monitoring of iodine status while tracking salt-consumption patterns to adjust the recommended iodine content of edible salt.

Keywords: iodine schoolchildren; urine iodine; goitre; iodised salt; water iodine; iodine pregnant women

1. Introduction

Iodine is a micronutrient that primarily acts through the thyroid gland and its two hormones (thyroxine and triiodothyronine), and it is vital to the integrity of many physiological functions in the human body [1,2]. Iodine deficiency may affect multiple aspects of human development (including intrauterine physical and neurological development), linear growth, and physiological organ function. Organs such as the brain and nervous system are particularly vulnerable in their formative stages during intrauterine life [1,2]. Fortunately, iodine deficiency is relatively easy and inexpensive to prevent through universal iodisation of all edible salt. This is a pure food-chain effect, beginning with soil erosion and leading to environmental iodine deficiency, and a lack of iodine sources in our typical diet. Iodised salt was first introduced in Switzerland in 1922 [2,3] and has been used in many previously iodine-deficient countries with good results [4]. The restoration of iodine sufficiency in many of these countries has been a major public-health triumph facilitated by the United Nations Children's Fund (UNICEF), World Health Organisation (WHO), and International Council of Control Iodine Deficiency Disorders (ICCIDD, now named Iodine Global Network (IGN)). Statutory regulations enforcing universal salt iodisation (USI) were implemented by regulatory authorities in each country [5]. Sri Lanka is one such country that has successfully adopted a USI programme since 1995.

History of Iodine Deficiency and Its Management in Sri Lanka

Bennet and Pridham first referred to the existence of endemic goitre along the coast of Galle in the southern province of Sri Lanka in 1849 [6]. However, the link between poor iodine consumption and endemic goitre was first recognised only in the 20th century in a WHO study that confirmed high goitre rates, an iodine-poor diet, and low iodine concentrations in drinking water in 1950 [7]. Mahadeva and his group in 1960 identified a "goitre belt" extending across the western, central, southern, sabaragamuwa, and uva provinces in Sri Lanka [8]. The high annual rainfall in these regions led experts to believe that iodine was "leeched" from the soil, leading to iodine deficiency. At that stage, almost no goitre had been identified in the northern, eastern, and north-western provinces [9]. However, in 1986, Fernando et al. described a high goitre rate of 18.8% in schoolchildren in 17 of 24 districts in Sri Lanka—a variable prevalence of 6.5% in the Matale district and 30.2% in the Kalutara district [10]. This study used palpation as the method of goitre assessment, and was the first to recognise iodine deficiency as a major public-health problem.

USI was introduced nationwide by the government in 1995 by statutory regulation [11]. This legislation banned the sale of non-iodised salt for human consumption, thus ensuring access to iodised salt to all consumers in the country. Potassium iodate was used as the vehicle of iodine supplementation, and added to salt at an optimal concentration of 50 ppm at producer level and 25 ppm at consumer level. The national reference laboratory for monitoring USI was established at the Medical Research Institute (MRI) in 2000 with the aid of UNICEF. This laboratory has the dual role of monitoring USI and of assessing its clinical impact by performing periodic national iodine surveys (NISs). External quality control is linked to the EQUIP programme of the Centers for Disease Control (CDC), Atlanta, Georgia, USA [12].

We review and describe the iodine-nutrition status in Sri Lanka by utilising serial datasets from the four national iodine surveys carried out by the MRI between 2000 and 2016. We assessed the success of USI in Sri Lanka in relation to global indicators of population iodine status, i.e., median urine iodine concentration (mUIC), total goitre prevalence rates (TGRs), and household salt iodine (HHIS) consumption.

2. Methods

2.1. Available Data Sources for Analysis

mUIC, TGRs, and HHIS were available for analysis from 4 national iodine surveys (NISs) between 2000 and 2016—NIS2000, NIS2005, NIS2010, and NIS2016 [13–16]. These NIS used a two-stage stratified cluster-sampling technique as specified by the WHO, UNICEF, and IGN [17,18]. During each NIS, the same team of field investigators visited all nine administrative provinces of the country to detect goitres by palpation, and collected urine from 6–12-year–old schoolchildren, and salt from their households and drinking-water samples from the household or school locality. Figure 1 illustrates the map of Sri Lanka demarcating 9 provinces. All four national studies were carried out to ascertain provincial variation. A total of 16,910 schoolchildren of 6–12 years of age were studied in the four surveys and included in the final analysis (Table 1). Furthermore, we had available data for analysis from the national micronutrient study in pregnant women in 2015 (MNSPM2015) (Table 2) [19].

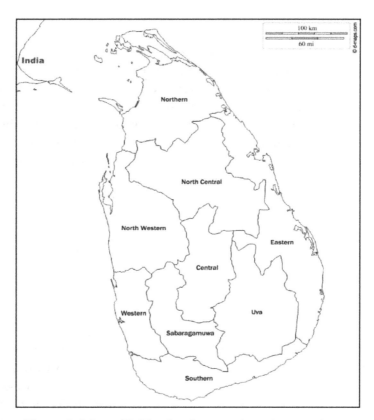

Figure 1. Map of Sri Lanka demarcating nine provinces.

Table 1. Median urine iodine concentration (mUIC), goitre prevalence, and household salt iodine consumption in schoolchildren aged 6–12 years in 2000–2016. TGR, total goitre prevalence rate; HHIS, household salt iodine; IQR, interquartile range.

Surveys	UIC (µg/L)		TGR [3]	HHIS (%) [4]			
	% < 50 [1]	Median (IQR) [2]	%	<5	5–14.9	15–30	>30
NIS–2016 (n = 5000)	1.6	232.5 (159.3–315.8)	1.9	3.1	18.4	63.5	15.0
NIS–2010 (n = 7401)	6.7	163.4 (99.1–245.1)	4.4	4.6	27.1	52.5	16.1
NIS–2005 (n = 1879)	7.4	154.4 (90.3–252.6)	3.8	0.0	8.7	47.7	43.5
NIS–2000 (n = 2628)	2.7	145.3 (84.6–315.8)	18.0	–	–	–	–

Note: [1–4] $p = 0.000$. (- No data)

Table 2. Median UIC in pregnant women in three trimesters (national micronutrient study in pregnant women in 2015, NNMSPM2015).

Trimesters	UIC (µg/L)		No
Period of Amenorrhea (POA)	% <50 [1]	Median (IQR) [2]	
First trimester (≤12 weeks of POA)	17.0	102.3 (61.7–147.1)	447
Second trimester (13–28 weeks of POA)	6.2	217.5 (115.6–313.0)	339
Third trimester (>28 weeks of POA)	0.0	273.1 (228.9–337.6)	176
Overall	**10.1**	**157.7 (91.2–256.4)**	**962**

[1,2] $p = 0.000$.

2.2. Indicators of Population Iodine Status

Three primary indicators of population iodine status were considered, and we used the methodology described below to assess the outcomes of the USI programme: (i) mUIC was measured by ammonium persulfate digestion with spectrophotometric detection of the Sandell–Kolthoff reaction in a laboratory certified by the EQUIP programme [20–22]; (ii) TGR—the grading of goitres was done by palpation by the same team utilising the classification recommended by the WHO, UNICEF, and IGN [3,18]: (a) "no goitre"—thyroid not palpable or visible; (b) "goitre present"—thyroid palpable not visible or palpable and visible; and (iii) iodine content in salt: titration method to measure the iodine content of salt certified by a regional iodine laboratory [3,18]. Geographical location (province), iodine in drinking water, and household salt were measured to estimate their influence on optimal iodine consumption. Iodine levels in drinking water at the household level and school localities were tested using ammonium persulfate oxidation [20].

3. Data Analysis

The following definitions were used for classifying population iodine nutrition status [22]. (i) Median UIC: (a) adequate mUIC—150–299 µg/L (pregnant women) and 100–299 µg/L (schoolchildren); (b) excessive mUIC—$\geq$300 µg/L; and (c) iodine sufficiency—<20% samples should have mUIC of <50 µg/L. (ii) Household salt iodine (HHIS) content: we classified salt iodine content as follows. (a) <5 mg/kg—non-iodised; (b) 5–14.9 mg/kg—inadequately iodised; (c) 15–30 mg/kg—adequately iodised; and (d) >30 mg/kg—over-iodised. (iii) Iodine content in drinking water: iodine in drinking water was classified as follows. (a) <5 mg/kg—no iodine; (b) 5–14.9 mg/kg—low iodine; (c) 15–30 mg/kg—moderate iodine; and (d) >30 mg/kg—high iodine [23,24].

Statistical analysis was performed using SPSS (IBM version 24). Data that were not normally distributed were expressed as median and interquartile range (IQR) unless otherwise stated. The Mann–Whitney U–test was used to compare data between the two groups. The Kruskal–Wallis test (nonparametric analysis of variance (ANOVA)) was used to assess the significance of differences between more than two groups. Categorical variables were analysed using the chi-squared test for trend; a p–value of <0.05 was considered statistically significant.

4. Results

(i) mUIC was consistently in the adequate or iodine-sufficient range in all four national iodine surveys of 2000–2016. There has been a significant increase in mUIC, but still within the adequate range in surveys between 2000 (145.3 (84.6–240.4)) and 2016 (232.5 (159.3–315.8)); $p = 0.000$). There has also been a significant reduction in the percentage of schoolchildren with mUIC < 50 µg/L (2.7% in 2000 vs 1.6% in 2016; $p = 0.000$). As shown in Table 2, the mUIC of pregnant women was also in the adequate or iodine-sufficient range (157.7 (228.9–337.6) µg/L) at the national level, and in the second and third trimesters 217.5 (115.6–313.0), and 273.1 (228.9–337.6) µg/L; p < 0.000). Table 3 shows there is regional variability in mUIC levels in children of 6–12 years of age (297.3 *vs.* 178.8 µg/L in 2016; $p = 0.000$). It was significantly higher in the northern and north–central provinces when compared to the rest of the country since 2005.

Table 3. Regional variations of key indicators of population iodine nutrition in 2000–2016.

Province	Median Iodine Content in Salt (IQR; mg/kg)			Adequately Iodised HHIS (%)			Median UIC (IQR) (µg/dL)			
	2005 [1]	2010 [2]	2016 [3]	2005 [4]	2010 [5]	2016 [6]	2000 [7]	2005 [8]	2010 [9]	2016 [10]
Western	28.5 (22.3–37.9)	21.2 (13.2–27.5)	19.0 (14.8–25.4)	96.1	70.0	71.6	151.4 (92.8–238.1)	142.2 (96.7–197.7)	168.4 (11.7–231.5)	233.1 (166.7–313.3)
Southern	32.7 (23.2–41.7)	21.2 (11.6–27.5)	21.2 (13.8–25.4)	94.4	66.7	70.2	122.4 (74.2–178.9)	111.0 (69.9–189.5)	123.3 (74.3–203.0)	201.3 (121.5–289.9)
Central	27.5 (20.6–34.9)	22.2 (14.8–27.5)	27.5 (21.2–34.9)	97.4	74.0	91.0	96.2 (61.6–149.1)	144.7 (83.8–211.9)	168.2 (104.1–247.4)	220.7 (168.3–286.4)
Northern	19.0 (14.8–26.9)	14.8 (7.4–23.3)	22.2 (18.0–26.5)	74.3	48.3	83.6	139.5 (74.1–247.4)	283.4 (182.8–403.1)	203.8 (124.6–292.1)	297.3 (230.4–355.4)
Eastern	29.0 (21.6–45.9)	23.3 (16.9–28.6)	23.3 (20.1–26.5)	90.6	78.5	91.2	231.3 (152.9–328.3)	160.4 (94.5–250.9)	173.2 (110.9–241.7)	233.8 (159.5–323.5)
North Western	28.0 (22.7–35.8)	19.0 (9.4–25.4)	19.3 (12.7–24.3)	93.6	60.6	68.1	122.5 (76.6–190.9)	152.8 (98.7–221.3)	151.7 (93.4–228.1)	229.4 (155.9–318.6)
North Central	28.6 (20.4–40.7)	21.2 (12.7–27.5)	18.0 (12.2–24.3)	90.1	67.7	64.1	135.9 (76.9–204.9)	229.9 (135.2–332.0)	237.9 (164.6–328.7)	278.0 (186.3–327.2)
Uva	28.5 (23.8–30.1)	23.3 (13.8–28.6)	21.2 (16.9–25.4)	94.6	72.9	81.5	181.1 (106.0–320.1)	108.5 (68.4–186.4)	129.3 (78.9–198.1)	178.8 (126.5–259.1)
Sabaragamuwa	32.0 (22.7–41.2)	22.2 (12.7–29.6)	22.2 (18.0–27.5)	92.4	70.7	82.0	194.4 (117.6–304.0)	109.0 (69.3–205.8)	121.1 (69.7–187.0)	217.5 (148.7–305.0)
Sri Lanka	28.0 (20.6–38.6)	21.2 (11.6–27.5)	21.2 (15.9–26.5)	91.4	67.6	78.0	145.3 (84.6–240.4)	154.4 (90.3–252.6)	163.5 (99.1–245.1)	232.5 (159.3–315.8)

Note: [1–10] $p = 0.000$.

(ii) There was significant reduction in TGR by palpation between surveys done in 2000 (18.0%) and 2016 (1.9%; $p = 0.000$; Table 1).

(iii) The iodine content of HHIS was only measured since 2005, and since that time, over 95% of all HHIS has contained at least some iodine (>5 mg/kg). The percentage of HHIS with adequate iodine concentrations (defined as 15–30 mg/kg) showed a significant increase—47.7% in NIS2005 vs. 63.5% in NIS2016 ($p = 0.000$). Furthermore, only 3.1% had a salt content of <5 mg/kg (non-iodised) in the last survey in 2016. The prevalence of over-iodised salt (>30mg/kg) significantly fell from 43.5% in 2005 to 15.0% in 2016 ($p = 0.000$; Table 1). HHIS was less than 90% at the national level, and in all provinces in 2010 and 2016 except for the central and eastern provinces. In 2016, the interprovincial difference of median iodine content in HHIS was between 18.0 and 27.5 mg/kg (Table 3).

(iv) Median iodine content of drinking water was 33.4 (12.3–66.8) µg/L. Wide variation was observed between provinces (8.3 (4.6–29.0) vs 75.5 (48.4–102.5) µg/L; $p = 0.000$) in the uva and north–central provinces, respectively (Table 4).

Table 4. Regional variations of median iodine content of drinking water in 2016.

Province	No	Median (IQR) µg/L
Western	67	15.6 (4.1–29.1)
Southern	70	19.1 (15.3–29.9)
Central	68	18.0 (5.7–44.6)
Northern	78	53.4 (28.9–79.4)
Eastern	189	33.3 (17.0–69.6)
North Western	122	39.9 (9.4–61.4)
North Central	170	75.5 (48.4–102.5)
Uva	62	8.3 (4.6–50.4)
Sabaragamuwa	108	31.3 (15.1–50.4)
Sri Lanka	934	33.4 (12.3–66.8)

Note: $p = 0.000$.

Figure 2 provides a graphical representation of the data on median UIC of children aged 6–12 years in 2016, stratified by the iodine content in HHIS and in drinking water. These data are noteworthy since the mUIC was within the optimal range in all subgroups, including those households of which the iodine content in HHIS was <5 ppm or in the range of 5–14.9 ppm, suggesting that the consumed iodine in HHIS is not the exclusive diet source of iodine. There was a significant increase in median UIC with increasing iodine concentrations in drinking water ($p = 0.000$).

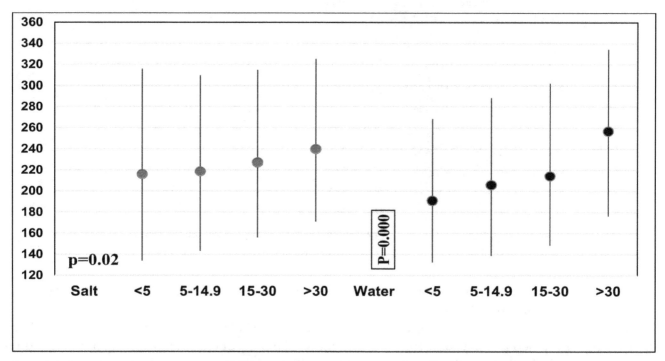

Figure 2. Median urine iodine concentration (IQR) and its relationship with iodine concentrations in household salt and drinking water in school children aged 6–12 years in 2016.

5. Discussion

USI was first implemented in Sri Lanka in 1995. We demonstrated in this retrospective review of data from four national iodine surveys of over more than two decades of continuous salt iodisation that (i) mUIC has consistently been in the adequate range with a sequential increase within safe and recommended limits; (ii) the goitre-prevalence rate to palpation in children between 6–12 years significantly decreased between 2000 and 2016 (18.0% to 1.9%; $p = 0.000$); and (iii) the percentage of adequately iodised household salt samples significantly increased during this period (47.7% in 2005 *vs.* 63.3% in 2016; $p = 0.000$), and its household consumption remains satisfactory (Tables 1 and 3).

These indices of population iodine nutrition favourably reflect the success of the USI programme enforced by successive governments of Sri Lanka, having adequate iodine status at the national level and in most provinces (Tables 1 and 3). Furthermore, there has been a recurrence of iodine deficiency in several countries where iodine-deficiency disorders (IDDs) were eliminated with USI because of inadequate monitoring of their USI programmes [25–29]. Strict monitoring is essential in sustaining proper iodine nutrition in countries that adopt USI [28].

However, there is a need for caution. (a) The median UIC of pregnant women is only marginally above the recommended cut off of 150 μg/L, and iodine-insufficient in the first trimester (102.3 (61.7–147.1) μg/L (Table 2)). There was a remarkable improvement in the iodine status of pregnant women compared to 2011 (113.7 μg/L) [30]. There was also a significant minority of pregnant women (nearly 10%) who had a median UIC of <50 μg/L. This is an important population group, and inadequate iodine delivery to this group may have important long-term consequences, particularly regarding the intrauterine development of the brain, central nervous system, and physical growth [29]. (b) The median UIC of schoolchildren in the northern and north–central provinces in 2016 approached 300 μg/L. In these two areas at risk of iodine excess, iodine content in drinking water was the highest among those provinces (Table 4). Other countries' experience with high iodine content in drinking water should be reviewed [31,32]. (c) Some regional variability in mUIC was observed over the course of the programme, but in the most recent survey, the range was between 178.8 and 297.3 µg/L, all within the optimal range. The reasons for regional variability of median UIC have not been investigated in detail, but need to be noted (Table 2). There is a clear need, therefore, to closely monitor these groups in the future, with periodic well-designed and more elaborate studies. However, we acknowledge that these UIC assessments were done on single "spot" samples of urine and may not be truly representative of the iodine-nutrition status of each individual in these communities [28].

We also showed that the supervision and monitoring of salt iodisation has improved over two decades of USI. The percentage of samples delivering adequate levels of salt at the consumer level (i.e., 15–30 mg/kg) increased from 47.5% in NIS2005 to 63.3% in NIS2016 ($p = 0.000$), while at the same time, the percentage of over-iodised salt samples has significantly decreased ($p = 0.000$; Table 1). The percentage of households using adequately iodised salt was less than 90% (the WHO goal for USI) at the national level and in seven out of nine provinces (Table 3). However, it showed that the median HHIS content in provinces was between 18.0 and 27.5 mg/kg, confirming that household iodised salt was providing a significant amount of iodine to the diet [33].

Despite a <90% of households consuming adequately iodised salt, there has been an increase in mUIC, and some provinces in the country consistently showed a high level of mUIC. Daily mean per capita salt intake of Sri Lankans was reported as 8.3 g (CI: 7.9, 8.8) in 2012 [34]. We also need to be aware of the contribution of other sources of iodine contributing to population iodine nutrition, e.g., drinking water, processed foods, or condiments, which are being manufactured with iodised salt, as well as some iodine in foods. Our results indicated a positive association between iodine status in schoolchildren and water iodine concentration, although the major contributor to iodine intake is iodised salt in the diet (Figure 2). In fact, over 95% of households have consistently had access to iodised salt since 2005. A similar contribution was observed in other countries [24,32]. There is a need to adjust the recommended level of HHIS, and to explore the iodine supply through different dietary sources and the geological assessment of soil iodine content for future monitoring.

IGN/UNICEF recommends that the optimal iodine intake, as measured by the median UIC for school-age children, should be <300 µg/L, while the mUIC among pregnant women should be <500 µg/L [22]. Thus, the current salt-iodisation programme is having its desired impact and not placing the Sri Lankan population at risk for iodine excess, as described in the previous study [33]. The salt-iodisation programme needs to be consistently monitored so that the level of iodine in all edible salt, including that used at the household level as well as in processed foods and condiments, leads to an optimal intake. As salt-reduction efforts are implemented, there may be a decline in overall salt consumption, in which case the government may need to accordingly adjust the recommended salt iodine level to ensure that public-health strategies of iodine-deficiency prevention, salt reduction, and reduction in NCDs are realised.

Despite adequate iodine nutrition among schoolchildren, iodine nutrition among pregnant women remains just above the cut-off levels in the country. There is a need to focus on pregnant women for continuous monitoring while sustaining the iodised-salt programme.

This study has several strengths. (a) Data availability from a large number of 6–12-year-old schoolchildren (16,910 in total); (b) uniform methodology for UIC assessments over the period of review in a single laboratory with stringent external quality control; (c) permanent health staff used as a single team in all four studies and goitre palpation; (d) minimising variability in urine- and salt-assay methodology using the same protocols developed by the UNICEF, WHO, and IGN. However, the unavailability of pre-USI data for comparison was an inherent shortcoming of this study.

6. Conclusions

The iodine nutrition of the population has remained optimal and stable in Sri Lanka during more than two decades of continuous salt iodisation after its introduction in 1995. However, we recommend the close and careful monitoring of pregnant women and schoolchildren in view of the data we presented.

The delivery of salt to consumers has improved and is adequate in the majority. The contribution of dietary sources other than salt needs to be assessed in well-planned studies.

Author Contributions: R.J. analysed datasets; R.J., J.G., L.D.P., J.H.L., and O.E.O. conceptualised, designed, and wrote the paper. All authors read the manuscript, made a substantial contribution to the revision, and approved the final manuscript. All authors have read and agreed to the published version of the manuscript.

Acknowledgments: We thank the staff of the Department of Nutrition, Medical Research Institute, Ministry of Health, Sri Lanka for conducting the national survey, and all the participants of the study. We would like to thank Dulitha Fernando, Pierre Boudex, and the late Meliyanthi Gunathilaka for supporting us in every step. Adikari, Morina Hossein, Aberra Bekele, Moazzem Hossaine from UNICEF, Colombo and Chandrakant Pandav for all their support from the beginning. This research received no specific grant from any funding agency in the public, commercial, or not-for-profit sectors.

References

1. Stanbury, J.B.; Hetzel, B.S. *Endemic Goitre and Endemic Cretinism, Iodine Nutrition in Health and Disease;* John Wiley and Sons: New York, NY, USA, 1980.

2. World Health Organization. *Iodine and Health—Eliminating Iodine Deficiency Disorders Safely through Salt Iodisation;* A statement by the WHO; WHO: Geneva, Switzerland, 1994.

3. World Health Organization. *Assessment of Iodine Deficiency Disorders and Monitoring Their Elimination: A Guide for Programme Managers,* 3rd ed.; WHO: Geneva, Switzerland, 2007.

4. Iodine Global Network (IGN). Global Scorecard of Iodine Nutrition in 2019. Available online: https://www.ign.org/cm_data/Global_Scorecard_2019_SAC.pdf (accessed on 14 March 2020).

5. World Health Organization. Recommended Iodine Levels in Salt and Guidelines for Monitoring their Adequacy and Effectiveness. Based on a Joint WHO/UNICEF/ICCIDD Consultation. World Health Organization: Geneva, Switzerland, 8–9 July 1996. Available online: https://apps.who.int/iris/bitstream/handle/10665/63322/WHO_NUT_96.13.pdf (accessed on 14 March 2020).

6. Greenwald, I. Some notes on the history of goitre in Ceylon. *Ceylon Med J.* **1953**, *2*, 140. [PubMed]

7. Wilson, D.C. Goitre in Ceylon and Nigeria. *Br. J. Nutr.* **1954**, *8*, 90–99. [CrossRef] [PubMed]

8. Mahadeva, K.; Seneviratne, D.A.; Jayatilleke, D.B.; Shanmuganathan, S.S.; Premachandra, P.; Nagarajah, M. Further studies on the problem of goitre in Ceylon. *Br. J. Nutr.* **1968**, *22*, 527–534. [CrossRef] [PubMed]

9. Deo, M.G.; Subramanian, T.A.V. Iodine metabolism in children and women with goitre in Ceylon. *Br. J. Nutr.* **1971**, *25*, 97–105. [CrossRef] [PubMed]

10. Fernando, M.A.; Balsuriya, S.; Herath, K.B.; Katugampola, S. Endemic Goitre in Sri Lanka. *Asia Pac. J. Public Health* **1989**, *3*, 11–18. [CrossRef] [PubMed]

11. Government of Sri Lanka. *Food (Iodization of Salt) Regulations under Section 32 of the Food Act, No. 26 of 1980;* Department of Government Printing: Colombo, Sri Lanka, 1995.

12. Centers for Diseases Control and Prevention (CDC). The Challenge of Iodine Deficiency Disorders. EQIP 10 Years Anniversary. Atlanta, USA. 2011. Available online: https://www.cdc.gov/labstandards/pdf/equip/EQUIP_Booklet.pdf (accessed on 14 March 2020).

13. Jayatissa, R.; Gunathilaka, M.; Fernando, D. Iodine nutrition status among schoolchildren after salt iodisation. *Ceylon Med. J.* **2005**, *50*, 144–148. [CrossRef] [PubMed]

14. Jayatissa, R.; Gunathilaka, M.; Fernando, D. *Second National Iodine Survey;* Medical Research Institute: Colombo, Sri Lanka, 2006. Available online: http://www.mri.gov.lk/assets/Nutrition/2005-Second-National-IDD-Survey-.pdf (accessed on 21 March 2020).

15. Jayatissa, R.; Gunathilaka, M.; Fernando, D. *Third National Iodine Survey;* Medical Research Institute: Colombo, Sri Lanka, 2010. Available online: https://www.ign.org/cm_data/2017_Sri_Lanka.pdf (accessed on 21 March 2020).

16. Jayatissa, R.; Fernando, D.; De Silva, H. *Fourth National Iodine Survey;* Medical Research Institute: Colombo, Sri Lanka, 2016. Available online: http://www.mri.gov.lk/assets/Nutrition/2016-Fourth-National-IDD-survey-.pdf (accessed on 21 March 2020).

17. Gorstein, J.S.K.; Parvanta, I.; Begin, I. *Indicators and Methods for Cross-Sectional Surveys of Vitamin and Mineral Status of Populations*; The Micronutrient Initiative: Ottawa, ON, Canada; Center of Disease Surveillance: Atlanta, GA, USA, 2007.

18. World Health Organisation. *Indicators for Assessing Iodine Deficiency Disorders and their Control through Salt Iodizaton*; WHO/NUT/94.6; WHO; UNICEF; ICCIDD: Geneva, Switzerland, 1994; pp. 1–55.

19. Jayatissa, R.; Fernando, D.; De Silva, H. *National Nutrition and Micronutrient Survey of Pregnant Women in Sri Lanka: 2015*; Medical Research Institute/UNICEF/WFP: Colombo, Sri Lanka, 2017. Available online: https://www.wfp.org/publications/national-nutrition-and-micronutrient-survey-pregnant-women-sri-lanka (accessed on 21 March 2020).

20. Ohashi, T.; Yamaki, M.; Pandav, C.S.; Karmarkar, M.G.; Irie, M. Simple microplate method for determination of urinary iodine. *Clin. Chem.* **2000**, *46*, 529–536. [CrossRef] [PubMed]

21. Delange, F.; de Benoist, B.; Burgi, H.; ICCIDD Working Group. At what median urinary iodine concentration is a population iodine suffcient? *IDD News Lett.* **2001**, *17*, 10–11.

22. United Nation of Independent Children's Fund (UNICEF). *Guidance on the Monitoring of Salt Iodization Programmes and Determination of Population Iodine Status*; UNICEF: New York, NY, USA, 2019.

23. World Health Organization. *Iodine in Drinking Water*; WHO: Geneva, Switzerland, 2003.

24. Lv, S.; Wang, Y.; Xu, D.; Rutherford, S.; Chong, Z.; Du, Y.; Jia, L.; Zhao, J. Drinking water contributes to excessive iodine intake among children in Hebei, China. *Eur. J. Clin. Nutr.* **2013**, *67*, 961–965. [CrossRef] [PubMed]

25. Markou, K.B.; Georgopoulos, A.; Makri, M.; Anastasiou, E.; Vlasopoulou, B.; Lazarou, N.; Veizis, A.; Sakellaropoulos, G.; Vagenakis, A.G. Iodine deficiency in Azerbaijan after the discontinuation of an iodine prophylaxis program: Reassessment of iodine intake and goiter prevalence in schoolchildren. *Thyroid* **2001**, *11*, 1141–1146. [CrossRef] [PubMed]

26. Li, M.; Ma, G.; Boyages, S.C.; Eastman, C.J. Re-emergence of iodine deficiency in Australia. *Asia Pac. J. Clin. Nutr.* **2001**, *10*, 200–203. [CrossRef] [PubMed]

27. Zimmermann, M.B.; Wegmüller, R.; Zeder, C.; Torresani, T.; Chaouki, N. Rapid relapse of thyroid dysfunction and goiter in school age children after withdrawal of salt iodization. *Am. J. Clin. Nutr.* **2004**, *79*, 642–645. [CrossRef] [PubMed]

28. Zimmermann, M.B. Assessing iodine status and monitoring progress of iodised salt programs. *J. Nutr.* **2004**, *134*, 1673–1677. [CrossRef] [PubMed]

29. Lazarus, J.H.; Bestwick, J.P.; Channon, S.; Paradice, R.; Maina, A.; Rees, R.; Chiusano, E.; John, R.; Guaraldo, V.; George, L.M. Antenatal thyroid screening and childhood cognitive function. *N. Engl. J. Med.* **2012**, *366*, 493–501. [CrossRef]

30. Jayatissa, R.; Gunathilaka, M.M.; Ranbanda, J.M.; Peiris, P.; Jayasingha, J.; Ekanayaka, P.; Kulathunga, H. Iodine status of pregnant women in Sri Lanka. *Sri Lanka J. Diabetes Endocrinol. Metab.* **2013**, *3*, 4–7. [CrossRef]

31. Zimmermann, M.B.; Ito, Y.; Hess, S.Y.; Fujieda, K.; Molinari, L. High thyroid volume in children with excess dietary iodine intakes. *Am. J. Clin. Nutr.* **2005**, *81*, 840–844. [CrossRef]

32. Shen, H.; Liu, S.; Sun, D.; Zhang, S.; Su, X.; Shen, Y.; Han, H. Geographical distribution of drinking water with high iodine level and association between high iodine level in drinking water and goitre: A Chines national investigation. *Br. J. Nutr.* **2011**, *106*, 243–247. [CrossRef] [PubMed]

33. Jayatissa, R.; Fernando, D.N. Supplementation of micronutrients in children and food fortification initiatives in Sri Lanka: Benefits versus risks. *Ann. N. Y. Acad. Sci.* **2018**, 1–14. [CrossRef] [PubMed]

34. Jayatissa, R.; Yamori, Y.; De Silva, A.H.; Mori, M.; De Silva, P.C. Estimation of salt intake, potassium intake and sodium-to-potassium ratio by 24-hour urinary excretion: An urban rural study in Sri Lanka. **2012**, in press. [CrossRef]

Nutraceuticals in Thyroidology: A Review of in Vitro and in Vivo Animal Studies

Salvatore Benvenga [1,2], **Silvia Martina Ferrari** [3], **Giusy Elia** [3], **Francesca Ragusa** [3], **Armando Patrizio** [3], **Sabrina Rosaria Paparo** [3], **Stefania Camastra** [3], **Daniela Bonofiglio** [4], **Alessandro Antonelli** [3,*] **and Poupak Fallahi** [5]

[1] Master Program on Childhood, Adolescent and Women's Endocrine Health, Department of Clinical and Experimental Medicine, University of Messina, 98125 Messina; s.benvenga@live.it

[2] Interdepartmental Program of Molecular & Clinical Endocrinology, and Women's Endocrine Health, University Hospital, Policlinico Universitario G. Martino, 98125 Messina, Italy

[3] Department of Clinical and Experimental Medicine, University of Pisa, 56126 Pisa, Italy; sm.ferrari@int.med.unipi.it (S.M.F.); e.giusy_87@hotmail.it (G.E.); francescaragusa86@gmail.com (F.R.); armandopatrizio125@gmail.com (A.P.); sabrinapaparo@gmail.com (S.R.P.); stefania.camastra@unipi.it (S.C.)

[4] Department of Pharmacy, Health and Nutritional Sciences, University of Calabria, 87036 Arcavacata di Rende (CS), Italy; daniela.bonofiglio@unical.it

[5] Department of Translational Research and New Technologies in Medicine and Surgery, University of Pisa, 56126 Pisa, Italy; poupak.fallahi@unipi.it

* Correspondence: alessandro.antonelli@med.unipi.it

Abstract: Nutraceuticals are defined as a food, or parts of a food, that provide medical or health benefits, including the prevention of different pathological conditions, and thyroid diseases, or the treatment of them. Nutraceuticals have a place in complementary medicines, being positioned in an area among food, food supplements, and pharmaceuticals. The market of certain nutraceuticals such as thyroid supplements has been growing in the last years. In addition, iodine is a fundamental micronutrient for thyroid function, but also other dietary components can have a key role in clinical thyroidology. Here, we have summarized the in vitro, and in vivo animal studies present in literature, focusing on the commonest nutraceuticals generally encountered in the clinical practice (such as carnitine, flavonoids, melatonin, omega-3, resveratrol, selenium, vitamins, zinc, and inositol), highlighting conflicting results. These experimental studies are expected to improve clinicians' knowledge about the main supplements being used, in order to clarify the potential risks or side effects and support patients in their use.

Keywords: nutraceuticals; thyroid; carnitine; flavonoids; melatonin; omega-3; resveratrol; selenium; vitamins; zinc

1. Introduction

The term "nutraceutical" is placed in an area among food, food supplements, and pharmaceuticals [1]. Nutraceuticals are considered complementary medicines, defined as a "food, or parts of a food, that provide medical or health benefits, including the prevention and treatment of disease" [2]. Most nutraceuticals are normal human metabolites (i.e., dehydroepiandrosterone (DHEA) and S-adenoylmethionine (SAMe), carnitine, creatine, coenzyme Q10, lipoic acid, melatonin), or bioactive plant dietary components [2]. Food categories and supplements are both described in the European regulation (No. 1924/2006 of the European Parliament and of the Council, updated by EU Regulation 2015/2283), even if an official mention or recognition of the term "nutraceutical" does not exist [3]. The European Food Safety Authority (EFSA) does not distinguish clearly the terms "food supplements" and "nutraceuticals, while in America "medical foods" and "dietary supplements" are regulatory terms, although "nutraceuticals" and "functional foods" are determined according to consumer trends [1].

In the last years, interest and knowledge in nutraceuticals have been growing. Nutraceuticals can be considered for the prevention of different pathological conditions, including thyroid diseases and associated disorders [4–6].

In addition to iodine, which is a fundamental nutrient for thyroid function, other dietary components (such as carnitine, flavonoids, melatonin, omega-3, resveratrol, selenium, vitamins, zinc, and inositol) were found to have some role in thyroid homeostasis, so that they could have a role in clinical thyroidology. The principal issue about the appropriateness and effectiveness of nutraceuticals in prevention and treatment depends on the lack or scarcity of clinical data [1]. Moreover, there is the problem of the not uncommon discrepancy between the concentration reported in the label and the real one [1]. Conventional medicines are usually submitted to quality control to ensure that they contain the claimed dose of active constituents, and that they have suitable disintegration characteristics and bioavailability, enabling absorption in the gut tract. Composition of nutraceuticals is increasingly being evaluated, the results of the analyses being that composition sometimes fails the relevant standards, or the label claims are not respected [2].

Here, we aim to review various nutraceuticals that can influence human thyroid homeostasis, addressing on the in vitro, and in vivo experimental animal studies reported in literature. We will focus on nutraceuticals, other than iodine, that are more likely to be encountered in the clinical practice.

2. Search of the Literature

A PubMed search, run on March 2020, using the word "nutraceuticals" as the entry, yielded 74,935 results, indicating the great interest in general for this emerging class of natural compounds that makes the line between food and drugs to fade. Interestingly, using the entry "nutraceuticals AND thyroid" a total of 6622 published papers were obtained, highlighting that the scientific interest of nutraceutical area covers the thyroid research field. Indeed, different nutraceuticals possibly influence human thyroid function and/or thyroid tumor biology that will be reviewed and commented upon. Particularly, using the filter "humans" to exclude "other animals", and the filter "other animals" in order to exclude "humans", we have meticulously screened the in vitro and in vivo experimental studies on thyroid and carnitine ("carnitine AND thyroid"), flavonoids ("flavonoids AND thyroid"), isoflavonoids ("isoflavonoids AND thyroid"), soy ("soy AND thyroid"), melatonin ("melatonin AND thyroid"), omega-3 polyunsaturated fatty acids ("omega-3 polyunsaturated fatty acids AND thyroid"), resveratrol ("resveratrol AND thyroid"), selenium ("selenium AND thyroid"), vitamins ("vitamins AND thyroid"), zinc ("zinc AND thyroid"), and inositol ("inositol AND thyroid") (Table 1).

Table 1. Summary of number of articles on given nutraceuticals retrievable on PubMed as of 21 March 2020 *.

n. of Items.	Entry	Humans	Other Animals
1	nutraceuticals	55,737	31,391
2	nutraceuticals AND thyroid	522 (0.9%)	224 (0.9%)
3	carnitine	8134	8778
4	carnitine AND thyroid	71 (0.8%)	95 (1.1%)
5	flavonoids	44,187	49,719
6	flavonoids AND thyroid	222 (0.5%)	248 (0.5%)
7	isoflavonoids	404	281
8	isoflavonoids AND thyroid	4 (0.9%)	4 (1.4%)
9	soy	7965	6531
10	soy AND thyroid	93 (1.2%)	75 (1.1%)

Table 1. *Cont.*

n. of Items.	Entry	Humans	Other Animals
11	melatonin	11,142	14,477
12	melatonin AND thyroid	200 (1.8%)	364 (2.5%)
13	omega-3 polyunsaturated fatty acids	17,168	12,783
14	omega-3 polyunsaturated fatty acids AND thyroid	37 (0.21%)	38 (0.3%)
15	resveratrol	5823	5961
16	resveratrol AND thyroid	54 (0.9%)	42 (0.7%)
17	selenium	13,794	13,888
18	selenium AND thyroid	600 (4.3%)	372 (2.7%)
19	vitamin A	32,637	22,296
20	vitamin A AND thyroid	495 (1.5%)	593 (2.7%)
21	vitamin D	61,418	20311
22	vitamin D AND thyroid	1280 (2.1%)	554 (2.7%)
23	vitamin E	22,004	18,811
24	vitamin E AND thyroid	96 (0.4%)	123 (0.6%)
25	zinc	58,247	50,628
26	zinc AND thyroid	503 (0.86%)	401 (0.7%)
27	inositol	17,144	27,226
28	inositol AND thyroid	147 (0.86%)	205 (0.75%)

* The PubMed search was run using the filter "humans" to exclude "other animals", and the filter "other animals" in order to exclude "humans". Note how thyroidal studies account for a tiny fraction of total studies for any listed nutraceutical, and with comparable percentages in humans and animals. For instance, "resveratrol AND thyroid" accounted for 54 of 5823 studies in humans (0.9%) and 42 of 5961 studies in other animals (0.7%).

3. Carnitine

The naturally occurring quaternary amine, carnitine, is ubiquitous in mammalian tissues, and according to studies of about 40 years ago, it was considered a peripheral antagonist of thyroid hormone (TH) action [7].

Old studies published in German language showed that carnitine is capable of contrasting TH-induced changes associated with the nitrogen balance in rats and metamorphosis of tadpoles [8,9]. In the more recent of such papers, carnitine contrasted the thyroxine (T4)-induced liver and circulating concentration of both alanine aminotransferase (ALT) and aspartate aminotransferase (AST) [9]. Tissue culture experiments on human skin fibroblasts, human hepatoma cells HepG2, and mouse neuroblastoma cells NB 41A3 demonstrated that L-carnitine inhibits cell entry, and overall nuclear entry, of triiodothyronine (T3) and T4 [7]. There was no inhibition on TH efflux from cells, and no inhibition of TH binding to isolated nuclei. These data confirm that carnitine is a peripheral antagonist of TH action, and that one level of inhibition occurs at the nuclear envelope or before it [7].

Four experimental groups were formed starting from 21 male Sprague Dawley rats: hyperthyroidism ($n = 5$), hyperthyroidism plus low dose L-carnitine (100 mg/kg/d for 10 days; $n = 5$), hyperthyroidism plus high dose L-carnitine (500 mg/Kg/d for 10 days; $n = 5$), and controls (0.2 mL/100 g body weight, subcutaneously, of 0.9% NaCl solution; $n = 6$) [10]. The injection of levothyroxine (L-T4) in a dose of 250 µg/kg body weight per day for 20 consecutive days was able to induce hyperthyroidism in rats. The treatment with either dose of L-carnitine was by intraperitoneal injection, and it started on the 10th day of hyperthyroidism continuing for the following 10 days. Activities of one marker of oxidative stress (malondialdehyde (MDA)) and activities of three markers of antioxidant defense (namely, the antioxidant enzymes catalase (CAT), glutathione peroxidase (GPX), and myeloperoxidase (MPO)) were measured in liver homogenates. MDA activity was increased by 59% in the carnitine-untreated hyperthyroid group, but it decreased significantly and to levels comparable to the control rats in either group of hyperthyroid rats receiving L-carnitine. Activities of the three enzymes were 21% to 76% lower in the carnitine-untreated hyperthyroid rats with respect to the control group. Treatment of hyperthyroid rats with either low or high dose of L-carnitine increased strongly the liver activities of the antioxidant enzymes (with dose-dependency absent for CAT, moderate for GPX and great for MPO), indicating that even a low dose of L-carnitine was enough to prevent the oxidative stress induced in the rat liver by L-T4 [10].

Some experimental data are available in the neoplastic setting of the thyroid. L-carnitine, the biologically active form of carnitine, transports long-chain acyl groups from fatty acids into the mitochondrial matrix to generate metabolic energy in living cells. Although, it has been reported that treatment with L-carnitine efficiently induced ATP generation in normal cells, it has been found to selectively inhibit cancer cell growth in vitro and in vivo models [11].

Controversially, the expression of the enzyme involved in this transport, the carnitine palmitoyltransferase 1C (Cpt1c), has been detected at higher levels in papillary thyroid tissues compared with normal ones and Cpt1c up-regulation has been found to promote cancer cell growth and metastasis in human papillary thyroid carcinomas cell lines [12].

Recently, carnitine has been reported as a potential candidate biomarker able to discriminate between normal and thyroid cancer cells, however, further studies are needed to confirm carnitine as the thyroid cancer diagnostic oncometabolite [13]. Of interest, a recent Turkish study [14] used 40 guinea pigs to assess the protective effects of amifostine (200 mg/kg ip), L-carnitine (200 mg/kg ip), or vitamin E (40 mg/kg im) against high dose radioactive iodine (131I) treatment-induced salivary gland damage. Control animals received ^{131}I was administered intraperitoneally at doses (555–660 MBq) that ablate the thyroid and impair the parenchymal function of the salivary glands. The damage of the salivary glands was evaluated one month after treatment, by salivary gland scintigraphy and histopathology, in 40 guinea pigs. The three molecules gave different levels of protection against radioactive iodine treatment injury in salivary glands; however, none of the agents could provide absolute protection.

4. Flavonoids, Isoflavonoids, Soy

Flavonoids are the most common group of polyphenolic compounds in the human diet and are widespread in plants [15], and they can be classified into flavonoids or bioflavonoids; isoflavonoids; and neoflavonoids. It has been reported that flavonoids can interfere with thyroperoxidase (TPO) activity, reducing TH synthesis with subsequent raise of thyroid-stimulating hormone (TSH) levels and potential development of goiter. Goiter occurrence has been described among infants fed with soy formula, while the thyroid profile was normal in post-menopausal women with regular soy diet. Moreover, flavonoids seem to impair the peripheral action of TH, by the inhibition of deiodinase or displacing T4 from transthyretin [16]. Recently, the debate on soy foods and diet has earned attention among the healthcare and general public.

Since isoflavones from soy and other legumes showed to act on estrogen pathway, they are also proposed as nutraceutical products to relieve women from symptoms of menopause [17]. However, data regarding the impact of isoflavones on endogenous estrogens levels in women are still controversial. To date, no health issue on isoflavones has been ratified by EFSA because of insufficient scientific evidence, while the available human studies ruled out the hypothesis of adverse effects of isolated isoflavones on mammary gland, uterus or thyroid health among postmenopausal women. Nevertheless, there are many divergences to consider in term of metabolism of isoflavones, developmental stage at time of consumption and in their temporarily restricted uptake during certain stages of life, that make animal models not reliable for humans. Thus, potential adverse effects cannot be completely ignored, especially among women with unknown diseases status (i.e., undetected precancerous lesions in the mammary gland) [17].

In 2014, a review explored 5 health benefits-relieves of menopausal symptoms and prevention of breast cancer, heart disease, osteoporosis, and prostate cancer, and 5 health risks-increased risk of breast cancer, hypothyroidism, male hormonal and fertility problems, antinutrient content, and harmful processing by-products [18]. The authors considered in their analysis prospective human trials, systematic reviews of human trials, observational human studies, in vitro studies, laboratory analyses of soy components, and animal studies. They noticed that isoflavones and soy foods may wane menopausal symptoms and protect from breast cancer and heart disease, but not from osteoporosis. The impact on male fertility and reproduction was controversial. With regard to thyroid activity, data are conflicting and there is uncertainty, demonstrating that soy may have unpredictable effect on thyroid physiology [18].

In a study, adult female cynomolgus monkeys (Macaca fascicularis) were randomized in 2 groups, according to diet: One to consume casein-lactalbumin ($n = 44$) and the other soy protein with isoflavones ($n = 41$) [19]. All animals were ovariectomized after 34 months, and then, for other 34 months, half of the monkeys from each diet treatment group continued to receive their preovariectomy diet. The remaining animals were not considered furtherly. The authors concluded that soy protein and isoflavones do not adversely affect thyroid function in females [19].

Anyway, studies of soy isoflavones in experimental animals suggest possible adverse effects as well (i.e., anti-thyroid effects, modulation of endocrine function, and enhancement of reproductive organ cancer) [20].

A study showed that rats fed with a diet containing soy (20% defatted soy bean) had a severe hypothyroid state (low T4, increased TSH and thyroid weight), with evidence for increased thyroid cell proliferation. This hypothyroidism was induced only when a dietary condition of iodine deficiency was added [21].

Another paper indicated a dramatic synergism between soy intake and iodine deficiency on the induction of thyroid hyperplasia in rats [22]. Female F344 rats were randomized into 8 groups, and for a 5-week period received a diet containing: 1) 0.2% soy isoflavone mixture (SI); 2) 0.2% SI + iodine deficiency (ID); 3) 0.04% SI; 4) 0.04% SI + ID; 5) 20% defatted soybean (DS) alone; 6) 20% DS + ID; 7) ID alone; 8) basal diet alone. In the group receiving 20% DS, serum T4 and TSH levels increased inducing thyroid growth in rats exposed also to the ID diet. In the ID diet groups, proliferating cell nuclear antigen labeling indices (%) were elevated and increased by DS, but not SI, suggesting that isoflavones may not participate in the mechanisms underlying the synergistic goitrogenic effect of soybean with iodine deficiency [22].

Genistein (4′,5,7-trihydroxyflavone) is a phytoestrogen that belongs to the class of soy isoflavones and is effective to treat osteoporosis, menopausal vasomotor symptoms, cardiovascular diseases, as well as a variety of cancers. Little is known about the action of isoflavones on thyroid integrity in humans, even if it seems that genistein does not act negatively on thyroid safety in euthyroid humans [23]. Recently, it has been demonstrated that genistein has antineoplastic effects, but it does not induce genotoxic effects whereas it decreases oxidative-induced DNA damage in human primary thyroid cells from papillary thyroid cancer, supporting its potential use in therapeutic intervention [24].

A study evaluated the biological effects of genistein in rats receiving genistein aglycone in soy-free feed fortified at 0, 5, 100, and 500 ppm, beginning in utero through 20 weeks [24]. In rat serum, the genistein content was of 8 μM, and it increases in thyroid tissues up to 1 pmol/mg both in male and female rats. The activity of TPO was reduced by up to 80% dose-dependently in rats of both gender. Male and female rats receiving a standard soy-based rodent diet had TPO activity ~50% lower than rats consuming a soy-free diet. Comparing treated and untreated groups, there were no differences in T3, T4, and TSH serum levels, thyroid weights, and histopathology. The reported data suggested that, even if normal rats lose partial activity of TPO when they receive soy isoflavone, thyroid homeostasis is guaranteed by remaining enzymatic activity [25].

Quercetin is the most abundant dietary flavonoid in fruit and vegetables, and it has different therapeutic actions, i.e., the induction of apoptosis in cancer cells, and antioxidant, antiviral, anti-proliferative, and anti-inflammatory effects [26]. Regarding the thyroid, many studies have shown anti-thyroid and goitrogenic effects of flavonoids, different according to each specific flavonoid [16].

As a pretreatment for Wistar rats, quercetin was administered orally at the dose of 10 mg/kg for 7 days, and it protected them from myocardial infarction induced by subcutaneous injection of isoproterenol. The ST-segment elevation was lowered and levels of lipid peroxidation products were decreased in plasma and heart [27]. Moreover, the pretreatment with quercetin reduced significantly the levels of total cholesterol, triglycerides and free fatty acids in serum, heart, and heart mitochondria and serum phospholipids, and it lowered levels of serum LDL and very LDL cholesterol, while raised significantly serum HDL [27].

When quercetin was given (0.1%; w/w in diet) to human CRP transgenic mice, a humanized inflammation model, and ApoE*3Leiden transgenic mice, a humanized atherosclerosis model, it halted IL-1b-induced CRP expression in the first and lowered the burden of atherosclerosis (40%) in the second through a reduction of circulating inflammatory markers, "serum amyloid A proteins" and fibrinogen. The quercetin plasma levels (13–19 mM) were similar among both groups and to those measured in rodents treated with the same doses (0.1%, w/w) [28].

In 2008, quercetin was shown to halt the spread in FRTL-5 thyroid cells dose- and time-dependently, by inhibiting insulin-regulated Akt kinase action [29]. Quercetin interferes with TSH-dependent NIS gene expression and I- transport in FRTL-5 cells. These observations may help us to understand the molecular mechanism of the antithyroid effect of quercetin on cell growth and function. Even if collected from an in vitro, hormonally controlled, functioning thyroid cell line, that does not have the characteristics of a transformed cell, these results led to evaluate quercetin as an antithyroid drug in hyperfunctioning states [29].

In recent studies, quercetin seems to reduce the expression of the thyrotropin receptor, TPO and thyroglobulin (Tg) genes [30]. The antithyroid impact of quercetin was further evaluated in vivo: Quercetin was administered (50 mg/kg) to a Sprague–Dawley rat and after 14 days of treatment, radioiodine uptake decreased significantly demonstrating that quercetin may act as a thyroid disruptor [30].

Apigenin, a plant-derived flavonoid, has been also considered able to increase the iodide influx through Akt inhibition in thyroid cells under acute TSH stimulation [31]. Radioiodide accumulation thanks to apigenin-mediated Akt inhibition was also described in PCCl3 rat thyroid cells overexpressing BRAF(V600E) and in primary thyroid tumor cells from TRβ(PV/PV) mice. These results suggest that the outcome of radioiodine therapy for thyroid cancer can be improved by apigenin and other Akt inhibitors given as food supplements [31].

Soy extracts suppressed iodine uptake and increased the protein content of a known autoimmunogenic Tg fragment in Fischer rat thyroid cells (FRTL). These effects might be responsible for the association between higher incidence of Soy consumption with thyroid disorders such as hypothyroidism, goiter, and autoimmune thyroid disease [32].

Among flavonoids, epigallocatechin-3 gallate (EGCG), a catechin abundant in green tea, when administrated to male rats at doses of 25, 50, and 100 mg/kg body weight showed antithyroidal effects as emerged by decreased activity of thyroid peroxidase and 5'-deiodinase I and increased thyroidal Na^+/K^+ ATPase activity. In addition, serum T3 and T4 levels were reduced, while serum TSH was elevated in rats, showing in vivo goitrogenic potential [33].

Moreover, the effect of EGCG (10, 40, 60 μM) was also tested on the proliferation and motility of human thyroid papillary (FB-2) and follicular (WRO) carcinoma cell lines. EGCG treatment inhibited thyroid cancer cell growth, reduced cell motility and migration with concomitant loss of epithelial-to-mesenchymal cell transition markers [34].

5. Melatonin

Melatonin is an indoleamine with different activities in animals and plants, such as anti-aging, antioxidant, circadian rhythm controlling, antiproliferative, or immunomodulatory [35].

In a paper published in 1991, both in the Results ("As shown in Table 2, in surviving mice at 19 and 23 months, melatonin treatment resulted in a significant decrease in night levels of T3 and T4 after 7 ... ") and in the Discussion ("chronic night treatment with melatonin in the drinking water in aging mice significantly lowers night levels of T3 and T4 in peripheral blood (Table 2) and thus affects aging related thyroid dysfunction by a mechanism yet to be elucidated"), the authors stated that both T3 and T4 decreased after 7 months of melatonin treatment [36]. However, inspection of their Table 2 (see the following Table 2 that was redrawn by S. Benvenga), shows that only the reduction of T3 was statistically significant. Incidentally, another inaccuracy is that such reductions are lower (-20% for T3 and -23% for T4) than those shown in their Table 2 (-25% and -30%).

Table 2. Table redrawn from reference #36. In that paper [36], this table was Table 2, and its heading was "Chronic (night) treatment with melatonin modifies night levels of thyroid hormones in serum and maintains the delayed-type hypersensitivity (DTH) response of aging C57BL/6 male mice".

Groups	Age (Months)	Melatonin (Duration of Treatments, Months)	T3 (ng/mL)	T4 (µg/dL)
Untreated ($n = 10$)	19	—————	0.854 ± 0.165	5.48 ± 1.09
Treated ($n = 10$)	19	3	0.873 ± 0.160 ($+ 2.2\%$) $P > 0.05$ (NS)	5.46 ± 1.51 ($- 0.36\%$) $P > 0.05$ (NS)
Untreated ($n = 4$)	23	—————	0.850 ± 0.028	4.94 ± 1.10
Treated ($n = 8$)	23	7	0.682 ± 0.049 ($- 19.8\%$) * $P < 0.001$	3.79 ± 1.37 ($- 23.3\%$) § $P > 0.05$ (NS)

* In the original Table, the Authors wrote "(-25%)". Having noted this error, S. Benvenga wished to repeat statistical analysis with the same test used by the Authors (two-tailed Student's t test). He obtained, $t = 6.199$, which is significant at a $P < 0.001$, confirming the tabulated P value. § In the original table, the authors wrote "(-30%)". Having noted this error, S. Benvenga wished to repeat statistical analysis with the same test used by the Authors (two-tailed Student's t test). He obtained, $t = 1.450$, which is insignificant ($P > 0.10$), thus confirming the tabulated value.

One note of caution comes from preliminary experiments by the same group in C3H/He female mice that started to be treated with melatonin (10 µg/mL in the drinking water) at 1 year of age. "Melatonin not only failed to prolong the life span of the mice, but, on the contrary, induced a high number of tumors primarily affecting the reproductive tract (lympho- or reticulosarcoma, carcinoma of ovarian origin; histology not shown here) and thus adversely affected the health and survival of melatonin-treated mice" [36]. Indeed, as stated in the Discussion "It was not surprising, in this study, that ovarian tumors developed following chronic melatonin administration, as Kikuchi et al. found that melatonin stimulated in vitro proliferation of a human ovarian KF cell line" [36]. Instead, "a remarkable prolongation of life was seen when NZB mice were chronically given melatonin in the drinking water at night, while no effect was seen when melatonin was given during the day. In spite of the effect of melatonin, the common causes of death in all melatonin-treated or control NZB mice were autoimmune hemolytic anemia, nephrosclerosis and development of systemic or localized type A or B reticulum cell neoplasia" [36]. "A repetition of our experiments by night administration of melatonin in older, aging C57BL/6 male mice resulted again in a significant prolongation of their survival" [36].

At the end of a 4-week duration study in adult male rats, pinealectomy was associated with increased levels of serum FT3 and FT4 levels compared to control rats and, to a greater extent, compared to zinc-deficient rats [37]. The same Turkish team [38] showed that, at the end of a 4-week treatment period with 3 mg/kg/day of zinc and/or melatonin, melatonin has a thyroid function suppressing action, just the opposite to the effect of zinc. However, when zinc is administered along with melatonin, the thyroid function suppression exerted by melatonin is lowered. Just recently, in rats with experimentally-induced thyroid dysfunction, Baltaci et al. [39] found that both melatonin and zinc levels are increased in hyperthyroidism and decreased in hypothyroidism.

In cultured rat thyroid follicular cells, melatonin increases directly Tg expression, thus regulating TH biosynthetic activity. On the other hand, it has also been reported that thyroid C-cells synthesize melatonin suggesting in the meantime a paracrine role for this molecule in the regulation of thyroid activity [35].

Interestingly, melatonin was found to suppress cell viability, migration and to induce apoptosis in thyroid cancer cell lines in vitro and reduce tumor growth in the subcutaneous mouse model in vivo. In addition, melatonin could enhance sensitivity of thyroid cancer cells to irradiation in vitro and in vivo, suggesting that this molecule may have clinical benefits in thyroid cancer [40].

6. Omega-3 Polyunsaturated Fatty Acids (Or Fish Oil)

Omega-3 (ω-3) polyunsaturated fatty acids (PUFAs) are docosapentaenoic acid (DPA), α-linolenic acid (ALA), stearidonic acid (SDA), docosahexaenoic acid (DHA), and eicosapentaenoic acid (EPA). Several clinical trials and animal models have suggested that ω-3 possess multiple effects, such as reduction of lipid levels, direct interactions with cytosolic or membrane bound proteins, metabolic effects, alteration of membrane fluidity (after being incorporated into the phospholipid bilayer) or cardiac tissue remodeling and cell-to-cell communications, even if the data demonstrating improvement remain contradictory [41].

Some Authors demonstrated the anti-apoptotic action of ω-3-fatty acids (ω-3 FAs) on cerebellar organogenesis in a murine model of hypothyroidism-induced neuronal apoptosis [42]. Pregnant and lactating rats were first made hypothyroid by methimazole (MMI) administration and then received ω-3 FAs as a mixture of DHA and EPA. Serum levels of T3, T4, TSH, and the cerebellum of postnatal pups at 16 days of age were evaluated. Compared with the euthyroid pups, serum T4 and T3 levels were significantly lower in the untreated hypothyroid and ω-3 FA-treated hypothyroid pups. Thus, ω-3 FA-supplementation caused no significant change in serum T4 and T3 levels in the hypothyroid d16 pups. Compared with the euthyroid and untreated hypothyroid pups, the percentages of EPA and DHA in total cerebellar FAs rose significantly in the ω-3 FA-treated hypothyroid pups. The weight of the cerebellum decreased significantly in untreated hypothyroid pups compared to euthyroids, which was totally recovered upon ω-3 FA treatment of hypothyroids. The cerebellar weight in untreated hypothyroids was about 16% lower than euthyroids and ω-3 FA-treated hypothyroids. The percentage of apoptotic cells in the cerebellum was significantly higher in hypothyroid than in euthyroid pups. However, the apoptotic index of the ω-3 FA-treated hypothyroid pups was not significantly different from that of the euthyroids, but was significantly lower than untreated hypothyroid pups. There was a significantly impaired DNA fragmentation and caspase-3 activation in the developing cerebellum of hypothyroid pups. Upon ω-3 FA treatment the cleaved caspase-3 levels attenuated significantly compared to untreated hypothyroids, nearly reaching the levels of euthyroids. The levels of pro-apoptotic basal cell lymphoma protein-2 (Bcl-2)-associated X protein (Bax) were significantly higher and Bcl-2 and Bcl-extra large (Bcl-xL) were significantly lower in the cerebellum of hypothyroids than in euthyroids. In the cerebellum of ω-3 FA-treated hypothyroids, there was significantly lower expression of Bax and significantly higher expression of Bcl-2 and Bcl-xL compared to untreated hypothyroids. Finally, ω-3 FA-supplementation restored levels of cerebellar phospho (p)-AKT, phospho-extracellular regulated kinase (p-ERK) and phospho-c-Jun N-terminal kinase (p-JNK), all of these molecules being downregulated in hypothyroidism, with no impact on the expression of myelin basic protein, a TH responsive gene. These findings suggest a protective role of ω-3 FAs against cerebellum and brain injury due to fetal hypothyroidism [42].

Another study investigated in adult male rats the effect of hypothyroidism on spatial learning and memory, the underlying mechanisms and the potential therapeutic role of ω-3 supplementation [43]. A subdivision into 3 groups was done starting from 30 male rats: Control, hypothyroid and ω-3 treated. ω-3 FAs supplementation improved memory deficits, increased serum total antioxidant capacity, and also a diminished expression of Cav1.2 protein (the voltage dependent LTCC alpha 1c subunit), together with reduced structural changes, were observed. The data showed that ω-3 FAs could be a useful neuroprotective agent against the cognitive damage that hypothyroidism can induce [43].

TH also have impact on lipid metabolism. For this reason, it has been explored the effect of ω-3 FAs (at dose of 200 mg/kg of body weight/day for 6 weeks) on lipid metabolism among euthyroid, hyperthyroid or hypothyroid Lewis male rats [44]. Hyperthyroid rats had higher fasting blood glucose and plasma postprandial triglycerides levels compared to euthyroid and hypothyroid animals. In contrast, hypothyroid rats had higher levels of total cholesterol, LDL, and HDL cholesterol [44].

A large body of evidence reveals that ω-3 PUFAs have general anti-inflammatory activities and antineoplastic properties. For instance, they act through different mechanisms including alteration of membrane fluidity and cell surface receptor function, modulation of COX activity and increased cellular oxidative stress. The anti-cancer activities exerted by ω-3 PUFAs are also due to their ability to bind the tumor suppressor Peroxisome Proliferator-Activated Receptor gamma (PPARγ) [45,46].

Ligand activation of PPARγ induces growth inhibition and apoptosis in different thyroid cell lines, including anaplastic thyroid cancer cells [47–49]. Activation of PPARγ could represent a novel treatment option for anaplastic thyroid cancer in order to extend life duration thus warranting a good quality of life [50,51].

7. Resveratrol

Resveratrol (3,5,4'-trihydroxy-trans-stilbene) is a stilbenoid polyphenol that can be found in various vegetables and fruit, including peanuts, peanut sprouts and grapes. As it seems to have a significant role as either a chemo-preventive and therapeutic agent to treat different diseases [52,53], resveratrol has recently obtained more attention among health professionals and other nutrition experts.

Resveratrol has antioxidant, anti-inflammatory, and antidiabetic effects, in particular its cardiovascular protective actions are associated with various molecular targets, including apoptosis, inflammation, oxidative stress, angiogenesis, mitochondrial dysfunction, and platelet aggregation [53].

In a rat model of subclinical hypothyroidism (SCH), in which SCH is caused by hemi-thyroid electrocauterization, the effect and potential mechanism of resveratrol on memory and spatial learning were studied [54]. The treatment with resveratrol (15 mg/kg) and L-T4 in SCH rats demonstrated an inversion of learning and memory impairment in behavioral test. Resveratrol treatment of SCH rats caused reduced expression of the hypothalamic thyrotropin releasing hormone (TRH) mRNA and decreased plasma TSH. This could indicate that resveratrol treatment would reverse the hypothalamic–pituitary–thyroid (HPT) axis imbalance in SCH rats. Furthermore, resveratrol treatment of SCH rats up-regulated the hippocampal levels of syt-1 and BDNF. In brief, resveratrol treatment improves spatial learning and memory of SHC rats [54].

In another study, by the same team, the possible antidepressant effect of resveratrol was evaluated, after having previously shown that this rat model develops a depression-like behavior [55]. In SCH rats, the over-expression of the hypothalamic TRH mRNA and the high concentration of TSH were decreased to control levels by resveratrol treatment. Compared to SCH rats, resveratrol-treated SCH rats showed a higher preference for sucrose in the sucrose preference test, an increase in breeding frequency and distance in the open field test and a reduced immobility in the forced swimming test. Resveratrol-treated SCH rats had lower plasma corticosterone levels, adrenal gland weight in relation to bodyweight, and expression of the hypothalamic corticotrophin release hormone (CRH) mRNA. In addition to this, resveratrol, on the one hand, adjusted negatively the relative ratio of phosphorylated-β-catenin (p-β-catenin)/β-catenin and expression of GSK3β, and on the other, adjusted positively the relative ratio of phosphorylated-GSK3β (p-GSK3β)/GSK3β and protein levels of p-GSK3β, cyclin D1, and c-myc, in the hippocampus [55]. Altogether, these results indicate that the canonical Wnt pathway was activated in the hippocampus of the untreated model rats and that activation was ameliorated by the resveratrol treatment [36]. The authors concluded that resveratrol exerts anxiolytic- and antidepressant-like effect in SCH rats by downregulating hyperactivity of the HPA axis and regulating both the HPT axis and the Wnt/β-catenin pathway [55].

Fluoride is the most abundant anion in groundwater, creating problems in drinking water and causing metabolic, functional, and structural damage in several organ systems, including structural abnormalities of the thyroid follicles. It was shown that resveratrol supplementation in fluoride-exposed animals prevented metabolic toxicity caused by fluoride, and restored the functional status and the ultra-structural organization of the thyroid [56]. Hence, this study shows therapeutic efficacy of resveratrol as a natural antioxidant in thyroprotection against toxic insult caused by fluoride [37].

The antiproliferative effect of resveratrol depends on the induction of ERK1/2- and p53-dependent antiproliferation in tumoral cells, binding to a specific receptor on plasma membrane integrin $\alpha v \beta 3$, and the accumulation of resveratrol-induced nuclear COX-2; in turn, COX-2 combined with ERK1/2, and ultimately with p53, generates a transcriptionally active complex [57]. To date there are conflicting opinions on the preventive and therapeutic abilities of resveratrol. Physiological concentrations of TH (especially T4) interfere with the antiproliferative/anticancer action of resveratrol. This suggests that the in vivo block of the surface receptor for TH on cancer cells, as well as the reduction of circulating levels of T4 and the substitution of T3 (to maintain a condition of euthyroidism), could be used as strategies to recover or potentiate the clinical effectiveness of resveratrol in tumor treatment [57,58].

Resveratrol has been reported to inhibit sodium/iodide symporter (NIS) gene expression and function in FRTL-5 cells, decreasing cellular iodide uptake after 48-h treatment and this effect was also confirmed in in vivo Sprague–Dawley rats [59].

Recently, resveratrol has been investigated for its antithyroid effects in vitro and in vivo models. Specifically, in FRTL-5 cells resveratrol has been found to reduce the expression of thyroid-specific genes, such as Tg, TPO, TSHR, NKX2-1, Foxe1, and PAX8 while in rats treated with resveratrol 25 mg/kg body weight intraperitoneally for 60 days a significant increase in thyroid size along with higher serum TSH levels compared with control rats were found [60].

Regarding the role of resveratrol as antineoplastic agent, it has been recently reported that this compound inhibits cell proliferation through STAT3 signaling involvement [61] and reverses retinoic acid resistance of anaplastic thyroid cancer cells [62].

More importantly, resveratrol sensitizes selectively thyroid cancer cells to 131-iodine toxicity, while it exhibited radioprotective effects on normal cells, thus for these beneficial actions, resveratrol might improve the treatment of patients with thyroid cancer during radioiodine therapy [63].

In the thyroid setting, the proliferation of thyroid tumoral cells can be stopped by resveratrol, due to the resveratrol-induced increases the quantity and phosphorylation of p53 [1]. Resveratrol also has an action on iodine trapping, for which it appears to be a promising anti-thyroid drug. Overall, the in vitro and in vivo data indicate that resveratrol may act as a thyroid disruptor and a goitrogen, which should be taken into account for potential therapeutic use of resveratrol or as a supplement.

8. Selenium

The chemical non-metal element selenium is an essential micronutrient necessary for cellular function. Selenium exerts its nutritional functions in the form of the amino acid selenoCysteine (SeCys) inserted into a group of proteins known as selenoproteins, some of which are the antioxidant enzymes, glutathione peroxidase (GSH-Px) and thioredoxin reductase, and the three deiodinases of thyroid hormones [64]. The major sources of selenium intake are meat and meat products (31%), fish and shellfish (20%), pasta and rice (12%), and bread and breakfast cereals (11%), while the largest selenium concentrations (1 mg/kg) are found in Brazil nuts and offal [64].

One study investigated the improving effects of selenium on cerebrum and cerebellum impairments caused by the MMI-induced hypothyroidism in suckling rats [65]. Pregnant rats were randomized into 4 groups to receive control diet, MMI alone, MMI plus selenium, or selenium alone. Treatments were given from the 14th day of pregnancy until day 14 after delivery. Following the treatment with MMI, a reduction in plasma levels of FT3 and FT4, protein, DNA and RNA contents in cerebrum and cerebellum was observed, in comparison to controls. These parameters improved after cotreatment with selenium. Furthermore, antioxidant enzyme activities (SOD, CAT, GSH-Px) decreased significantly in the group treated with MMI, while malonaldialdehyde (MDA) levels in cerebrum and cerebellum raised. Co-administration of selenium restored these parameters to near normal values. The authors concluded that selenium improved the cerebral and cerebellar damages induced by MMI in suckling rats, and because of such neuroprotection selenium could be used as a dietary supplement against brain impairments [65].

Laureano-Melo and colleagues [66] evaluated potential behavioral alterations in offspring of female rats supplemented with sodium selenite during pregnancy and lactation. Selenium supplementation raised T3 and T4 serum levels, decreased tryptophan hydroxylase 2 expression and cholinesterase activity, and increased tyrosine hydroxylase expression in the hippocampus. In childhood, the selenium-supplemented offspring had a decrease in anxiety-like behavior; in adulthood, the locomotor activity and rearing episodes increased in selenium-treated pups. These findings demonstrated that maternal supplementation by sodium selenite induced psychobiological alterations during childhood and adulthood, probably caused by neurochemical changes generated by TH during the critical period of the central nervous system ontogeny [66].

One study evaluated the effect of selenium on CD4(+)CD25(+)Foxp3(+) regulatory T cells (Treg) by using an iodine-induced AIT model [67]. This study aimed to explain clinical observations concerning decreased serum levels of thyroid autoantibodies in patients with autoimmune thyroiditis (AIT). NOD.H-2(h4) mice received 0.005% sodium iodine (NaI) water for 8 weeks, and AIT was induced. The group of selenium-treated mice were fed 0.3 mg/L sodium selenite in drinking water. AIT mice showed fewer Treg cells and lower Foxp3 mRNA expression in splenocytes compared to controls ($P < 0.01$). However, both Treg cells and Foxp3 mRNA expression increased after the treatment with selenium, in comparison to untreated AIT mice ($P < 0.05$). Moreover, selenium-treated AIT mice had lower serum Tg antibody (TgAb) titers and reduced lymphocytic infiltration in the thyroid than untreated AIT mice. These findings suggested that selenium supplementation, through the up-regulation of the Foxp3 mRNA expression, can restore normal levels of CD4(+)CD25(+) T cells in mice with AIT [67].

In the thyroid oncology setting, data are available for human cell lines of thyroid malignancy ARO (anaplastic), NPA (BRAF positive papillary), WRO (BRAF negative papillary), and FRO (follicular) cells treated with 150 microM seleno-l-methionine (SM) were assessed for viability at 24, 48, and 72 h. Seleno-methionine treatment was found to inhibit thyroid cancer cell proliferation through the overexpression of GADD (growth arrest and DNA damage inducible) family genes and cell cycle arrest in S and G2/M phases [68].

Although these data are intriguing, the available evidence on the relationship between selenium and thyroid cancer is yet inconclusive [69].

9. Vitamins

9.1. Vitamin A

Vitamin A deficiency (VAD) and iodine deficiency (ID) are major global public health problems, affecting more than 30% of the population worldwide. VAD can adversely affect thyroid metabolism [70]. A study investigated the effect of concurrent vitamin A and ID on the thyroid-pituitary axis in rats [70]. Weaning rats received for 30 days a diet deficient in vitamin A (VAD group), iodine (ID group), vitamin A and iodine (VAD+ID group), or sufficient in both vitamin A and iodine (control). Serum retinol levels were ~35% lower in the VAD and VAD+ID groups ($P < 0.001$), in comparison to controls and ID groups. No significant differences in TSH, TSH-beta mRNA, thyroid weight, or TH levels, were observed in the VAD and control groups, while they were higher in the VAD+ID and ID groups, and FT4 and TT4 were lower compared to controls. The authors concluded that moderate VAD alone has no measurable effect on the pituitary-thyroid axis, and that concurrent ID and VAD produce more severe primary hypothyroidism than ID alone [70]. Repletion studies in VAD and ID animals suggested: a) In animals with concurrent moderate VAD and ID, primary hypothyroidism does not reduce the effectiveness of high doses of oral Vitamin A; b) VAD does not lower the effectiveness of dietary iodine to correct pituitary-thyroid axis dysfunction due to ID; c) without iodine repletion, high-dose Vitamin A alone in combined VAD and ID could decrease both thyroid hyperstimulation and the risk for goiter [71].

One Chinese study [72] moved from the fact that the interconnections among neural tube defects (NTDs) and TH or vitamin A have been investigated previously but the interaction between the TH and vitamin A pathways were not elucidated. The authors measured the expression levels of TH signaling genes in human fetuses with spinal NTDs associated with maternal hyperthyroidism, and the levels of retinoic acid (RA) signaling genes in mouse fetuses exposed to an overdose of RA on spinal cord tissues [72]. The promoters of cellular retinoic acid-binding protein 1 (CRABP1) and retinoic acid receptor beta (RARB) (both being RA signaling genes) were ectopically occupied by elevated retinoid X receptor gamma (RXRG) and retinoid X receptor beta (RXRB), but had lowered levels of inhibitory histone modifications, indicating that elevated TH signaling improperly induces RA signaling genes. On the contrary, the observed decrease in deiodinase type 3 (Dio3) expression in the mouse model could be explained by raised levels of inhibitory histone modifications in the Dio3 promoter region, indicating that overactive RA signaling could ectopically derepress TH signaling. These data led to hypothesize a potential improper cross-promotion in vivo between two different hormonal signals through their common RXRs, and then histone modifications recruitment [72].

In FRTL-5 cells, all-trans retinoic acid (ATRA) exerts protective role attenuating endoplasmic reticulum (ER) stress-induced alteration of NIS by modulating the phosphorylation of p38 MAPK [73].

ATRA has been also known to induce in vitro radioiodine uptake and to inhibit cell proliferation and invasion of human thyroid carcinoma cells [74,75], thus making this molecule a promising drug able to improve the isotope sensitivity of the most aggressive thyroid carcinoma.

9.2. Vitamin D

Cholecalciferol (or vitamin D3) is synthetized in the skin upon the exposure to ultraviolet B radiation, and it is also introduced from few dietary sources (such as fatty fish). Ergocalciferol (vitamin D2) is synthesized by plants and fungi. Both forms are hydroxylated to 25-hydroxyvitamin D in the liver [76].

Mice, previously sensitized with porcine Tg, and injected intraperitoneally with/without calcitriol (0.1–0.2 µg/kg body weight/die), showed a minor severity of thyroid inflammation vs mice treated with placebo [77]. This effect was even higher in the case of injection with calcitriol and cyclosporine [78].

In another study, mice were pre-treated with intra-peritoneal injection of calcitriol (5 µg/kg every 48 h) before sensitization with porcine Tg. The thyroid did not show the standard inflammation signs compared to controls, indicating a protective role of vitamin D in preventing thyroiditis [79].

The effect of vitamin D was also investigated in animal models of Graves' disease (GD) [80]. By immunization with adenovirus encoding the A-subunit of thyrotropin receptor, BALB/c mice became model of GD. Hyperthyroid BALB/mice fed with a vitamin D deficient diet showed fewer splenic B cells, decreased interferon-gamma responses to mitogen and lack of memory T-cell responses to A-subunit protein, with respect to mice fed with a regular diet. No differences in TSHR antibody levels were observed. Furthermore, vitamin D deficient BALB/c mice had lower pre-immunization T4 levels and developed persistent hyperthyroidism, indicating that vitamin D is able to modulate thyroid function in this animal model [80].

A study investigated the potential pathophysiological mechanisms for hypocalcaemia in hyperthyroid cats [81]. Hyperthyroid cats had lower ionized calcium levels than healthy geriatric cats, and ionized calcium concentrations were higher in hyperthyroid cats with concomitant or masked chronic kidney disease than non-uremic hyperthyroid cats. Moreover, hyperthyroid cats had higher plasma calcitriol concentrations than control cats. In hyperthyroid cats, hypocalcaemia was not associated with concomitant or masked chronic kidney disease or reduced plasma calcitriol levels. Elevated TH concentrations might influence ionized calcium levels independently from the control by parathyroid hormone and calcitriol [81].

Evidence suggests that vitamin D can negatively regulate the entire process of tumorigenesis, from initiation to metastasis by multiple mechanisms including the regulation of growth factors, cell cycle and signaling pathways [82]. Indeed, it has been largely reported the antineoplastic activities of vitamin D alone and/or in combination with other agents on thyroid cancer cells [83–85]. These findings suggest that the activation of vitamin D signaling could be a promising strategy for prevention, as well as treatment of thyroid cancer.

9.3. Vitamin E

Due to its ability to scavenge free radicals, vitamin E is considered an antioxidant. Vitamin E is also very active in the antioxidative protection of thyroid cells membranes, and it is concentrated in the thyroid in control rats, and increased two fold in goiters. Acute and excessive iodine supplementation can cause iodine-induced thyroid cyto-toxicity, that is probably due to an excessive oxidative stress. A study aimed to investigate whether vitamin E could improve iodine-induced thyroid cytotoxicity [86]. Rats received a low-iodine (LI) diet for 12 weeks and developed goiter. A 50-fold vitamin E dose could attenuate two fold iodine-induced thyroid cytotoxicity, even if weight or relative weight of the iodine-induced involuting gland was not diminished by its supplementation, showing that excess iodine can cause thyroid damage and vitamin E can improve in part the iodine-induced thyroid cytotoxicity [86].

In Sprague–Dawley rats, the oxidative stress status of the serum and hippocampus in hypothyroidism, and the effect on cognitive deficit, of L-T4 replacement therapy with vitamin E supplementation, were evaluated. It was shown that L-T4 replacement therapy with vitamin E can improve cognitive deficit in propylthiouracil (PTU)-induced hypothyroidism by decreasing the oxidative stress status [87]. Another study confirmed that L-T4 replacement therapy in combination with vitamin E reduces hippocampus cellular apoptosis index by ameliorating oxidative stress, suggesting that in a hypothyroid rat model the mechanisms of hippocampus tissue damage are associated with hippocampus apoptosis caused by a marked oxidative stress [88].

The role of vitamin E and curcumin has been investigated on hyperthyroidism-induced mitochondrial oxygen consumption and oxidative damage to lipids and proteins of rat liver [89]. Adult male rats received 0.0012% L-T4 in their drinking water and became hyperthyroid, and vitamin E (200 mg/kg body weight) and curcumin (30 mg/kg body weight) for 30 days. Both vitamin E and curcumin have differential regulation on complexes I and II mediated-mitochondrial respiration and were protective against hepatic dysfunction and oxidative stress induced by L-T4 [89].

Another study, conducted in Labeo rohita juveniles fed normal or increased levels of vitamin E and tryptophan for 60 days and then exposed to sub-lethal nitrite for another 45 days without changing their diet, reported that the negative impact on steroidogenesis exercised by environmental nitrites could be bypassed by supplementation of high levels of vitamin E and to a lesser extent of tryptophan [90].

Recently, vitamin E has been found in combination with curcumine and piperine to exert inhibitory effect on cell proliferation through influencing cell cycle regulators such as β-catenin, cyclin D1 and p53 in human thyroid papillary carcinoma cells; however, further studies are necessary to candidate vitamin D as alternative cancer therapy [91].

10. Zinc

The negative effect of zinc deficiency and positive effect of zinc supplementation on thyroid function of adult male rats (as measured by serum FT3 and FT4 levels) have been mentioned above [36,37]. In these rats, circulating zinc levels are increased in hyperthyroidism and decreased in hypothyroidism [38].

In adult male rats, thyroid function has been slightly damaged by the oral administration of 3 mL 30% ethanol [92]. The moderate decrease in serum T3 and T4 and increase in serum TSH was reversed by the 8-week administration of zinc (Zinc sulfate, 227 mL in the drinking water). Of note, serum Zn levels were low upon ethanol feeding, but they were restored to normal levels after Zn supplementation.

In contrast with the above data on adult male rats [36,37], there are findings from obese mice [93] and from small ruminants [94]. Obese mice and lean controls received a basal diet or a zinc-supplemented diet (200 mg/kg diet) for 8 weeks. After the basal diet, obese mice had lower serum and hepatic T4 and T3 levels than lean mice ($P < 0.05$). Zinc supplementation diminished significantly circulating T4 levels in both groups [93]. A total of 24 healthy male ruminants (12 lambs and 12 goats) were subdivided in 2 groups: Control or Zn group [94]. Control lambs and goats received basal rations alone (40 mg/kg and 35 mg/kg in dry matter, respectively). Both species of animals in the Zn group received a basal ration added with zinc sulphate up to a dose of 250 mg Zn/kg. The treatment lasted for 12 weeks in lambs and 8 weeks in goats. Animals receiving Zn showed more elevated plasma Zn levels than controls during all the experimental period, excluding the 4th week in goats. Compared to controls, the levels of serum total T4 and total T3 were lower in lambs and goats receiving Zn, except in the 4th week. Furthermore, circulating total TH levels of the goats were higher at the 4th week than at the 8th week. Even if a decrease (vs. controls) in the levels of free T4 and free T3 of both small ruminant species in the Zn groups was present, it was not statistically significant [94].

In another study, adult male rats were supplemented for 45 days with either zinc (227 mg/L) or magnesium (100 mg/Kg body weight) and then treated with daily intraperitoneal injection of 100 mg/kg body weight of alloxan for 15 days (days 46 to 60) to induce diabetes mellitus. Circulating total cholesterol, triglyceride, and glucose levels were higher while serum T3 and T4 were lower in diabetic rats than controls. Zinc supplementation did not change any parameter in diabetic rats, whereas magnesium decreased the elevated total cholesterol and triglyceride levels of the diabetic rats to the control level [95].

FRTL-5 cell model, derived from a Fischer rat thyroid and displaying follicular cell phenotype, was used to study the effect of zinc depletion, upon the zinc-specific chelator N,N,N0,N0-tetrakis (2-pyridylmethyl) ethylene-diamine, on thyroid function. In this experimental setting which would mimic the in vivo condition, Tg secretion was decreased. Proteomic analyses performed comparing data from zinc depleted/repleted thyroid cells have identified 108 proteins modulated by intracellular zinc status with important physiopathological implications for this endocrine tissue [96].

11. Inositol

Inositol is a water-soluble compound strictly related to the vitamin B group (also called vitamin B8). Its most abundant form is myo-inositol [97].

That myo-inositol plays an important role in the thyroid gland can be inferred by the evidence, in male rats, that radioactive myo-inositol is accumulated rapidly (within 1 h) by the thyroid [98]. A previous study in primary cultures of sheep and human thyrocytes demonstrated the TSH regulates myo-inositol transport through an increased phospholipase A2-mediated turnover of phosphatidylinositol and a simultaneous increase in arachidonic acid turnover [99]. Biosynthesis of myo-inositol has been investigated in hypophysectomized and thyroidectomized male rats [100]. It was shown that inositol-1-phosphate synthase is controlled by the pituitary in the reproductive organs and by the thyroid in the liver [100].

Myo-inositol is the precursor for the synthesis of phosphoinositides, implicated in the phosphatidylinositol (PtdIns) signal transduction pathway, and it is involved in different cellular processes. In the thyroid cells, PtdIns takes part in the intracellular TSH signaling, via Phosphatidylinositol (3,4,5)-trisphosphate (PtdIns(3,4,5)P3) (PIP-3) [101].

In a recent systematic review on metabolite profile alterations of thyroid cells myo-inositol has been suggested as a thyroid cancer oncometabolite [13].

The effects of inositol supplementation on serum levels of thyroid hormones were evaluated in dairy cows [102]. The supplementation decreased circulating T3 and FT3 concentrations, but not T4 and FT4 concentrations [102].

In humans, it has been shown that the increased levels of TSH declined in patients with AIT and subclinical hypothyroidism, treated with myo-inositol and seleno-methionine. The concentration of both TPOAb and TgAb decreased in both groups. The supplementation with seleno-methionine alone was not able to promote the same reduction [103].

Another paper first showed an immune-modulatory effect of myo-inositol in association with seleno-methionine in patients with euthyroid AIT [104].

A paper reported the beneficial effects of myo-inositol, seleno-methionine or their combination on peripheral blood mononuclear cells (PBMC) exposed in vitro to hydrogen peroxide (H2O2)-induced oxidative stress in both control and women with Hashimoto's thyroiditis (HT) [105]. PBMC, from 8 HT women and 3 controls, were cultured in the presence of H2O2 alone, or with subsequent addition of myo-inositol, seleno-methionine, or their combination. H2O2 alone decreased PBMC proliferation, and it decreased furtherly and dose-dependently in either group. Moreover, H2O2 alone reduced vitality both in controls and HT women, but vitality was rescued by the three additions, contrasting also genotoxicity. Chemokines levels were increased by H2O2 alone (more in HT women than in controls), and each addition dose-dependently decreased these concentrations in either group, particularly with Myo+SelMet [105].

Another study investigated whether myo-inositol alone, or its combination with seleno-methionine, is effective in protecting thyrocytes from the effects given by cytokines, or H2O2 [106]. H2O2 had a toxic effect in primary thyrocytes increasing the apoptosis, and decreasing the proliferation, slightly reducing cytokines-induced CXCL10 secretion. The interferon(IFN)-γ + tumor necrosis factor alpha(TNF)-α induced secretion of CXCL10 was reduced by myo-inositol+seleno-methionine, in both the presence or absence of H2O2. Seleno-methionine alone had no effect. These findings suggested a protective effect of myo-inositol on thyroid cells [106].

Finally, the beneficial effects of myo-inositol, either alone (2.5 g/kg/day in the drinking water) or administered in association with T3 (30 micrograms.kg-1.day-1 s.c.), were investigated on the cardiac lipid content and function of streptozocin-induced diabetic (STZ-D) rats [107]. The elevations in both plasma and myocardial lipids associated with diabetes were prevented by myo-inositol treatment. Moreover, a partial improvement in cardiac performance of STZ-D rats was observed in the group treated with myo-inositol alone and the group treated with myo-inositol plus T3 [107].

12. Conclusions

Nutraceuticals have a place in complementary medicines, defined as a "food, or parts of a food, that provide medical or health benefits, including the prevention and treatment of disease" [2], for the prevention of different pathological conditions, including thyroid diseases. Thyroid supplements have gained lots of attention in the last years. Iodine is the major nutrient for thyroid function, but also other dietary components can have a key role in clinical thyroidology. In this review, we have summarized the cell cultures and animal studies present in literature, focusing on the commonest nutraceuticals generally encountered in the clinical practice (such as carnitine, flavonoids, melatonin, omega-3, resveratrol, selenium, vitamins, zinc, inositol), highlighting conflicting results (Table 3 and Figure 1). These experimental studies are expected to improve the clinicians' knowledge about the main supplements being used, in order to clarify the potential risks or side effects and support patients in their use.

Table 3. Summary of the main findings.

Compounds	Main Findings	References
carnitine	antagonism of thyroid hormone action, thyroid diagnostic oncometabolite	[9] [13]
flavonoids, isoflavonoids, soy	inhibition of deiodinase or displacing T4 from transthyretin, decreased activity of thyroid peroxidase anti-thyroid effects goitrogenic effect antineoplastic effects	[16,33] [20,29–31] [22] [24,34]
melatonin	regulation of thyroid activity antineoplastic effects	[37–39] [40]
omega-3 poly-unsaturated fatty acids	neuroprotection against fetal hypothyroidism antineoplastic effects	[42,43] [45]
resveratrol	improvement of spatial learning and memory antidepressant effect inhibition of sodium/iodide symporter expression and function antineoplastic effects	[54] [55] [59] [57,58,61–63]
selenium	neuroprotection against fetal hypothyroidism immunoregulation antineoplastic effects	[65,66] [67] [68]
vitamin A	antigoitrogenic effect regulation thyroid hormone signaling antineoplastic effects	[71] [72] [73–75]
vitamin D	immunoregulation antineoplastic effects	[77–80] [82]
vitamin E	antioxidative protection antineoplastic effects	[86–89] [91]
zinc	modulation thyroid function	[36–38,92–96]
inositol	involvement in the intracellular TSH signaling, via PIP-3 inositol supplementation decreased circulating T3 and FT3 concentrations thyroid diagnostic oncometabolite the treatment, in combination with seleno-methionine, declined the elevated levels of TSH in patients with AIT and subclinical hypothyroidism immune-modulatory effect of myo-inositol in association with seleno-methionine in patients with euthyroid AIT beneficial effects of myo-inositol, seleno-methionine or their combination on PBMC exposed in vitro to H2O2-induced oxidative stress in both control and women with HT protective effect of myo-inositol on thyroid cells myo-inositol, either alone or in association with T3 improved cardiac lipid content and function of streptozocin-induced diabetic rats	[101] [102] [13] [103] [104] [105] [106] [107]

AIT, autoimmune thyroiditis; H2O2, hydrogen peroxide; HT, Hashimoto's thyroiditis; PIP-3, Phosphatidylinositol (3,4,5)-trisphosphate (PtdIns(3,4,5)P3); PBMC, peripheral blood mononuclear cells.

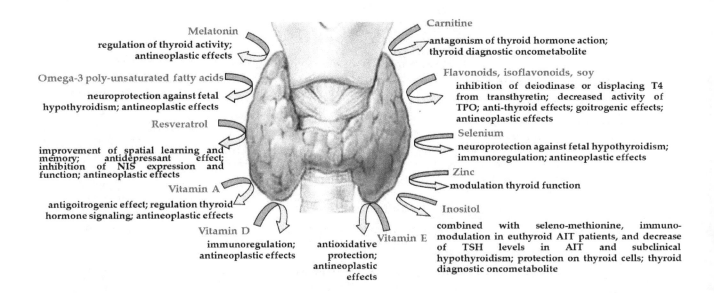

Figure 1. Summary of the main findings. NIS, sodium/iodide symporter; TPO, thyroid peroxidase; AIT, autoimmune thyroiditis.

Author Contributions: Conceptualization, S.B. and A.A.; methodology, G.E., F.R., A.P., S.R.P., S.C.; writing—original draft preparation, S.B., A.A., D.B. and S.M.F.; writing—review and editing, S.B., A.A., D.B., and P.F.; supervision, S.B., A.A., D.B. All authors have read and agreed to the published version of the manuscript.

Acknowledgments: Nothing to declare.

References

1. Benvenga, S.; Feldt-Rasmussen, U.; Bonofiglio, D.; Asamoah, E. Nutraceutical Supplements in the Thyroid Setting: Health Benefits beyond Basic Nutrition. *Nutrients* **2019**, *11*, 2214. [CrossRef] [PubMed]

2. Lockwood, G.B. The quality of commercially available nutraceutical supplements and food sources. *J. Pharm. Pharmacol.* **2011**, *63*, 3–10. [CrossRef] [PubMed]

3. European Parliament. Regulation EU 2015/2283 of the European Parliament and of the Council of 25 November 2015 on Novel Foods, Amending Regulation (EU) No 1169/2011 of the European Parliament and of the Council and Repealing Regulation (EC) No 258/97 of the European Parliament and of the Council and Commission Regulation (EC) No 1852/2001. Available online: https://eur-lex.europa.eu/legal-content/en/TXT/?uri=CELEX%3A32015R2283 (accessed on 13 March 2020).

4. Galetta, F.; Franzoni, F.; Bernini, G.; Poupak, F.; Carpi, A.; Cini, G.; Tocchini, L.; Antonelli, A.; Santoro, G. Cardiovascular complications in patients with pheochromocytoma: A mini-review. *Biomed. Pharmacother.* **2010**, *64*, 505–509. [CrossRef] [PubMed]

5. Galetta, F.; Franzoni, F.; Fallahi, P.; Tocchini, L.; Braccini, L.; Santoro, G.; Antonelli, A. Changes in heart rate variability and QT dispersion in patients with overt hypothyroidism. *Eur. J. Endocrinol.* **2008**, *158*, 85–90. [CrossRef]

6. Antonelli, A.; Ferrari, S.M.; Frascerra, S.; Di Domenicantonio, A.; Nicolini, A.; Ferrari, P.; Ferrannini, E.; Fallahi, P. Increase of circulating CXCL9 and CXCL11 associated with euthyroid or subclinically hypothyroid autoimmune thyroiditis. *J. Clin. Endocrinol. Metab.* **2011**, *96*, 1859–1863. [CrossRef]

7. Benvenga, S.; Lakshmanan, M.; Trimarchi, F. Carnitine is a naturally occurring inhibitor of thyroid hormone nuclear uptake. *Thyroid* **2000**, *12*, 1043–1050. [CrossRef]

8. Rotzsch, W.; Strack, E. Umstaz Und Wirkung des Carnitins im Tierkorper. *Int. Abstr. Biol. Sci.* **1958**, *11*, 80.

9. Hellthaler, G.; Wenzel, K.W.; Rotzsch, W. Aminotransferasen unter thyroxin und Karnitin. *Acta Biol. German* **1967**, *19*, 641–652.

10. Yildirim, S.; Yildirim, A.; Dane, S.; Aliyev, E.; Yigitoglu, R. Dose-dependent protective effect of L-carnitine on oxidative stress in the livers of hyperthyroid rats. *Eurasian J. Med.* **2013**, *45*, 1–6. [CrossRef]

11. Huang, H.; Liu, N.; Guo, H.; Liao, S.; Li, X.; Yang, C.; Liu, S.; Song, W.; Liu, C.; Guan, L.; et al. L-Carnitine Is an Endogenous HDAC Inhibitor Selectively Inhibiting Cancer Cell Growth In Vivo and In Vitro. *PLoS ONE* **2012**, *7*, e49062. [CrossRef]

12. Wang, R.; Cheng, Y.; Su, D.; Gong, B.; He, X.; Zhou, X.; Pang, Z.; Cheng, L.; Chen, Y.; Yao, Z. Cpt1c regulated by AMPK promotes papillary thyroid carcinomas cells survival under metabolic stress conditions. *J. Cancer* **2017**, *8*, 3675–3681. [CrossRef] [PubMed]

13. Khatami, F.; Payab, M.; Sarvari, M.; Gilany, K.; Larijani, B.; Arjmand, B.; Tavangar, S.M. Oncometabolites as biomarkers in thyroid cancer: A systematic review. *Cancer Manag. Res.* **2019**, *11*, 1829–1841. [CrossRef] [PubMed]

14. Torun, N.; Muratli, A.; Serim, B.D.; Ergulen, A.; Altun, G.D. Radioprotective Effects of Amifostine, L-Carnitine and Vitamin E in Preventing Early Salivary Gland Injury due to Radioactive Iodine Treatment. *Curr. Med. Imag. Rev.* **2019**, *15*, 395–404. [CrossRef]

15. Spencer, J.P. Flavonoids: Modulators of brain function? *Br. J. Nutr.* **2008**, *99*, ES60–ES77. [CrossRef]

16. de Souza Dos Santos, M.C.; Gonçalves, C.F.; Vaisman, M.; Ferreira, A.C.; de Carvalho, D.P. Impact of flavonoids on thyroid function. *Food Chem. Toxicol.* **2011**, *49*, 2495–2502. [CrossRef]

17. Lehmann, L.; Soukup, S.T.; Gerhäuser, C.; Vollmer, G.; Kulling, S.E. [Isoflavone-containing dietary supplements]. *Bundesgesundheitsblatt Gesundheitsforschung Gesundheitsschutz* **2017**, *60*, 305–313. [CrossRef]

18. D'Adamo, C.R.; Sahin, A. Soy foods and supplementation: A review of commonly perceived health benefits and risks. *Altern. Ther. Health Med.* **2014**, *20*, 39–51.

19. Silverstein, M.G.; Kaplan, J.R.; Appt, S.E.; Register, T.C.; Shively, C.A. Effect of soy isoflavones on thyroid hormones in intact and ovariectomized cynomolgus monkeys (Macaca fascicularis). *Menopause* **2014**, *21*, 1136–1142. [CrossRef]

20. Doerge, D.R.; Chang, H.C. Inactivation of thyroid peroxidase by soy isoflavones, in vitro and in vivo. *J. Chromatogr. B* **2002**, *777*, 269–279. [CrossRef]

21. Ikeda, T.; Nishikawa, A.; Imazawa, T.; Kimura, S.; Hirose, M. Dramatic synergism between excess soybean intake and iodine deficiency on the development of rat thyroid hyperplasia. *Carcinogenesis* **2000**, *21*, 707–713. [CrossRef]

22. Son, H.Y.; Nishikawa, A.; Ikeda, T.; Imazawa, T.; Kimura, S.; Hirose, M. Lack of effect of soy isoflavone on thyroid hyperplasia in rats receiving an iodine-deficient diet. *Jpn. J. Cancer Res.* **2001**, *92*, 103–108. [CrossRef] [PubMed]

23. Marini, H.; Polito, F.; Adamo, E.B.; Bitto, A.; Squadrito, F.; Benvenga, S. Update on genistein and thyroid: An overall message of safety. *Front. Endocrinol.* **2012**, *3*, 94. [CrossRef] [PubMed]

24. Ferrari, S.M.; Antonelli, A.; Guidi, P.; Bernardeschi, M.; Scarcelli, V.; Fallahi, P.; Frenzilli, G. Genotoxicity Evaluation of the Soybean Isoflavone Genistein in Human Papillary Thyroid Cancer Cells. Study of Its Potential Use in Thyroid Cancer Therapy. *Nutr. Cancer* **2019**, *71*, 1335–1344. [CrossRef] [PubMed]

25. Chang, H.C.; Doerge, D.R. Dietary genistein inactivates rat thyroid peroxidase in vivo without an apparent hypothyroid effect. *Toxicol. Appl. Pharmacol.* **2000**, *168*, 244–252. [CrossRef] [PubMed]

26. Russo, M.; Spagnuolo, C.; Tedesco, I.; Bilotto, S.; Russo, G.L. The flavonoid quercetin in disease prevention and therapy: Facts and fancies. *Biochem. Pharmacol.* **2012**, *83*, 6–15. [CrossRef]

27. Prince, P.S.; Sathya, B. Pretreatment with quercetin ameliorates lipids, lipoproteins and marker enzymes of lipid metabolism in isoproterenol treated cardiotoxic male Wistar rats. *Eur. J. Pharmacol.* **2010**, *635*, 142–148. [CrossRef]

28. Kleemann, R.; Verschuren, L.; Morrison, M.; Zadelaar, S.; van Erk, M.J.; Wielinga, P.Y.; Kooistra, T. Antiinflammatory, anti-proliferative and anti-atherosclerotic effects of quercetin in human in vitro and in vivo models. *Atherosclerosis* **2011**, *218*, 44–52. [CrossRef]

29. Giuliani, C.; Noguchi, Y.; Harii, N.; Napolitano, G.; Tatone, D.; Bucci, I.; Piantelli, M.; Monaco, F.; Kohn, L.D. The flavonoid quercetin regulates growth and gene expression in rat FRTL-5 thyroid cells. *Endocrinology* **2008**, *149*, 84–92. [CrossRef]

30. Giuliani, C.; Bucci, I.; Di Santo, S.; Rossi, C.; Grassadonia, A.; Piantelli, M.; Monaco, F.; Napolitano, G. The flavonoid quercetin inhibits thyroid-restricted genes expression and thyroid function. *Food Chem. Toxicol.* **2014**, *66*, 23–29. [CrossRef]

31. Lakshmanan, A.; Doseff, A.I.; Ringel, M.D.; Saji, M.; Rousset, B.; Zhang, X.; Jhiang, S.M. Apigenin in combination with Akt inhibition significantly enhances thyrotropin-stimulated radioiodide accumulation in thyroid cells. *Thyroid* **2014**, *24*, 878–887. [CrossRef]

32. Tran, L.; Hammuda, M.; Wood, C.; Xiao, C.W. Soy extracts suppressed iodine uptake and stimulated the production of autoimmunogen in rat thyrocytes. *Exp. Biol. Med.* **2013**, *238*, 623–630. [CrossRef] [PubMed]

33. Chandra, A.K.; De, N. Goitrogenic/antithyroidal potential of green tea extract in relation to catechin in rats. *Food Chem. Toxicol.* **2010**, *48*, 2304–2311. [CrossRef] [PubMed]

34. De Amicis, F.; Perri, A.; Vizza, D.; Russo, A.; Panno, M.L.; Bonofiglio, D.; Giordano, C.; Mauro, L.; Aquila, S.; Tramontano, D.; et al. Epigallocatechin gallate inhibits growth and epithelial-to-mesenchymal transition in human thyroid carcinoma cell lines. *J. Cell Physiol.* **2013**, *228*, 2054–2062. [CrossRef]

35. Garcia-Marin, R.; Fernandez-Santos, J.M.; Morillo-Bernal, J.; Gordillo-Martinez, F.; Vazquez-Roman, V.; Utrilla, J.C.; Carrillo-Vico, A.; Guerrero, J.M.; Martin-Lacave, I. Melatonin in the thyroid gland: Regulation by thyroid-stimulating hormone and role in thyroglobulin gene expression. *J. Physiol. Pharmacol.* **2015**, *66*, 643–652. [PubMed]

36. Pierpaoli, G.; Dall'Ara, A.; Pedrinis, E.; Regelson, W. The pineal control of aging: The effects of melatonin and pineal grafting on the survival of older mice. *Ann. N. Y. Acad. Sci.* **1991**, *621*, 291–313. [CrossRef]

37. Baltaci, A.K.; Mogulkoc, R.; Bediz, C.S.; Kul, A.; Ugur, A. Pinealectomy and zinc deficiency have opposite effects on thyroid hormones in rats. *Endocr. Res.* **2003**, *29*, 473–481. [CrossRef]

38. Baltaci, A.K.; Mogulkoc, R.; Kul, A.; Bediz, C.S.; Ugur, A. Opposite effects of zinc and melatonin on thyroid hormones in rats. *Toxicology* **2004**, *195*, 65–75. [CrossRef]

39. Baltaci, A.K.; Mogulkoc, R.; Leptin, N.P.Y. Melatonin and Zinc Levels in Experimental Hypothyroidism and Hyperthyroidism: The Relation to Zinc. *Biochem. Genet.* **2017**, *55*, 223–233. [CrossRef]

40. Zou, Z.W.; Liu, T.; Li, Y.; Chen, P.; Peng, X.; Ma, C.; Zhang, W.J.; Li, P.D. Melatonin suppresses thyroid cancer growth and overcomes radioresistance via inhibition of p65 phosphorylation and induction of ROS. *Redox Biol.* **2018**, *16*, 226–236. [CrossRef]

41. Soukup, T. Effects of long-term thyroid hormone level alterations, n-3 polyunsaturated fatty acid supplementation and statin administration in rats. *Physiol. Res.* **2014**, *63*, S119–S131.

42. Sinha, R.A.; Khare, P.; Rai, A.; Maurya, S.K.; Pathak, A.; Mohan, V.; Nagar, G.K.; Mudiam, M.K.; Godbole, M.M.; Bandyopadhyay, S. Anti-apoptotic role of omega-3-fatty acids in developing brain: Perinatal hypothyroid rat cerebellum as apoptotic model. *Int. J. Dev. Neurosci.* **2009**, *27*, 377–383. [CrossRef] [PubMed]

43. Abd Allah, E.S.; Gomaa, A.M.; Sayed, M.M. The effect of omega-3 on cognition in hypothyroid adult male rats. *Acta Physiol. Hung.* **2014**, *101*, 362–376. [CrossRef] [PubMed]

44. Rauchová, H.; Vokurková, M.; Pavelka, S.; Behuliak, M.; Tribulová, N.; Soukup, T. N-3 polyunsaturated fatty acids supplementation does not affect changes of lipid metabolism induced in rats by altered thyroid status. *Horm. Metab. Res.* **2013**, *45*, 507–512. [CrossRef] [PubMed]

45. Gani, O.A. Are fish oil omega-3 long-chain fatty acids and their derivatives peroxisome proliferator-activated receptor agonists? *Cardiovasc. Diabetol.* **2008**, *20*, 1–6. [CrossRef] [PubMed]

46. Yousefnia, S.; Momenzadeh, S.; Seyed Forootan, F.; Ghaedi, K.; Nasr Esfahani, M.H. The influence of peroxisome proliferator-activated receptor γ (PPARγ) ligands on cancer cell tumorigenicity. *Gene* **2018**, *649*, 14–22. [CrossRef] [PubMed]

47. Ohta, K.; Endo, T.; Haraguchi, K.; Hershman, J.M.; Onaya, T. Ligands for peroxisome proliferator-activated receptor gamma inhibit growth and induce apoptosis of human papillary thyroid carcinoma cells. *J. Clin. Endocrinol. Metab.* **2001**, *86*, 2170–2177. [CrossRef]

48. Hayashi, N.; Nakamori, S.; Hiraoka, N.; Tsujie, M.; Xundi, X.; Takano, T.; Amino, N.; Sakon, M.; Monden, M. Antitumor effects of peroxisome proliferator activate receptor gamma ligands on anaplastic thyroid carcinoma. *Int. J. Oncol.* **2004**, *24*, 89–95.

49. Bonofiglio, D.; Qi, H.; Gabriele, S.; Catalano, S.; Aquila, S.; Belmonte, M.; Andò, S. Peroxisome proliferator-activated receptor gamma inhibits follicular and anaplastic thyroid carcinoma cells growth by upregulating p21Cip1/WAF1 gene in a Sp1-dependent manner. *Endocr. Relat. Cancer* **2008**, *15*, 545–557. [CrossRef]

50. Antonelli, A.; Fallahi, P.; Ferrari, S.M.; Ruffilli, I.; Santini, F.; Minuto, M.; Galleri, D.; Miccoli, P. New targeted therapies for thyroid cancer. *Curr. Genom.* **2011**, *12*, 626–631. [CrossRef]

51. Antonelli, A.; Miccoli, P.; Derzhitski, V.E.; Panasiuk, G.; Solovieva, N.; Baschieri, L. Epidemiologic and clinical evaluation of thyroid cancer in children from the Gomel region (Belarus). *World J. Surg.* **1996**, *20*, 867–871. [CrossRef]

52. Rauf, A.; Imran, M.; Suleria, H.A.R.; Ahmad, B.; Peters, D.G.; Mubarak, M.S. A comprehensive review of the health perspectives of resveratrol. *Food Funct.* **2017**, *8*, 4284–4305. [CrossRef] [PubMed]

53. Limmongkon, A.; Janhom, P.; Amthong, A.; Kawpanuk, M.; Nopprang, P.; Poohadsuan, J.; Somboon, T.; Saijeen, S.; Surangkul, D.; Srikummool, M.; et al. Antioxidant activity, total phenolic, and resveratrol content in five cultivars of peanut sprouts. *Asian Pac. J. Trop. Biomed.* **2017**, *7*, 332–338. [CrossRef]

54. Ge, J.F.; Xu, Y.Y.; Li, N.; Zhang, Y.; Qiu, G.L.; Chu, C.H.; Wang, C.Y.; Qin, G.; Chen, F.H. Resveratrol improved the spatial learning and memory in subclinical hypothyroidism rat induced by hemi-thyroid electrocauterization. *Endocr. J.* **2015**, *62*, 927–938. [CrossRef]

55. Ge, J.F.; Xu, Y.Y.; Qin, G.; Cheng, J.Q.; Chen, F.H. Resveratrol Ameliorates the Anxiety- and Depression-Like Behavior of Subclinical Hypothyroidism Rat: Possible Involvement of the HPT Axis, HPA Axis, and Wnt/β-Catenin Pathway. *Front. Endocrinol.* **2016**, *7*, 44. [CrossRef]

56. Sarkar, C.; Pal, S. Ameliorative effect of resveratrol against fluoride-induced alteration of thyroid function in male wistar rats. *Biol. Trace Elem. Res.* **2014**, *162*, 278–287. [CrossRef]

57. Ho, Y.; Lin, Y.S.; Liu, H.L.; Shih, Y.J.; Lin, S.Y.; Shih, A.; Chin, Y.T.; Chen, Y.R.; Lin, H.Y.; Davis, P.J. Biological Mechanisms by Which Antiproliferative Actions of Resveratrol Are Minimized. *Nutrients* **2017**, *9*, 1046. [CrossRef]

58. Hercbergs, A.; Johnson, R.E.; Ashur-Fabian, O.; Garfield, D.H.; Davis, P.J. Medically induced euthyroid hypothyroxinemia may extend survival in compassionate need cancer patients: An observational study. *Oncologist* **2015**, *20*, 72–76. [CrossRef]

59. Giuliani, C.; Bucci, I.; Di Santo, S.; Rossi, C.; Grassadonia, A.; Mariotti, M.; Piantelli, M.; Monaco, F.; Napolitano, G. Resveratrol inhibits sodium/iodide symporter gene expression and function in rat thyroid cells. *PLoS ONE* **2014**, *9*, e107936. [CrossRef]

60. Giuliani, C.; Iezzi, M.; Ciolli, L.; Hysi, A.; Bucci, I.; Di Santo, S.; Rossi, C.; Zucchelli, M.; Napolitano, G. Resveratrol has anti-thyroid effects both in vitro and in vivo. *Food Chem. Toxicol.* **2017**, *107*, 237–247. [CrossRef]

61. Wu, J.; Li, Y.T.; Tian, X.T.; Liu, Y.S.; Wu, M.L.; Li, P.N.; Liu, J. STAT3 signaling statuses determine the fate of resveratrol-treated anaplastic thyroid cancer cells. *Cancer Biomark.* **2020**, *27*, 461–469. [CrossRef]

62. Liu, X.; Li, H.; Wu, M.L.; Wu, J.; Sun, Y.; Zhang, K.L.; Liu, J. Resveratrol Reverses Retinoic Acid Resistance of Anaplastic Thyroid Cancer Cells via Demethylating CRABP2 Gene. *Front. Endocrinol.* **2019**, *10*, 734. [CrossRef] [PubMed]

63. Hosseinimehr, S.J.; Hossein, S.A.H. Resveratrol Sensitizes Selectively Thyroid Cancer Cell to 131-Iodine Toxicity. *J. Toxicol.* **2014**, *2014*, 839597. [CrossRef] [PubMed]

64. Duntas, L.H.; Benvenga, S. Selenium: An element for life. *Endocrine* **2015**, *48*, 756–775. [CrossRef] [PubMed]

65. Ben Amara, I.; Fetoui, H.; Guermazi, F.; Zeghal, N. Dietary selenium addition improves cerebrum and cerebellum impairments induced by methimazole in suckling rats. *Int. J. Dev. Neurosci.* **2009**, *27*, 719–726. [CrossRef]

66. Laureano-Melo, R.; Império, G.E.; da Silva-Almeida, C.; Kluck, G.E.; Cruz Seara Fde, A.; da Rocha, F.F.; da Silveira, A.L.; Reis, L.C.; Ortiga-Carvalho, T.M.; da Silva Côrtes, W. Sodium selenite supplementation during pregnancy and lactation promotes anxiolysis and improves mnemonic performance in wistar rats' offspring. *Pharmacol. Biochem. Behav.* **2015**, *138*, 123–132. [CrossRef]

67. Xue, H.; Wang, W.; Li, Y.; Shan, Z.; Li, Y.; Teng, X.; Gao, Y.; Fan, C.; Teng, W. Selenium upregulates CD4(+)CD25(+) regulatory T cells in iodine-induced autoimmune thyroiditis model of NOD.H-2(h4) mice. *Endocr. J.* **2010**, *57*, 595–601. [CrossRef]

68. Kato, M.A.; Finley, D.J.; Lubitz, C.C.; Zhu, B.; Moo, T.A.; Loeven, M.R.; Ricci, J.A.; Zarnegar, R.; Katdare, M.; Fahey, T.J. 3rd. Selenium decreases thyroid cancer cell growth by increasing expression of GADD153 and GADD34. *Nutr. Cancer* **2010**, *62*, 66–73. [CrossRef]

69. de Oliveira Maia, M.; Batista, B.A.M.; Sousa, M.P.; de Souza, L.M.; Maia, C.S.C. Selenium and thyroid cancer: A systematic review. *Nutr. Cancer* **2019**, *22*, 1–9. [CrossRef]

70. Biebinger, R.; Arnold, M.; Koss, M.; Kloeckener-Gruissem, B.; Langhans, W.; Hurrell, R.F.; Zimmermann, M.B. Effect of concurrent vitamin A and iodine deficiencies on the thyroid-pituitary axis in rats. *Thyroid* **2006**, *16*, 961–965. [CrossRef]

71. Zimmermann, M.B. Interactions of vitamin A and iodine deficiencies: Effects on the pituitary-thyroid axis. *Int. J. Vitam. Nutr. Res.* **2007**, *77*, 236–240. [CrossRef]

72. Li, H.; Bai, B.; Zhang, Q.; Bao, Y.; Guo, J.; Chen, S.; Miao, C.; Liu, X.; Zhang, T. Ectopic cross-talk between thyroid and retinoic acid signaling: A possible etiology for spinal neural tube defects. *Gene* **2015**, *573*, 254–260. [CrossRef] [PubMed]

73. Lee, S.J.; Kim, S.H.; Kang, J.G.; Kim, C.S.; Ihm, S.H.; Choi, M.G.; Yoo, H.J. Effects of all-trans retinoic acid on sodium/iodide symporter and CCAAT/enhancer-binding protein-homologous protein under condition of endoplasmic reticulum stress in FRTL5 thyroid cells. *Horm. Metab. Res.* **2011**, *43*, 331–336. [CrossRef] [PubMed]

74. Lan, L.; Basourakos, S.; Cui, D.; Zuo, X.; Deng, W.; Huo, L.; Chen, H.; Zhang, G.; Deng, L.; Shi, B.; et al. ATRA increases iodine uptake and inhibits the proliferation and invasiveness of human anaplastic thyroid carcinoma SW1736 cells: Involvement of β-catenin phosphorylation inhibition. *Oncol. Lett.* **2017**, *14*, 7733–7738. [CrossRef] [PubMed]

75. Zhang, M.; Guo, R.; Xu, H.; Zhang, M.; Li, B. Retinoic acid and tributyrin induce in-vitro radioiodine uptake and inhibition of cell proliferation in a poorly differentiated follicular thyroid carcinoma. *Nucl. Med. Commun.* **2011**, *32*, 605–610. [CrossRef] [PubMed]

76. Nettore, I.C.; Albano, L.; Ungaro, P.; Colao, A.; Macchia, P.E. Sunshine vitamin and thyroid. *Rev. Endocr. Metab. Disord.* **2017**, *18*, 347–354. [CrossRef]

77. Fournier, C.; Gepner, P.; Sadouk, M.; Charreire, J. In vivo beneficial effects of cyclosporin A and 1,25-dihydroxyvitamin D3 on the induction of experimental autoimmune thyroiditis. *Clin. Immunol. Immunopathol.* **1990**, *54*, 53–63. [CrossRef]

78. Chen, W.; Lin, H.; Wang, M. Immune intervention effects on the induction of experimental autoimmune thyroiditis. *J. Huazhong Univ. Sci. Technol. Med. Sci.* **2002**, *22*, 343–345. [CrossRef]

79. Liu, S.; Xiong, F.; Liu, E.M.; Zhu, M.; Lei, P.Y. [Effects of 1,25- dihydroxyvitamin D3 in rats with experimental autoimmune thyroiditis]. *Nan Fang Yi Ke Da Xue Xue Bao* **2010**, *30*, 1573–1576.

80. Misharin, A.; Hewison, M.; Chen, C.R.; Lagishetty, V.; Aliesky, H.A.; Mizutori, Y.; Rapaport, B.; McLachlan, S.M. Vitamin D deficiency modulates Graves' hyperthyroidism induced in BALB/c mice by thyrotropin receptor immunization. *Endocrinology* **2009**, *150*, 1051–1060. [CrossRef]

81. Williams, T.L.; Elliott, J.; Berry, J.; Syme, H.M. Investigation of the pathophysiological mechanism for altered calcium homeostasis in hyperthyroid cats. *J. Small Anim. Pract.* **2013**, *54*, 367–373. [CrossRef]

82. Jeon, S.M.; Shin, E.A. Exploring vitamin D metabolism and function in cancer. *Exp. Mol. Med.* **2018**, *50*, 20. [CrossRef] [PubMed]

83. Clinckspoor, I.; Hauben, E.; Verlinden, L.; Van den Bruel, A.; Vanwalleghem, L.; Vander Poorten, V.; Delaere, P.; Mathieu, C.; Verstuyf, A.; Decallonne, B. Altered expression of key players in vitamin D metabolism and signaling in malignant and benign thyroid tumors. *J. Histochem. Cytochem.* **2012**, *60*, 502–511. [CrossRef] [PubMed]

84. Zhang, T.; He, L.; Sun, W.; Qin, Y.; Zhang, P.; Zhang, H. 1,25-Dihydroxyvitamin D3 enhances the susceptibility of anaplastic thyroid cancer cells to adriamycin-induced apoptosis by increasing the generation of reactive oxygen species. *Mol. Med. Rep.* **2019**, *20*, 2641–2648. [CrossRef] [PubMed]

85. Peng, W.; Wang, K.; Zheng, R.; Derwahl, M. 1,25 dihydroxyvitamin D3 inhibits the proliferation of thyroid cancer stem-like cells via cell cycle arrest. *Endocr. Res.* **2016**, *41*, 71–80. [CrossRef]

86. Yu, J.; Shan, Z.; Chong, W.; Mao, J.; Geng, Y.; Zhang, C.; Xing, Q.; Wang, W.; Li, N.; Fan, C.; et al. Vitamin E ameliorates iodine-induced cytotoxicity in thyroid. *J. Endocrinol.* **2011**, *209*, 299–306. [CrossRef]

87. Pan, T.; Zhong, M.; Zhong, X.; Zhang, Y.; Zhu, D. Levothyroxine replacement therapy with vitamin E supplementation prevents oxidative stress and cognitive deficit in experimental hypothyroidism. *Endocrine* **2013**, *43*, 434–439. [CrossRef]

88. Guo, Y.; Wan, S.Y.; Zhong, X.; Zhong, M.K.; Pan, T.R. Levothyroxine replacement therapy with vitamin E supplementation prevents the oxidative stress and apoptosis in hippocampus of hypothyroid rats. *Neuroendocrinol. Lett.* **2014**, *35*, 684–690.

89. Subudhi, U.; Das, K.; Paital, B.; Bhanja, S.; Chainy, G.B. Alleviation of enhanced oxidative stress and oxygen consumption of L-thyroxine induced hyperthyroid rat liver mitochondria by vitamin E and curcumin. *Chem. Biol. Interact.* **2008**, *173*, 105–114. [CrossRef]

90. Ciji, A.; Sahu, N.P.; Pal, A.K.; Akhtar, M.S. Nitrite-induced alterations in sex steroids and thyroid hormones of Labeo rohita juveniles: Effects of dietary vitamin E and L-tryptophan. *Fish Physiol. Biochem.* **2013**, *39*, 1297–1307. [CrossRef]

91. Esposito, T.; Lucariello, A.; Hay, E.; Contieri, M.; Tammaro, P.; Varriale, B.; Guerra, G.; De Luca, A.; Perna, A. Effects of curcumin and its adjuvant on TPC1 thyroid cell line. *Chem. Biol. Interact.* **2019**, *305*, 112–118. [CrossRef]

92. Pathak, R.; Dhawan, D.; Pathak, A. Effect of zinc supplementation on the status of thyroid hormones and Na, K, and Ca levels in blood following ethanol feeding. *Biol. Trace Elem. Res.* **2011**, *140*, 208–214. [CrossRef] [PubMed]

93. Chen, M.D.; Lin, P.Y.; Lin, W.H. Zinc supplementation on serum levels and hepatic conversion of thyroid hormones in obese (ob/ob) mice. *Biol. Trace Elem. Res.* **1998**, *61*, 89–96. [CrossRef] [PubMed]

94. Keçeci, T.; Keskin, E. Zinc supplementation decreases total thyroid hormone concentration in small ruminants. *Acta Vet. Hung.* **2002**, *50*, 93–100. [CrossRef] [PubMed]

95. Baydas, B.; Karagoz, S.; Meral, I. Effects of oral zinc and magnesium supplementation on serum thyroid hormone and lipid levels in experimentally induced diabetic rats. *Biol. Trace Elem. Res.* **2002**, *88*, 247–253. [CrossRef]

96. Guantario, B.; Capolupo, A.; Monti, M.C.; Leoni, G.; Ranaldi, G.; Tosco, A.; Marzullo, L.; Murgia, C.; Perozzi, G. Proteomic Analysis of Zn Depletion/Repletion in the Hormone-Secreting Thyroid Follicular Cell Line FRTL-5. *Nutrients* **2018**, *10*, 1981. [CrossRef]

97. Benvenga, S.; Antonelli, A. Inositol(s) in thyroid function, growth and autoimmunity. *Rev. Endocr. Metab. Disord.* **2016**, *17*, 471–484. [CrossRef]

98. Lewin, L.M.; Yannai, Y.; Sulimovici, S.; Kraicer, P.F. Studies on the Metabolic Role of Myo-Inositol. Distribution of Radioactive Myo-Inositol in the Male Rat. *Biochem. J.* **1976**, *156*, 375–380. [CrossRef]

99. Grafton, G.; Baxter, M.A.; Sheppard, M.C.; Eggo, M.C. Regulation of Myo-Inositol Transport During the Growth and Differentiation of Thyrocytes: A Link With Thyroid-Stimulating Hormone-Induced Phospholipase A2 Activity. *Biochem. J.* **1995**, *309*, 667–675. [CrossRef]

100. Hasegawa, R.; Eisenberg, F., Jr. Selective Hormonal Control of Myo-Inositol Biosynthesis in Reproductive Organs and Liver of the Male Rat. *Proc. Natl. Acad. Sci. USA* **1981**, *78*, 4863–4866. [CrossRef]

101. Fallahi, P.; Ferrari, S.M.; Elia, G.; Ragusa, F.; Paparo, S.R.; Caruso, C.; Guglielmi, G.; Antonelli, A. Myo-inositol in autoimmune thyroiditis, and hypothyroidism. *Rev. Endocr. Metab. Disord.* **2018**, *19*, 349–354. [CrossRef]

102. Gerloff, B.J.; Herdt, T.H.; Wells, W.W.; Nachreiner, R.F.; Emery, R.S. Inositol and Hepatic Lipidosis. II. Effect of Inositol Supplementation and Time from Parturition on Serum Insulin, Thyroxine and Triiodothyronine and Their Relationship to Serum and Liver Lipids in Dairy Cows. *J. Anim. Sci.* **1986**, *62*, 1693–1702. [CrossRef] [PubMed]

103. Nordio, M.; Pajalich, R. Combined treatment with Myo-inositol and selenium ensures euthyroidism in subclinical hypothyroidism patients with autoimmune thyroiditis. *J. Thyroid. Res.* **2013**, *2013*, 424163. [CrossRef] [PubMed]

104. Ferrari, S.M.; Fallahi, P.; Di Bari, F.; Vita, R.; Benvenga, S.; Antonelli, A. Myo-inositol and selenium reduce the risk of developing overt hypothyroidism in patients with autoimmune thyroiditis. *Eur. Rev. Med. Pharmacol. Sci.* **2017**, *21*, 36–42.

105. Benvenga, S.; Vicchio, T.; Di Bari, F.; Vita, R.; Fallahi, P.; Ferrari, S.M.; Catania, S.; Costa, C.; Antonelli, A. Favorable effects of myo-inositol, selenomethionine or their combination on the hydrogen peroxide-induced oxidative stress of peripheral mononuclear cells from patients with Hashimoto's thyroiditis: Preliminary in vitro studies. *Eur. Rev. Med. Pharmacol. Sci.* **2017**, *21*, 89–101. [PubMed]

106. Ferrari, S.M.; Elia, G.; Ragusa, F.; Paparo, S.R.; Caruso, C.; Benvenga, S.; Fallahi, P.; Antonelli, A. The protective effect of myo-inositol on human thyrocytes. *Rev. Endocr. Metab. Disord.* **2018**, *19*, 355–362. [CrossRef] [PubMed]

107. Xiang, H.; Heyliger, C.E.; McNeill, J.H. Effect of Myo-Inositol and T3 on Myocardial Lipids and Cardiac Function in Streptozocin-Induced Diabetic Rats. *Diabetes* **1988**, *37*, 1542–1548. [CrossRef]

Dietary Relationship with 24 h Urinary Iodine Concentrations of Young Adults in the Mountain West Region of the United States

Demetre E. Gostas [1], **D. Enette Larson-Meyer** [1,*], **Hillary A. Yoder** [2], **Ainsley E. Huffman** [3] and **Evan C. Johnson** [4]

[1]   Department of Family and Consumer Sciences, University of Wyoming, Laramie, WY 82071, USA; gostas1@uwyo.edu
[2]   Division of Kinesiology, University of Alabama, Tuscaloosa, AL 35487, USA; hayoder@crimson.ua.edu
[3]   University of Utah School of Medicine; Salt Lake City, UT 84108, USA; ainsley.huffman@hsc.utah.edu
[4]   Division of Kinesiology & Health, University of Wyoming; Laramie, WY 82070, USA; ejohns54@uwyo.edu
*   Correspondence: enette@uwyo.edu

Abstract: Background: Iodine deficiency is not seen as a public health concern in the US. However certain subpopulations may be vulnerable due to inadequate dietary sources. The purpose of the present study was to determine the dietary habits that influence iodine status in young adult men and women, and to evaluate the relationship between iodine status and thyroid function. Methods: 111 participants (31.6 ± 0.8 years, 173.2 ± 1.0 cm, 74.9 ± 1.7 kg) provided 24 h urine samples and completed an iodine-specific Food Frequency Questionnaire (FFQ) for assessment of urinary iodine content (UIC) as a marker of iodine status and habitual iodine intake, respectively. Serum Thyroid Stimulating Hormone (TSH) concentration was evaluated as a marker of thyroid function. Spearman correlational and regression analysis were performed to analyze the associations between iodine intake and iodine status, and iodine status and thyroid function. Results: 50.4% of participants had a 24 h UIC < 100 μg/L). Dairy ($r = 0.391$, $p < 0.000$) and egg intake ($r = 0.192$, $p = 0.044$) were the best predictors of UIC, accounting for 19.7% of the variance ($p \leq 0.0001$). There was a significant correlation between UIC and serum TSH ($r = 0.194$, $p < 0.05$) but TSH did not vary by iodine status category ($F = 1.087$, $p = 0.372$). Discussion: Total dairy and egg intake were the primary predictors of estimated iodine intake, as well as UIC. Iodized salt use was not a significant predictor, raising questions about the reliability of iodized salt recall. These data will be useful in directing public health and clinical assessment efforts in the US and other countries.

Keywords: Iodine Status; Food Frequency Questionnaire; iodized salt; iodine intake; dairy intake; adults

1. Introduction

Iodine is an essential trace mineral that forms the building blocks of the thyroid hormones thyroxine and triiodothyronine, which are critical regulators of metabolic activity [1]. Iodine's major environmental source is the ocean [2], with seafood and seaweed providing significant dietary sources. The iodine content of most other foods, however, is low and dependent on soil content and agriculture practices [3]. Exceptions include dairy products, which may be richer sources due to livestock iodine supplementation and use of iodophors for cleaning milk udders [4–6]. Insufficient iodine intake leads to iodine deficiency, which can manifest as hypothyroidism and endemic goiter in adults [3,7]. Iodine deficiency is of particular concern in women of reproductive age, as many pregnancies are unplanned [8], and deficiency can impair fetal cognitive and physical development [3,7].

Although iodine deficiency is a worldwide concern, with nearly one-third of the global population thought to be deficient [9], the iodine status of the US population has been viewed as adequate since the widespread iodization of salt in the late 1920s [10]. Urinary iodine concentration (UIC) measured over 24 h is a commonly used biomarker to assess iodine status in populations [3,11]. The most recent data from the National Health and Nutrition Examination Survey (NHANES 2005–2006 and 2007–2008) [12] show median UIC as adequate at 164 μg/L, with just under 10% of the population categorized as severely deficient [12]. Still, some subpopulations of the US may be vulnerable to deficiency due to food selection patterns or avoidance of iodized salt. These at-risk subpopulations include vegans/vegetarians [13], those who avoid seafood and/or dairy [14], and those follow a sodium restricted diet [15–17] or eat local foods in regions with iodine-depleted soils [2,3]. The Institute of Medicine [18] and the American Heart Association [19] have advocated for decreasing sodium intake to less than 2300 mg per day [18] and, more prudently, to less than 1500 mg per day [19], which could be reducing Americans' intake of iodized salt. Additionally, apparent trends toward local and plant-based diets may negatively influence iodine status depending on food selection patterns and habits (e.g., avoidance of seafood and dairy) and the content of local soils. Therefore, despite the labeling of the US populations' iodine intake as adequate, certain dietary choices, including strict adherence to dietary recommendations to restrict salt intake [20], may directly influence iodine status and indirectly influence thyroid function.

The present study was a pilot study that aimed to assess iodine intake and status in a sample of young adult men and women and determine the dietary patterns and habits that influence the observed iodine status. Twenty-four hour UIC was used as a reference standard for estimation of iodine status [7,21] although there is no consensus on the biomarker to use for the assessment of individual iodine status [22,23]. We hypothesized, based on the above, that we would observe at least some individuals with a low 24 h UIC (<100 μg/L), and that UIC would be associated with dietary factors such as the frequency of milk, fish and seafood intake, multivitamin and iodized salt use, and vegetarian status. A secondary purpose was to explore the relationship between iodine status and hypothyroidism using the thyroid stimulating hormone (TSH) as a general marker of thyroid function.

2. Materials and Methods

This study was conducted concurrently as part of a larger study evaluating urine color as a marker of change in daily water intake [24] conducted over a 13 month period beginning in the spring of 2016. Male and female participants between the age of 18 and 45 years were recruited from the Laramie, Wyoming community. To be eligible, participants had to be in good overall health and not have a health condition that could influence study results (e.g., anemia, diabetes, cystic fibrosis, cancer autoimmune disorders). Exclusionary criteria are previously published [24] and include: inability to understand and write English (for ability to complete written survey instruments); evidence of clinically relevant metabolic, cardiovascular, hematologic, hepatic, gastrointestinal, renal, pulmonary, endocrine or psychiatric history of disease (based on the medical history questionnaire); pregnancy or breast-feeding; regular prescription drug treatment within 15 days prior to start of the study; inability to discontinue use of specific dietary/herbal supplements (calcium, chromium, vitamin C, cat's claw, chaparral, cranberry, creatine, ephedra, germanium, hydrazine, licorice, l-lysine, pennyroyal, thunder god vine, willow bark, wormwood oil, yellow oleander, yohimbe); currently exercising >4 h per week; changes in diet or in body mass of >2.5 kg (~5 lbs) in the past month; or recent relocation from low altitude to Laramie within the past three months. The study was approved by the Institutional Review Board of the University of Wyoming. Volunteers were informed that the urine samples collected to assess hydration status would also be used to establish the iodine status of a healthy population of individuals through measurement of iodine levels in urine and if these levels are related to specific dietary or lifestyle factors. They were also informed of any possible risks prior to giving written formal consent to participate in the study.

2.1. Overview of Testing

This analysis was performed on 111 of the 125 total participants enrolled in the study, who had complete data on 24 h urinary iodine concentrations (UIC) and valid responses from a food frequency questionnaire (FFQ). Reasons for exclusion of 14 of the 125 participants included: voluntary withdrawal prior to completion, not following study protocol instructions, not providing adequate urine for analysis or not turning in complete dietary data. At study initiation (baseline), participants completed a dietary habits survey and an iodine-specific food-frequency questionnaire (FFQ). Height and weight were measured on a stadiometer (Health o meter ®, Model 201 HR) and digital weight scale (Seca, Model 780 2321138), respectively, with body mass index (BMI) calculated as kg/m². Physical activity was estimated using the International physical Activity Questionnaire (IPAQ) [25].

2.2. Measurement of Urinary Iodine Concentration and Iodine Status

As part of an 11 day collection protocol, participants collected a 24 h urine sample for the purpose of UIC measurement on the morning of day two. Participants were asked to void and discard the first morning urine sample and then collect all subsequent samples for 24 h, ending with the first sample upon waking on day three. Food and fluid intake were ad libitum during this 24 h urine collection. Iodine in urine was measured by a commercial laboratory (Mayo Clinic, Rochester, MN) using an inductively coupled plasma-mass spectrometry using tellurium as an internal standard and an aqueous acid calibration. The repeated tolerance acceptability was 10 ng/mL or 10%. Twenty-four hour UIC was defined using the following criteria: <20 μg/L (severe iodine deficiency), 20–49 μg/L (moderate iodine deficiency), 50–99 μg/L (mild iodine deficiency), 100–199 μg/L (adequate iodine nutrition), 200–299 μg/L (more than adequate iodine intake), ≥300 μg/L (excessive iodine intake) [15]. UIC was also entered into the equation of Zitterman, which incorporates body mass to estimate intake [26,27]. Urinary iodine (μg/L) × 0.0235 × body weight (kg) = Daily Iodine Intake.

2.3. Iodine Intake, Frequency of Iodine Containing Foods and Dietary Habits

The iodine-specific FFQ (Appendix A) evaluated the frequency of consumption of 43 food items known to have significant iodine content (e.g., seafood, seaweed, dairy—see Table 1). Frequency was evaluated according to the following responses: (a) never or less than one time per month; (b) one to three times per month; (c) one time per week; (d) two to four times per week; (e) five to six times per week; (f) one time per day; (g) two to three times per day; (h) four to five times per day; (i) or six or more times per day). Daily intake of iodine was estimated by multiplying the frequency midpoint by the average content of each vitamin D-containing food and expressed as IU/day (assuming 30 days per month), as previously outlined by Halliday et al. [28]. As iodine content is not available in food composition tables or databases, iodine content of the food items in the FFQ was derived from several sources (Table 1), with a majority of the data coming from the ongoing Total Diet Study (TDS) [29]. Iodine content in the TDS is listed per 100 g of the selected food item. Iodine content was recalculated from the TDS to iodine per serving size, to match the household measured listed in the FFQ. The iodine content in other sources was also converted to adjust given units to iodine per serving size. For ease of analysis, iodine intake from specific categories of foods were combined, which included estimates of iodine intake from total dairy (fluid milk plus yogurt), total fish (all types of fish) and total seafood (total fish plus all types of shellfish).

The Dietary Habits Survey (Appendix B) addressed questions regarding the frequency of table salt use in salting and cooking foods, and the type of table salt typically consumed (iodized, non-iodized). It also addressed whether participants followed a vegetarian diet, frequented a farmer's market for local food purchases, were a member of a Community Supported Agriculture program (CSA), or maintained a home garden for growing food, based on Yes, Sometimes, or NO responses (Appendix B). Both instruments were developed for the current study and have not yet been validated.

Table 1. Iodine content of foods deduced from current available resources.

Food Item	Estimated Iodine Level (μg per Serving)	Serving Size
Milk (fluid)	90.86 [a]	1 cup
Soy Milk	2.2 [b]	1 cup
Soy Protein Bar	20 [c]	1 bar
Soy Protein Powder	0 [d]	1 scoop
Soy Sauce	0 [d]	1 Tbsp
Non-dairy Milk	2.2 [b]	1 cup
Orange Juice	0 [a]	1 cup
Cereal	1.62 [a]	$\frac{3}{4}$ cup
Bread	1.18 [a]	1 slice (26 g)
Subway Sandwich	4.14 [a]	6-inch sandwich
Bagel	4.312 [a]	1 bagel (95 g)
Yogurt	87 [a]	1 cup
Cheese	13.33 [a]	2 oz
Egg	21.42 [a]	1 egg (50 g)
Margarine	0 [a]	1 tsp
Liver	11 [a]	100 g (3.5 oz)
Cod	93 [e]	3.5 oz
Grouper	84 [f]	3.5 oz
Haddock	224 [e]	3.5 oz
Halibut	9.9 [e]	3.5 oz
Herring	84 [f]	3.5 oz
Mackerel	84 [f]	3.5 oz
Perch	10.89 [e]	3.5 oz
Salmon	10.43 [e]	3.5 oz
Sardines	6.69 [g]	3.5 oz
Seabass	84 [f]	3.5 oz
Swordfish	19.8 [e]	3.5 oz
Tukaoua	84 [f]	3.5 oz
Tuna Albacore	6.69 [a]	3.5 oz
Tuna Light	6.69 [a]	3.5 oz
Walleye	84 [f]	3.5 oz
Other Fish	22 [h]	3.5 oz
Clams	74.8 [e]	4 oz
Crabmeat	42.56 [e]	4 oz
Lobster	209.67 [e]	4 oz
Mussels	9.14 [i]	4 oz
Oysters	135 [e]	4 oz
Scallops	9.14 [e]	4 oz
Shimp	8.184 [a]	4 oz
Seaweed	34.56 [j]	2.6 g (1 sheet)
Iodized Table Salt	68 [k]	1.5 g (1/4 tsp)
Other Salt	0 [l]	1.5 g
Multivitamin-(Iodine-Containing)	150 [m]	1 tablet
Kelp Supplement	225 [c]	1 capsule

Sources: [a] Total Diet Study 2006–2013 [29], [b] Bath et al. [30], [c] Popular product nutrient labels, [d] American Thyroid Association [31], [e] United States Department of Agriculture (USDA) National Food and Nutrient Analysis Program [32], [f] Inferred from other fish values from USDA's National Food and Nutrient Analysis Program, [g] Inferred from Canned Tuna TDS 2006–2013, [h] Inferred from the average of multiple fish types from USDA's National Food and Nutrient Analysis Program, [i] Inferred from the scallop value from USDA's National Food and Nutrient Analysis Program, [j] Teas et al. 2004 [33], [k] Total Diet Study 1982–1991 [34], [l] Dasgupta et al. 2008 [35], [m] Summation of observation of popular multivitamins available at local grocery stories and pharmacies.

2.4. Assessment of Thyroid Function

A blood sample was obtained on the morning of day three for measurement of TSH via immunometric assay, (Regional West, Scotts Bluff, NE). Daily quality control at different representative levels was evaluated across the measurement range, as precision changed with concentration for 112 replicates. The CV was 3.4% when the mean was 50 μg I per 24 h, and 1.3% when the mean was 191 μg I per 24 h. The presence of hypothyroidism (TSH > 4.68 mIU/L) and hyperthyroidism (TSH < 0.47 mIU/L) was evaluated based on standard laboratory ranges (normal TSH = 0.47 to 4.68 mIU/L) as well as using recent, more conservative criteria for subclinical hypothyroidism (TSH > 2.5) [36].

2.5. Statistical Analysis

Data were analyzed using IBM SPSS statistics software (SPSS Inc., Chicago, IL; version 24.0). Analysis of Variance (ANOVA) was used to compare differences in iodine intake, iodine status, thyroid function and other key variables by sex (male vs. female). Correlation coefficients (Pearson or Spearman Rank) were used to evaluate the associations between iodine status (i.e., UIC) and gross iodine intake, or iodine intake from specific foods or supplements (dairy, seafood, seaweed, iodized salt, multivitamin intake, etc.). Pearson correlations were also used for the evaluation of UIC and serum TSH relationships. In most cases, Spearman Rank Coefficients were used instead of Pearson Correlation Coefficients, due to the general non-normal distribution of intake data. Multiple linear Regression Models (Backwards Regression) were created to determine which dietary source(s) were the largest contributors to iodine intake and iodine status. ANOVA was also used to determine whether there were differences in iodine intake and status by the items indicated on the dietary habits survey, which included following a vegetarian diet, frequenting farmer's markets for local food purchases, being CSA members or maintaining a home garden for growing food. Data are expressed as means ± SEM unless otherwise specified. Significance was set as an alpha < 0.05.

3. Results

3.1. Subject Characteristics

The characteristics of the 111 participants are shown in Table 2. BMI and reported physical activity varied widely among participants. Men were taller, heavier, and had a higher BMI than women ($p < 0.05$). The sample size is provided in parenthesis in the case of occasional missing datapoints, attributed to inadequate samples for analysis or missing responses on questionnaires.

Table 2. Descriptive characteristics of Participants and Frequency of Overweight, Smoking and Physical Activity by Sex.

	Mean ± SEM		n
Age	31.6 ± 0.8		111
Height (cm)	173.2 ± 1.0		111
Body Mass (kg)	74.9 ± 1.7		111
BMI (kg/M^2)	24.8 ± 0.4		111
Hematocrit (%)	45.1 ± 0.28		110
TSH (mIU/L)	2.1 ± 0.11		107
	Male (n)	Female (n)	
Sex	59	52	111
BMI Underweight	1	0	1
BMI Normal	25	36	61
BMI Overweight	26	13	39
BMI Obese	7	3	10
Smokers	4	0	4
IPAQ Low	10	7	17
IPAQ Moderate	21	30	51
IPAQ High	22	14	36

3.2. 24 h UIC and Iodine Status

Twenty-four hour UIC ranged between 15 and 714 µg/L. The median value was 98.0 µg/L (interquartile range = 60.0–180.0), with no difference by sex ($p = 0.36$). The frequency of the various categories of iodine status based on WHO criteria is shown in Figure 1.

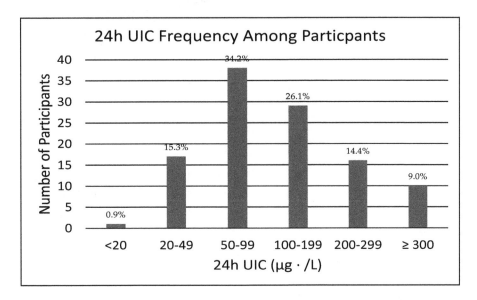

Figure 1. Iodine status based on the World Health Organization (WHO) criteria for urinary iodine concentration (UIC) [15]: <20 µg/L (Severe Deficiency); 20–49 µg/L (Moderate Deficiency); 50–99 µg/L (Mild Deficiency); 100–199 µg/L (Adequate); 200–299 µg/L (More than Adequate); ≥300 µg/L (Excessive).

Body Mass Index (BMI) and International Physical Activity Questionnaire (IPAQ) [37] scales were used in classifications. BMI classifications are as follows: Underweight (<18.5), Normal weight (18.5–24.9), Overweight (25.0–29.9), Obese (>30.0). IPAQ classifications are as follows: Low (not meeting criteria for Moderate or High), Moderate (likely doing 30 min moderate intensity physical activity on most days), High (likely doing at least 1 h of moderate intensity physical activity per day) [25].

3.3. Estimated Daily Iodine Intake and Frequency of Intake of Iodine-Containing Foods

Frequency of consumption of selected iodine-containing foods along with supplements is shown in Table 3. Overall, estimated daily iodine intake ranged from 36.4 to 1113.3 µg/day. Daily intake averaged 327.7 µg (SD: 21.0; median 291.4) and was not different by sex ($p = 0.49$). While the mean and median iodine intake was higher than the U.S. Recommended Dietary Allowance (RDA) for adults of 150 µg/day, 21.6% ($n = 24$) had estimated intakes less than the RDA, and 1.8% ($n = 2$) had intakes greater than the Upper Limit of 1100 µg/day. The estimated average daily iodine intakes from contributing foods are as follows) total dairy (100.0 µg ± 8.6), eggs (18.7 µg ± 2.3), total fish (4.4 µg ± 1.3), total seafood (includes fish plus shellfish; 8.4 µg ± 1.7), iodized table salt (33.7 µg ± 5.1), multivitamin (47.61 µg ± 9.0), and seaweed (0.81 µg ± 0.25). Using Spearman rank correlation coefficients, the total estimated iodine intake from the FFQ was correlated with reported total milk intake (r = 0.769, $p < 0.001$), dairy intake (milk plus yogurt) (r = 0.716, $p < 0.01$), egg consumption (r = 0.295, $p = 0.002$), total fish intake (r = 0.191, $p = 0.044$) and multivitamin use (r = 0.460, $p < 0.01$) but not with total seafood consumption (r = 0.169, $p = 0.08$), seaweed consumption (r = −0.050, $p = 0.6$), or iodized salt intake (r = 0.141, $p = 0.14$).

A linear regression model was created to determine which food source was the biggest determinant of estimated iodine intake. Dietary sources that were significantly correlated with total intake by simple correlation analysis (total dairy, egg consumption, total fish and multivitamin use) were entered, along with iodized table salt and seaweed. As shown in Table 4, all sources remained significant contributors to estimated iodine intake.

Table 3. Frequency of major sources of reported dietary iodine by serving.

Food Serving Size	Iodine (μg per Serving)	Frequency
Milk (1 cup fluid) (n = 110 *)	90.86	0 or <1 times·month^{-1} = 17 1–3 times·month^{-1} = 12 1 time·week^{-1} = 10 2–4 times·week^{-1} = 26 5–6 times·week^{-1} = 15 1 time·day^{-1} = 17 2–3 times·day^{-1} = 11 4–5 times·day^{-1} = 2
Yogurt (1 cup) (n = 111 *)	87	0 or <1 month^{-1} = 26 1–3 times·month^{-1} = 17 1 time·week^{-1} = 15 2–4 times·week^{-1} = 24 5–6 times·week^{-1} = 18 1 time·day^{-1} = 9 2–3 times·day^{-1} = 2 4–5 times·day^{-1} = 0
Eggs (1 whole) (n = 109 *)	21.42	0 or <1 month^{-1} = 16 1–3 times·month^{-1} = 8 1 time·week^{-1} = 15 2–4 times·week^{-1} = 29 5–6 times·week^{-1} = 18 1 time·day^{-1} = 6 2–3 times·day^{-1} = 11 4–5 times·day^{-1} = 6
Total Seafood (3.75 oz) (n = 110 *)	61	0 or <1 month^{-1} = 28 1–3 times·month^{-1} = 48 1 time·week^{-1} = 22 2–4 times·week^{-1} = 9 5–6 times·week^{-1} = 1 1 time·day^{-1} = 2 2–3 times·day^{-1} = 0 4–5 times·day^{-1} = 0
Iodized Table Salt (1.5 g) (n = 108 *)	68	0 or <1 month^{-1} = 28 1–3 times·month^{-1} = 18 1 time·week^{-1} = 12 2–4 times·week^{-1} = 12 5–6 times·week^{-1} = 12 1 time·day^{-1} = 14 2–3 times·day^{-1} = 10 4–5 times·day^{-1} = 2
Multivitamin (1 tablet) (n = 106 *)	150	0 or <1 month^{-1} = 67 1–3 times·month^{-1} = 8 1 time·week^{-1} = 3 2–4 times·week^{-1} = 4 5–6 times·week^{-1} = 4 1 time·day^{-1} = 17 2–3 times·day^{-1} = 2 4–5 times·day^{-1} = 1

* Number of participants who reported consuming each food source.

Table 4. Backwards Regression Model with Estimated iodine intake from food frequency questionnaire (FFQ) as the dependent variable and estimated iodine intake from various food categories as independent variables.

	R^2	SEE	Beta	Sig.
Model	0.991	21.81		0.005
Total Dairy	-	-	0.066	>0.001
Total Fish	-	-	0.108	>0.001
Multivitamin	-	-	0.034	>0.001
Iodized Table Salt	-	-	0.033	>0.001
Seaweed	-	-	0.122	>0.001
Egg	-	-	0.032	>0.001

SEE, standard error of the estimate.

3.4. Relationship between Iodine Intake and Iodine Status

Using Spearman Rank Correlations, the estimated total iodine intake from the FFQ was correlated with UIC (r = 0.310, p = 0.001) (Figure 2a). FFQ-estimated iodine intake was also correlated with predicted iodine intake using the equation of Zimmerman UIC (r = 0.327, p = 0.001) which incorporates UIC and body mass (Figure 2b) [26,27].

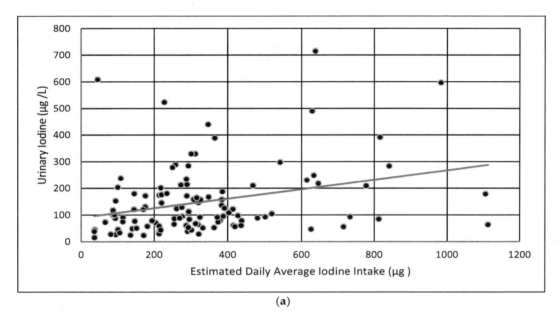

(a)

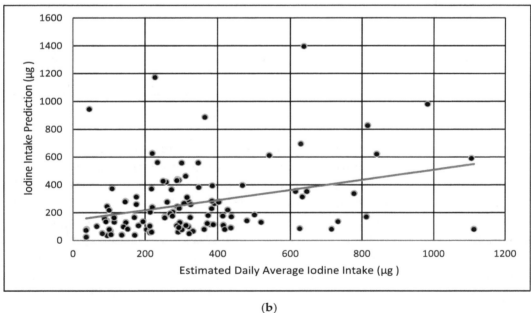

(b)

Figure 2. Estimated iodine intake by Food Frequency Questionnaire versus Urinary Iodine Concentration (**a**) and Iodine Intake Prediction (using the equation of Zimmerman) [26,27] where Daily Iodine Intake = Urinary iodine (μg/L) × 0.0235 × body weight (kg) (**b**).

By Spearman Rank Correlation Coefficients, UIC was correlated with reported total dairy intake (r = 0.391, p < 0.01), egg consumption (r = 0.192, p = 0.044) and seaweed consumption (r = −0.239, p = 0.011), but not with total fish intake (r = −0.003, p = 0.973), total seafood consumption (r = −0.055, p = 0.569), iodized table salt use (r = 0.044, p = 0.646) or multivitamin use (r = 0.031, p = 0.749).

A linear regression model was created to determine which food source(s) were the biggest determinant of 24 h UIC. Intake of iodine from dairy products, eggs, seaweed, fish, iodized salt and eggs were entered into the model. As shown in Table 5, only dairy and eggs remained significant contributors to UIC, explaining 19.7% of the variance ($p \leq 0.0001$). Total fish, iodized table salt, multivitamin use and seaweed consumption accounted for an additional 3.2% of the variance, but were not significant contributors ($p > 0.10$).

Table 5. Backwards regression models with urinary iodine concentration (UIC) as the dependent variable and estimated iodine intake from total dairy, total fish, multivitamin, iodized salt, seaweed and egg consumption entered as independent variables.

	R^2	SEE	Beta	Sig.
Model 1	0.229	118.1		0.001
Total Dairy	-	-	0.017	0.001
Total Fish	-	-	−0.033	0.249
Multivitamin	-	-	−0.006	0.128
Iodized Table Salt	-	-	0.003	0.704
Seaweed	-	-	0.111	0.455
Egg	-	-	0.037	0.032
Model 2	0.228	117.6		0.001
Total Dairy	-	-	0.017	0.001
Total Fish	-	-	−0.033	0.234
Multivitamin	-	-	−0.006	0.118
Seaweed	-	-	0.105	0.474
Egg	-	-	0.038	0.024
Model 3	0.224	117.3		0.001
Total Dairy	-	-	0.016	0.001
Total Fish	-	-	−0.033	0.234
Multivitamin	-	-	−0.006	0.125
Egg	-	-	0.040	0.016
Model 4	0.213	117.5		0.001
Total Dairy	-	-	0.016	0.001
Multivitamin	-	-	−0.006	0.136
Egg	-	-	0.041	0.013
Model 5	0.197	118.2		0.000
Total Dairy	-	-	0.016	0.000
Egg	-	-	0.039	0.018

3.5. Dietary Habits, Iodine Intakes and Intake Status

Twenty-one participants neglected to complete all questions on the Dietary Habits Survey. Complete data for those responding to questions addressing vegetarian status ($n = 94$), frequently visiting a farmer's market or food co-op for local food purchases ($n = 95$), having membership in a CSA ($n = 94$), and growing food in a home garden ($n = 95$) are shown in parentheses. Of those who completed the questions, five reported following a vegetarian or vegan diet, 49 reported regularly or sometimes frequenting a farmer's market for local food purchases, with 37 being members of a CSA or maintaining a home garden for growing food. Differences between estimated iodine intake or UIC were not observed according to whether participants reported following a vegetarian diet ($p = 0.52$ and 0.91), regularly or sometimes frequenting a farmer's market ($p = 0.60$ and 0.49), being a CAS member ($p = 0.44$ and 0.38) or maintaining a home garden (0.58 and 0.49) ($p > 0.05$).

3.6. Relationship between Iodine Status and Thyroid Function

The mean TSH ($n = 107$) was 2.07 ± 0.11 mIU/L. Based on standard laboratory criteria, four participants were classified with hypothyroidism (TSH > 4.68 mIU/L) and one was classified with hyperthyroidism (TSH < 0.47 mIU/L). Using more conservative criteria (TSH > 2.5), 24 were considered to have an underactive thyroid [36]. By Spearman rank correlation coefficients there was a correlation ($p < 0.05$) between serum TSH concentration and UIC (r = 0.194, $p = 0.045$). TSH concentration, however, did not differ by WHO iodine deficiency categories ($p = 0.372$). Notably, no differences in iodine intake or status were observed in those with TSH indicative of hypo- or hyperthyroid.

4. Discussion

The overall purpose of this pilot study was to evaluate iodine intake and status in a sample of young adult men and women and determine if intake and UIC, as a biomarker of status, are influenced by dietary patterns. Overall, we found that our sample, with a median UIC of 98.0 μg/L and with 16.2% with a UIC below <50 μg/L, may be borderline deficient. However, there was high intersubjective variability, providing an opportunity to explore dietary relationships with UICs. In contrast, 23.4% of participants had a 24 h UIC of >200 μg/L. These data suggest that some members of our population may be at risk of compromised or excessive iodine status if such patterns are consistently observed (e.g., are not based on a single 24 h UIC). Both inadequate and excess iodine intake can be linked to adverse health consequences [15,38]. These findings, however, are relevant only to the sample examined and cannot be extrapolated to, and are not necessarily representative of, the young adults in our town, the mountain west region or elsewhere in the US. However, the high intersubjective variability provided the opportunity to explore dietary relationships with UIC to estimate the dietary factors that may place individuals at risk of a single suboptimal 24 h UIC.

Total dairy and egg intake were the primary predictors of estimated iodine intake as well as UIC. Importantly, these two foods together predicted approximately 20% of the variance in UIC (Table 5). These results are in agreement with previous research showing a link between dairy and egg consumption and iodine status [39,40]. Dairy has been determined to be a reliable source due to iodine-fortified cattle feed [14] (which influences circulating iodine and the uptake of iodine by mammary epithelial cells and secretion into milk) [41] and the use of iodophor disinfecting agents on udders, although this can vary across the seasons and with industry practices [5,14,42]. In agreement with our study, a published review has suggested that milk and dairy contribute ~13% to 64% of the recommended daily iodine intake based on country-specific food intake data [6]. Eggs draw their iodine content from the laying hen's feed [43–46], which is increased with iodine supplementation. Dairy and eggs might be easier to recall compared to other sources such as iodized table salt, seafood or fish. Also, dairy is often a habitual food item, with yogurts and milk often complimenting popular breakfast and snacks such as ready-to-eat cereal with milk, yogurt with fruit, coffee with milk or a protein shake mixed with milk. Additionally, since eggs must be cracked or consumed individually, the physical nature of preparation could make serving frequency and size easier to recall.

In contrast, iodine intake from iodized table salt consumption was not found to be a primary predictor of iodine status within the present study. This finding is contrary to our hypothesis, as iodized salt is among the densest iodine sources, with more than threefold the amount of iodine per serving compared to an egg. This may be due to several factors. People may not know what iodized salt is or be aware of which sources of salt are iodized. This includes salt found in the kitchen, used in restaurants or used in processed foods. Iodization of salt, which was initiated in the United States in the late 1920s [10], is not currently mandated by the Food and Drug Administration. It is estimated that only 20% of the salt consumed in the United States is iodized [35]. Error may have been introduced if participants assumed that salt in processed foods or all salt in the saltshakers at restaurants is iodized. Additionally, it may be objectively difficult for participants to recall iodized salt use over a three month period. Salt is a seasoning that may be used sporadically in cooking and when salting foods to taste and, under these conditions, may contribute little to overall dietary intake. Finally, the amount of iodine found in iodized salt may vary considerably and depend on how long the salt has been on the grocery store shelf and in individual cupboards. One study found that iodine content varied among different brands of salt, and even within a single container [35]. Several others found that the iodine content of foods cooked with iodized salt depends on the food type and cooking method [47,48]. The increased popularity of blended salts (i.e., garlic salt) and artesian salts (i.e., Pink Himalayan, sea salt and Kosher rock salt) add another element of uncertainty as these products are typically not iodized [35], yet often share the same shelf space as iodized salt. As it is likely that habitual use of iodized salt does contribute to iodine status [49], future versions of our FFQ will consider the recall time of our FFQ as well as use of a photographic album during FFQ administration, along with more detailed and explicit questions related to salt intake, to help improve the accuracy of subjects' salt use recall.

Similar to table salt, seaweed consumption was also not found to be a positive contributor of iodine status, despite its known influence on status in countries including Korea, Japan and parts of coastal Alaska [50,51]. Our negative correlation between seaweed consumption and iodine status may be due to the low number of participants ($n = 26$) who reported eating seaweed and our use of a single value for seaweed by "serving" (Table 1). As different types of seaweed have different amounts of iodine [33], future versions of the FFQ should consider including better descriptions of the type of seaweed consumed to improve estimated iodine consumption. For example, one analysis of 12 common types of seaweed estimated that nori contained ~16 µg while processed kelp contained over 8000 µg per serving. Additionally, iodine status was not found to differ according to dietary patterns identified on the Dietary Habits Survey (vegetarian status, CSA membership, regular gardener, etc.). This is likely due to a low sample size of participants who identified with these specific dietary habits. Only about half of the subjects identified with at least one dietary preference ($n = 61$). Further studies could target these groups, as well as those adhering to AHA guidelines regarding reduced salt intake, to better analyze the influence of dietary habits on iodine status.

As both insufficient and excess iodine intake can affect thyroid function, a secondary purpose of this study was to explore the relationship between iodine status and serum TSH concentration as a marker of hypothyroidism and general thyroid function [7]. While we were expecting that participants with 24 h UICs in the WHO severe-to-moderate deficiency category would have high, normal or slightly elevated TSH concentrations, we instead found no relationship between thyroid function and WHO iodine deficiency category. In the typical hormone feedback scenario, serum TSH concentration should increase as iodine status drops [52], although the thyroid is very efficient at compensating for instances of low and excess iodine intake [53] and 24 h UIC may be more reflective of acute intake than long-term status (as discussed below). For example, a healthy adult stores ~15–20 mg of iodine, with 70–80% of these stores in the thyroid. These stores are in excess of the daily recommendation of 150 µg and can help prevent a drop in the synthesis of thyroid hormone (and subsequent increase in TSH) during periods of low iodine intake. The thyroid can also alter the efficiency of iodine organification or the incorporation of iodine into the thyroglobulin in times of excess iodine intake via 'the Wolff-Chaikoff effect' [54,55]. The weak but significant association between TSH and 24 h UIC ($r = 0.194$, $p = 0.045$) could be explained by a few participants that shifted the simple correlation in the positive direction in our sample, which had only a few subjects with TSH concentration falling in the hypo- (TSH > 4.68 mIU/L) or hyperthyroid (TSH <0.47 mIU/L) ranges, at 3.7% and 1%, respectively. The data may have also been influenced by the inclusion of participants with autoimmune disorders (as we did not measure thyroid autoantibodies) or the inclusion of four smokers.

The lack of a national database for iodine content in food was a major limitation of this study. The USDA is currently developing an iodine database for commonly consumed food products [56] which should greatly improve the assessment of iodine intake in relation to iodine status. However, the potential variability of the iodine content of foods due to iodine content of the soil in different regions [3] is likely to consistently complicate assessment of iodine intake and status. Further modification of our FFQ may also enhance its future use as a tool to estimate iodine intake and help determine the dietary habits that place an individual at risk of compromised iodine status. These include better clarification of iodized salt and specific fish and seaweed sources. Portion sizes may also be better quantified by allowing participants the opportunity to enter typical portion sizes or by including images and metaphors to visually clarify standard serving sizes (i.e., "3 oz"). A major strength of our study, however, was the creation of our own aggregated dietary iodine database for items in our FFQ. We combined multiple sources of the recent literature investigating iodine content in various foods (Table 1) and converted the listed units to iodine content per serving for better applicability to our FFQ and, ultimately, increased ease of analysis. The significant association between estimated dietary iodine intake from the FFQ and UIC further increased our confidence in our novel database. This database can be built upon for additional research until the USDA completes their official iodine database.

An additional limitation of our study and many others is the use of UIC as the biomarker of iodine status. Twenty-four hour UIC is a widely used biomarker for the assessment of iodine status, as approximately 90% of dietary iodine is excreted in the urine [57]. However, 24 h UIC is prone to collection and methodological errors and is thought to be more representative of acute (i.e., days) versus chronic iodine status [15], due to variations in 24 h UIC samples [58]. Some of this variability may be due to day-to-day differences in dietary iodine intake, but confounders such as circadian [59] and seasonal differences [60,61] also account for individual variability. Currently, there is no consensus on the biomarker to use for assessment of individual iodine status [22,23]. Additionally, in the current study, differences in the period of collection in our comparison of 24 h UIC and our FFQ, which addressed intake over three months, may have been a further limitation. While other biomarkers for assessment of this status have been suggested, including multiple 24 h UIC samples [22], age-adjusted iodine–creatine ratio [62], and serum thyroglobulin concentration [63], use of these markers are not without error and come with practical and logistics concerns when testing a large number of participants [64]. Thus, as mentioned previously, the results of the current study, particularly those related to UIC, are relevant only to the sample examined and cannot be extrapolated to, and are not necessarily representative of young adults, in our town, the mountain west region or elsewhere in the US. They do, however, support the need for continuous national iodine monitoring with emphasis on subgroups that may be susceptible to iodine deficiency [21] based on dietary choices.

5. Conclusions

The current study found an indication that our sample of healthy young individuals living in the mountain west region of the U.S. may be borderline deficient (based on a median 24 h UIC of 98 µg/L), although a high degree of variability in 24 h UIC was observed. These results, however, are indicative of the status of this sample only, and not of other, similar subsamples. Dairy and egg consumption were found to be significant predicators of 24 h UIC, whereas reported intake of iodized salt was not. Iodized salt consumption may either be difficult to assess reliably, or not as big a predictor of iodine status in iodine-replete areas. Development of a national dietary iodine database and better biomarkers for the assessment of iodine status in individuals will greatly improve understanding of the relationships between iodine intake, iodine status and thyroid function.

Author Contributions: Conceptualization, D.E.L.-M.; methodology, D.E.G., D.E.L.-M., H.A.Y., A.E.H. and E.C.J.; validation, D.E.G., D.E.L.-M. and E.C.J.; formal analysis, D.E.G. and D.E.L.-M.; investigation, D.E.G., H.A.Y., A.E.H. and E.C.J.; resources, D.E.L.M and E.C.J.; data curation, D.E.G., H.A.Y., A.E.H. and E.C.J.; writing—original draft preparation, D.E.G..; writing—review and editing, D.E.L.-M., H.A.Y. and E.C.J.; visualization, D.E.L.-M.; supervision, D.E.L.-M. and E.C.J.; project administration, E.C.J.; funding acquisition, E.C.J. All authors have read and agreed to the published version of the manuscript.

Acknowledgments: The investigators would like to thank, Shane McCullough, Joshua Loseke, and for assistance with data collection, and Sarah R. Rich for assistance with summation of iodine content of foods (Table 1).

Appendix A

Food Frequency Questionnaire (FFQ)
Instructions: For each food listed, check the box indicating how often on average you have used the amount specified during the last three months

Foods Consumed	Never or < 1 per mo.	1–3 per mo	1 per wk	2–4 per wk	5–6 per wk	1 per day	2–3 per day	4–5 per day	6+ per day
1.Milk, 1 cup									
2.Soy Milk, 1 cup									
3.Soy Protein bars, 1 bar									
4.Soy Protein powders, serving									
5.Soy Sauce, 1 Tablespoon									
6.Other non-dairy milks, Vit D fortified, 1 cup,									
7.Orange Juice, Vitamin D fortified (Tropicana), 1cup									
8.Cereal, Vitamin D fortified (Total Corn Flakes, Kelloggs Raisin Bran, Oat Bran, Cheerios), 3/4 cup									
9.Bread, commercial, not homemade									
10.Subway Sandwich, 6 inch									
11.Bagels, 1 each									
12.Yogurt, 1 cup									
13.Cheese, 2 ounce									
14.Egg, 1 whole									
15.Margarine, Vitamin D fortified (Promise, etc.), 1 teaspoon									
16.Liver, cooked, 3 ½ oz.									
17.Cod, cooked, 3 ½ oz									
18.Grouper cooked, 3 ½ oz									
19.Haddock cooked, 3 ½ oz									
20.Halibut, cooked, 3 ½ oz									
21.Herring, 3 1/2 oz.									
22.Mackerel, cooked, 3 ½ oz									
23. Perch, cooked, 3 ½ oz									
24.Salmon, cooked, 3 ½ oz									
25.Sardines, canned in oil, 3 ½ oz									
26.Sea Bass, cooked, 3 ½ oz									
27.Swordfish, cooked, 3 ½ oz									
28.Tukaoua, cooked, 3 ½ oz									
29.Tuna, Albacore, canned 3 ½ oz									
30.Tuna, light, canned, 3 ½ oz									
31.Walleye, cooked, 3 ½ oz									
32.Other fish, 3 ½ oz									
33.Clams, 4 oz									
34.Crabmeat, 4 oz									
35.Lobster, 4 oz									
36.Mussels, 4 oz									
37.Oysters, 4 oz									
38.Scallops, 4 oz									
39.Shrimp, 4 oz									

40.Sea weed (Nori, Komgu, Dulse, Wakame, Kelp)									
41.Iodized Table Salt									
42.Other Salt									

Supplements Consumed	Never or < 1 per mo.	1–3 per mo.	1 per wk	2–4 per wk	5–6 per wk	1 per day	2–3 per day	4–5 per day	6+ per day
1.Multiple Vitamin, 1 Tablet									
2.Calcium Vitamin, 1 Tablet									
3.Vitamin D , 1 Tablet									
(list amount _____)									
4.Calcium + Vitamin D (Viactiv), 1 Tablet									
5.Kelp (or other iodine supplement), 1 Tablet									
If you take any of the above , please list which you use, brand name, etc.									

Appendix B

Dietary Habits Survey

How frequently do you use the salt shaker to salt your foods?   Never   Sometimes   Usually

What type of salt do you use?

How frequently do you use salt in your cooking?   Never   Sometimes   Usually

What type of salt do you use?

Applicable Questions on the Dietary Preferences Survey

Do you follow a vegetarian Diet?   *Yes*   *No*

Do you shop at the Farmers Market or Food Coop)?   *Yes*   *No*   *Sometimes*

Do you belong to a CSA (Community Supported Agriculture)?   *Yes*   *No*

Do you have a garden and grow your own food?   *Yes*   *No*   *Sometimes*

Comments

References

1. Mariotti, S.; Beck-Peccoz, P. Physiology of the Hypothalamic-Pituitary-Thyroid Axis. In *Endotext*; Feingold, K.R., Anawalt, B., Boyce, A., Chrousos, G., Dungan, K., Grossman, A., Hershman, J.M., Kaltsas, G., Koch, C., Kopp, P., et al., Eds.; South Dartmouth, MA, USA, 2000; Available online: https://www.endotext.org/section/thyroiddiseasemanager/ (accessed on 15 July 2019).

2. Fuge, R.; Johnson, C.C. The geochemistry of iodine—A review. *Environ. Geochem. Health* **1986**, *8*, 31–54. [CrossRef]

3. Zimmermann, M.B. Iodine Deficiency. *Endocr. Rev.* **2009**, *30*, 376–408. [CrossRef]

4. Swanson, E.W.; Miller, J.K.; Mueller, F.J.; Patton, C.S.; Bacon, J.A.; Ramsey, N. Iodine in Milk and Meat of Dairy Cows Fed Different Amounts of Potassium Iodide or Ethylenediamine Dihydroiodide1. *J. Dairy Sci.* **1990**, *73*, 398–405. [CrossRef]

5. Galton, D.M.; Petersson, L.G.; Erb, H.N. Milk iodine residues in herds practicing iodophor premilking teat disinfection. *J. Dairy Sci.* **1986**, *69*, 267–271. [CrossRef]

6. van der Reijden, O.L.; Zimmermann, M.B.; Galetti, V. Iodine in dairy milk: Sources, concentrations and importance to human health. *Best Pract. Res. Clin. Endocrinol. Metab.* **2017**, *31*, 385–395. [CrossRef] [PubMed]

7. Niwattisaiwong, S. Iodine deficiency: Clinical implications. *Cleve Clin. J. Med.* **2017**, *84*, 236–244. [CrossRef] [PubMed]

8. Finer, L.B.; Henshaw, S.K. Disparities in rates of unintended pregnancy in the United States, 1994 and 2001. *Perspect. Sex. Reprod. Health* **2006**, *38*, 90–96. [CrossRef] [PubMed]

9. Zimmermann, M.B.; Andersson, M. Update on iodine status worldwide. *Curr. Opin. Endocrinol. Diabetes Obes.* **2012**, *19*, 382–387. [CrossRef]

10. Markel, H. "When it rains it pours": Endemic goiter, iodized salt, and David Murray Cowie, MD. *Am. J. Public Health* **1987**, *77*, 219–229. [CrossRef]

11. Gibson, R.S. *Principles of Nutritional Assessment*, 2nd ed.; Oxford University Press: New York, NY, USA, 2005; p. 908.

12. Caldwell, K.L.; Makhmudov, A.; Ely, E.; Jones, R.L.; Wang, R.Y. Iodine status of the US population, National Health and Nutrition Examination Survey, 2005–2006 and 2007–2008. *Thyroid* **2011**, *21*, 419–427. [CrossRef]

13. Krajčovičová-Kudláčková, M.; Bučková, K.; Klimeš, I.; Šeboková, E. Iodine Deficiency in Vegetarians and Vegans. *Ann. Nutr. Metab.* **2003**, *47*, 183–185. [CrossRef] [PubMed]

14. Pearce, E.N.; Pino, S.; He, X.; Bazrafshan, H.R.; Lee, S.L.; Braverman, L.E. Sources of Dietary Iodine: Bread, Cows' Milk, and Infant Formula in the Boston Area. *J. Clin. Endocrinol. Metab.* **2004**, *89*, 3421–3424. [CrossRef] [PubMed]

15. World Health Organization; The United Nations Children's Fund; International Council for Control of Iodine Deficiency Disorders. Assessment of iodine deficiency disorders and monitoring their elimination. In *A Guide for Programme Managers*; World Health Organization: Geneva, Switzerland, 2007.

16. Alderman, M.H.; Lamport, B. Moderate Sodium RestrictionDo the Benefits Justify the Hazards? *Am. J. Hypertens.* **1990**, *3*, 499–504. [CrossRef] [PubMed]

17. Tayie, F.A.K.; Jourdan, K. Hypertension, dietary salt restriction, and iodine deficiency among adults. *Am. J. Hypertens.* **2010**, *23*, 1095–1102. [CrossRef] [PubMed]

18. Boon, C.S.; Taylor, C.L.; Henney, J.E. *Strategies to Reduce Sodium Intake in the United States*; National Academies Press: Washington, DC, USA, 2010.

19. Appel, L.J.; Frohlich, E.D.; Hall, J.E.; Pearson, T.A.; Sacco, R.L.; Seals, D.R.; Sacks, F.M.; Smith, S.C., Jr.; Vafiadis, D.K.; Van Horn, L.V. The importance of population-wide sodium reduction as a means to prevent cardiovascular disease and stroke: A call to action from the American Heart Association. *Circulation* **2011**, *123*, 1138–1143. [CrossRef] [PubMed]

20. Dean, S. Medical Nutrition Therapy for Thyroid, Adrenal, and Other Endocrine Disorders. In *Krause's Food and the Nutrition Care Process*, 14th ed.; Mahn, L.K., Raymond, J.L., Eds.; Elsevier: Saint Louis, MO, USA, 2017; pp. 619–630.

21. National Instituesd of Health Office of Dietary Supplements. *Iodine Fact. Sheet for Health Professionals*; U.S. Department of Health & Human Services: Bethesda, MD, USA, 2019. Available online: https://ods.od.nih.gov/factsheets/Iodine-HealthProfessional/90/history/ (accessed on 2 April 2019).

22. König, F.; Andersson, M.; Hotz, K.; Aeberli, I.; Zimmermann, M.B. Ten repeat collections for urinary iodine from spot samples or 24-hour samples are needed to reliably estimate individual iodine status in women. *J. Nutr.* **2011**, *141*, 2049–2054. [CrossRef] [PubMed]

23. Skeaff, S.; Thomson, C.; Eastman, C. Iodine deficiency does exist but is difficult to assess in individuals. *N. Z. Med. J.* **2009**, *122*, 101–102.

24. Johnson, E.C.; Huffman, A.E.; Yoder, H.; Dolci, A.; Perrier, E.T.; Larson-Meyer, D.E.; Armstrong, L.E. Urinary Markers of Hydration during 3-day Water Restriction and Graded Rehydration. *Eur. J. Nutr.* **2019**, 1–11. [CrossRef]

25. Forde, C. Exercise Prescription for the Prevention and Treatment of Disease: Scoring the International Physical Activity Questionnaire (IPAQ). Available online: https://ugc.futurelearn.com/uploads/files/bc/c5/bcc53b14-ec1e-4d90-88e3-1568682f32ae/IPAQ_PDF.pdf (accessed on 2 April 2019).

26. Zimmermann, M.B. Iodine requirements and the risks and benefits of correcting iodine deficiency in populations. *J. Trace Elem. Med. Biol.* **2008**, *22*, 81–92. [CrossRef]

27. Trumbo, P.; Yates, A.A.; Schlicker, S.; Poos, M. Dietary reference intakes: Vitamin A, vitamin K, arsenic, boron, chromium, copper, iodine, iron, manganese, molybdenum, nickel, silicon, vanadium, and zinc. *J. Acad. Nutr. Diet.* **2001**, *101*, 294.

28. Halliday, T.M.; Peterson, N.J.; Thomas, J.J.; Kleppinger, K.; Hollis, B.W.; Larson-Meyer, D.E. Vitamin D status relative to diet, lifestyle, injury, and illness in college athletes. *Med. Sci. Sports Exerc.* **2011**, *43*, 335–343. [CrossRef] [PubMed]

29. Total Diet Study Elements Results Summary Statistics—Market Baskets 2006 through 2013. Available online: https://www.fda.gov/downloads/food...totaldietstudy/ucm184301.pdf (accessed on 4 March 2019).

30. Bath, S.C.; Hill, S.; Infante, H.G.; Elghul, S.; Nezianya, C.J.; Rayman, M.P. Iodine concentration of milk-alternative drinks available in the UK in comparison with cows' milk. *Br. J. Nutr.* **2017**, *118*, 525–532. [CrossRef] [PubMed]

31. Low Iodine Diet. Available online: https://www.thyroid.org/wp-content/uploads/patients/brochures/LowIodineDietFAQ.pdf (accessed on 4 March 2019).

32. Pehrsson, P.R.; Patterson, K.Y.; Spungen, J.H.; Wirtz, M.S.; Andrews, K.W.; Dwyer, J.T.; Swanson, C.A. Iodine in food-and dietary supplement–composition databases. *Am. J. Clin. Nutr.* **2016**, *104*, 868S–876S. [CrossRef] [PubMed]

33. Teas, J.; Pino, S.; Critchley, A.; Braverman, L.E. Variability of iodine content in common commercially available edible seaweeds. *Thyroid* **2004**, *14*, 836–841. [CrossRef]

34. Pennington, J.A.; Schoen, S.A. Total diet study: Estimated dietary intakes of nutritional elements, 1982–1991. *Int. J. Vitam. Nutr. Res.* **1996**, *66*, 350–362.

35. Dasgupta, P.K.; Liu, Y.; Dyke, J.V. Iodine Nutrition: Iodine Content of Iodized Salt in the United States. *Environ. Sci. Technol.* **2008**, *42*, 1315–1323. [CrossRef]

36. Baloch, Z.; Carayon, P.; Conte-Devolx, B.; Demers, L.M.; Feldt-Rasmussen, U.; Henry, J.F.; LiVosli, V.A.; Niccoli-Sire, P.; John, R.; Ruf, J. Laboratory medicine practice guidelines. Laboratory support for the diagnosis and monitoring of thyroid disease. *Thyroid Off. J. Am. Thyroid Assoc.* **2003**, *13*, 3.

37. Hagströmer, M.; Oja, P.; Sjöström, M. The International Physical Activity Questionnaire (IPAQ): A study of concurrent and construct validity. *Public Health Nutr.* **2006**, *9*, 755–762. [CrossRef]

38. Stanbury, J.B.; Ermans, A.E.; Bourdoux, P.; Todd, C.; Oken, E.; Tonglet, R.; Vidor, G.; Braverman, L.E.; Medeiros-Neto, G. Iodine-induced hyperthyroidism: Occurrence and epidemiology. *Thyroid* **1998**, *8*, 83–100. [CrossRef]

39. Hemken, R.W. Milk and meat iodine content: Relation to human health. *J. Am. Vet. Med Assoc.* **1980**, *176*, 1119–1121.

40. Kaufmann, S.; Wolfram, G.; Delange, F.; Rambeck, W.A. Iodine supplementation of laying hen feed: A supplementary measure to eliminate iodine deficiency in humans? *Z. Ernährungswiss.* **1998**, *37*, 288–293. [CrossRef] [PubMed]

41. Spitzweg, C.; Joba, W.; Eisenmenger, W.; Heufelder, A.E. Analysis of human sodium iodide symporter gene expression in extrathyroidal tissues and cloning of its complementary deoxyribonucleic acids from salivary gland, mammary gland, and gastric mucosa. *J. Clin. Endocrinol. Metab.* **1998**, *83*, 1746–1751. [CrossRef] [PubMed]

42. Hubble, I.B.; Mein, G.A. Effect of pre-milking udder preparation of dairy cows on milk quality. *Aust. J. Dairy Technol. (Aust.)* **1986**, *41*, 66–70.

43. Chandler, W.L. Iodine on the Poultry farm. *Poult. Sci.* **1926**, *6*, 31–35. [CrossRef]

44. Travnicek, J.; Kroupova, V.; Herzig, I.; Kursa, J. Iodine content in consumer hen eggs. *Vet. Med. Praha* **2006**, *51*, 93. [CrossRef]

45. Bourre, J.M.; Galea, F. An important source of omega-3 fatty acids, vitamins D and E, carotenoids, iodine and selenium: A new natural multi-enriched egg. *J. Nutr. Health Aging* **2006**, *10*, 371.

46. Michella, S.M.; Slaugh, B.T. Producing and marketing a specialty egg. *Poult. Sci.* **2000**, *79*, 975–976. [CrossRef]

47. Liu, L.; Li, X.; Wang, H.; Cao, X.; Ma, W. Reduction of iodate in iodated salt to iodide during cooking with iodine as measured by an improved HPLC/ICP-MS method. *J. Nutr. Biochem.* **2017**, *42*, 95–100. [CrossRef]

48. Meinhardt, A.K.; Muller, A.; Burcza, A.; Greiner, R. Influence of cooking on the iodine content in potatoes, pasta and rice using iodized salt. *Food Chem.* **2019**, *301*. [CrossRef]

49. Andersson, M.; de Benoist, B.; Rogers, L. Epidemiology of iodine deficiency: Salt iodisation and iodine status. *Best Pract. Res. Clin. Endocrinol. Metab.* **2010**, *24*, 1–11. [CrossRef]

50. Kim, J.Y.; Moon, S.J.; Kim, K.R.; Sohn, C.Y.; Oh, J.J. Dietary iodine intake and urinary iodine excretion in normal Korean adults. *Yonsei Med. J.* **1998**, *39*, 355–362. [CrossRef] [PubMed]

51.   Ballew, C. Final Report on the Alaska Traditional Diet Survey. Available online: http://anthctoday.org/epicenter/publications/Reports_Pubs/traditional_diet.pdf (accessed on 4 March 2019).

52.   Gershengorn, M.C.; Wolff, J.; Larsen, P.R. Thyroid-pituitary feedback during iodine repletion. *J. Clin. Endocrinol. Metab.* **1976**, *43*, 601–605. [CrossRef] [PubMed]

53.   Chung, H.R. Iodine and thyroid function. *Ann. Pediatric Endocrinol. Metab.* **2014**, *19*, 8–12. [CrossRef] [PubMed]

54.   Morton, M.E.; Chaikoff, I.L.; Rosenfeld, S. Inhibiting effect of inorganic iodide on the formation in vitro of thyroxine and diiodotyrosine by surviving thyroid tissue. *J. Biol. Chem.* **1944**, *154*, 381–387.

55.   Wolff, J.; Chaikoff, I.L. Plasma inorganic iodide as a homeostatic regulator of thyroid function. *J. Biol. Chem.* **1948**, *174*, 555–564. [PubMed]

56.   Ershow, A.; Skeaff, S.; Merkel, J.; Pehrsson, P. Development of databases on iodine in foods and dietary supplements. *Nutrients* **2018**, *10*, 100. [CrossRef] [PubMed]

57.   Hetzel, B.S.; Dunn, J.T. The iodine deficiency disorders: Their nature and prevention. *Annu. Rev. Nutr.* **1989**, *9*, 21–38. [CrossRef]

58.   Rasmussen, L.B.; Ovesen, L.; Christiansen, E. Day-to-day and within-day variation in urinary iodine excretion. *Eur. J. Clin. Nutr.* **1999**, *53*, 401. [CrossRef]

59.   Als, C.; Helbling, A.; Peter, K.; Haldimann, M.; Zimmerli, B.; Gerber, H. Urinary iodine concentration follows a circadian rhythm: A study with 3023 spot urine samples in adults and children. *J. Clin. Endocrinol. Metab.* **2000**, *85*, 1367–1369. [CrossRef]

60.   Als, C.; Haldimann, M.; Bürgi, E.; Donati, F.; Gerber, H.; Zimmerli, B. Swiss pilot study of individual seasonal fluctuations of urinary iodine concentration over two years: Is age-dependency linked to the major source of dietary iodine? *Eur. J. Clin. Nutr.* **2003**, *57*, 636. [CrossRef]

61.   Moreno-Reyes, R.; Carpentier, Y.A.; Macours, P.; Gulbis, B.; Corvilain, B.; Glinoer, D.; Goldman, S. Seasons but not ethnicity influence urinary iodine concentrations in Belgian adults. *Eur. J. Nutr.* **2011**, *50*, 285–290. [CrossRef] [PubMed]

62.   Bourdoux, P. Evaluation of the iodine intake: Problems of the iodine/creatinine ratio-comparison with iodine excretion and daily fluctuations of iodine concentration. *Exp. Clin. Endocrinol. Diabetes* **1998**, *106*, S17–S20. [CrossRef] [PubMed]

63.   Ma, Z.F.; Skeaff, S.A. Thyroglobulin as a biomarker of iodine deficiency: A review. *Thyroid* **2014**, *24*, 1195–1209. [CrossRef] [PubMed]

64.   Spencer, C.A.; Wang, C.-C. Thyroglobulin measurement: Techniques, clinical benefits, and pitfalls. *Endocrinol. Metab. Clin. N. Am.* **1995**, *24*, 841–863. [CrossRef]

The Joint Role of Thyroid Function and Iodine Status on Risk of Preterm Birth and Small for Gestational Age: A Population-Based Nested Case-Control Study of Finnish Women

Alexandra C. Purdue-Smithe [1], Tuija Männistö [2,3,4,5], Griffith A. Bell [6,7], Sunni L. Mumford [1], Aiyi Liu [8], Kurunthachalam Kannan [9], Un-Jung Kim [9], Eila Suvanto [2], Heljä-Marja Surcel [10,11], Mika Gissler [5,12] and James L. Mills [1,*]

[1]   Epidemiology Branch, Division of Intramural Population Health Research, *Eunice Kennedy Shriver* National Institute of Child Health and Human Development, National Institutes of Health, Bethesda, MD 20892, USA; alexandra.purdue-smithe@nih.gov (A.C.P.-S.); mumfords@mail.nih.gov (S.L.M.)

[2]   Northern Finland Laboratory Centre NordLab, 90120 Oulu, Finlan; Tuija.Mannisto@Nordlab.fi (T.M.); Eila.Suvanto@ppshp.fi (E.S.)

[3]   Department of Clinical Chemistry, University of Oulu, 90120 Oulu, Finland

[4]   Medical Research Center Oulu, Oulu University Hospital and University of Oulu, 90120 Oulu, Finland

[5]   Finnish Institute for Health and Welfare, 00290 Helsinki, Finland; mika.gissler@thl.fi

[6]   Ariadne Labs, Brigham and Women's Hospital, Harvard T.H. Chan School of Public Health, Boston, MA 02115, USA; griffith.bell@gmail.com

[7]   Harvard T.H. Chan School of Public Health, Department of Health Policy and Management, Boston, MA 02115, USA

[8]   Biostatistics and Bioinformatics Branch, Division of Intramural Population Health Research, *Eunice Kennedy Shriver* National Institute of Child Health and Human Development, National Institutes of Health, Bethesda, MD 20892, USA; liua@mail.nih.gov

[9]   Wadsworth Center, New York State Department of Health, Albany, NY 12201, USA; kurunthachalam.kannan@health.ny.gov (K.K.); changetm2011@gmail.com (U.-J.K.)

[10] Biobank Borealis of Northern Finland, Oulu University Hospital, 90120 Oulu, Finland; helja-marja.surcel@thl.fi

[11] Faculty of Medicine, University of Oulu, 90120 Oulu, Finland

[12] Karolinska Institute, 17177 Stockholm, Sweden

*   Correspondence: millsj@exchange.nih.gov

Abstract: Normal maternal thyroid function during pregnancy is essential for fetal development and depends upon an adequate supply of iodine. Little is known about how iodine status is associated with preterm birth and small for gestational age (SGA) in mildly iodine insufficient populations. Our objective was to evaluate associations of early pregnancy serum iodine, thyroglobulin (Tg), and thyroid-stimulating hormone (TSH) with odds of preterm birth and SGA in a prospective, population-based, nested case-control study from all births in Finland (2012–2013). Cases of preterm birth (n = 208) and SGA (n = 209) were randomly chosen from among all singleton births. Controls were randomly chosen from among singleton births that were not preterm (n = 242) or SGA (n = 241) infants during the same time period. Women provided blood samples at 10–14 weeks' gestation for serum iodide, Tg and TSH measurement. We used logistic regression to estimate odds ratios (ORs) and 95% confidence intervals (CIs) for preterm birth and SGA. Each log-unit increase in serum iodide was associated with higher odds of preterm birth (adjusted OR = 1.19, 95% CI = 1.02–1.40), but was not associated with SGA (adjusted OR = 1.01, 95% CI = 0.86–1.18). Tg was not associated with preterm birth (OR per 1 log-unit increase = 0.87, 95% CI = 0.73–1.05), but was inversely associated with SGA (OR per log-unit increase = 0.78, 95% CI = 0.65–0.94). Neither high nor low TSH (versus normal) were associated with either outcome. These findings suggest that among Finnish women, iodine status is not related to SGA, but higher serum iodide may be positively associated with preterm birth.

Keywords: iodine; thyroid hormones; thyroglobulin; thyroid stimulating hormone; pregnancy; preterm birth; small for gestational age

---

1. Introduction

Normal maternal thyroid function during pregnancy is essential for fetal development [1]. Hypothyroidism is associated with adverse pregnancy outcomes including pregnancy loss, preeclampsia, and preterm birth, as well as cognitive deficiencies and cretinism in the offspring [2]. Iodine, found in fish, eggs, dairy products, and iodized salt [3], plays an essential role in the production of thyroid hormones. Thyroid hormone production is regulated by the hypothalamic-pituitary-thyroid axis via thyroid-stimulating hormone (TSH) and requires the iodination of thyroglobulin (Tg) in the follicular lumen of thyrocytes [1]. Pregnant women are especially vulnerable to iodine deficiency due to fetal dependency on the maternal iodine supply and to a lesser extent, hemodilution, increased renal clearance of inorganic iodide, and estrogen-stimulated production of Tg, which collectively necessitate higher iodine intake [4].

Despite increased risk of iodine deficiency during pregnancy, even in developed countries [5,6], and ample data indicating that thyroid dysfunction is associated with adverse neonatal and obstetric outcomes, relatively few studies have evaluated how iodine status during pregnancy is related to preterm birth and infants being born small for gestational age (SGA), and the results are conflicting [7–13]. Importantly, previous studies were conducted in populations with high prevalence of other nutritional deficiencies and concurrent illnesses or included mostly iodine sufficient pregnant women [9,12]. Several of these studies also lacked information on thyroid hormones and therefore were unable to evaluate whether associations of iodine with preterm birth and SGA may be different among potentially hypo-or hyperthyroid women [9–11,13]. Additionally, prior studies used a single spot urinary iodine measurement to classify iodine status, which has been shown to have high intraindividual variability reflective of recent dietary intake, seasonal variation, urine dilution, and circadian rhythmicity [13–16]. Although urine iodine concentrations are useful for assessing the iodine status of whole populations, serum iodide may be less sensitive to recent dietary intake and may, therefore, better reflect individual long-term and bioavailable iodine status [17–19], reducing potential for misclassification.

The aim of the present study was to evaluate associations of serum iodide concentrations and thyroid hormones indicative of iodine status (i.e., Tg and TSH) with risk of preterm birth and SGA among pregnant Finnish women, a population considered to be mildly iodine deficient, but with relatively low prevalence of other nutritional deficiencies [3].

2. Materials and Methods

2.1. Study Population

We conducted a population-based, nested case-control study within the Finnish Maternity Cohort (FMC), using the Finnish Medical Birth Register (MBR) to ascertain pregnancy and perinatal outcome data. Beginning in 1983, the FMC has collected more than 2 million serum samples from more than 950,000 pregnant women living in Finland, which reflects ~98% coverage of the pregnant population. Blood samples were collected to screen for hepatitis B, human immunodeficiency virus (HIV), syphilis, and rubella antibodies. The samples were drawn in general between 10 and 14 weeks gestation at local maternity care units and sent to the prenatal serology laboratory of the Finnish Institute for Health and Welfare in Oulu. There, sera were separated by centrifugation, screening analyses were performed and the remaining serum (1–3 mL) was stored at −25 °C.

Biochemical data were linked to clinical data from the MBR via unique personal identification numbers given to all Finnish citizens and residents at birth or at time of permanent residence. The MBR includes data on all live births and stillbirths in Finland with a birth weight ≥500 g or a gestational age at birth ≥22 gestational weeks. Maternal data collected by the MBR includes age, height and weight, socioeconomic status based on self-reported occupation, marital status, pregnancy history, smoking status, and other factors. Data collected on infants included sex, gestational age at birth, and birth height and weight.

Women gave written informed consent for their samples to be used for research purposes. This study was approved by the steering committee of the FMC, the ethical review boards of the Northern Ostrobothnia Hospital District and the Finnish Institute for Health and Welfare, Oulu, Finland, and the Office of Human Subjects Research, National Institutes of Health, Bethesda, MD, USA (#13459).

2.2. Case and Control Ascertainment

We randomly selected 200 cases of preterm birth (defined as a live birth <37 weeks gestation) and 250 potential controls from among all singleton births in Finland between 2012 and 2013 with available serum samples in the FMC. Because the 250 potential controls were randomly selected without regard to case/control status, 8 control pregnancies were delivered preterm and were thus reclassified as cases. After reclassification, the final analytic sample included 208 cases and 242 controls. Similarly, we randomly selected 200 cases of SGA (defined as birthweight <10th percentile for gestational age), using the same control group. Nine control pregnancies were SGA and reclassified as such, resulting in 209 SGA cases and 241 controls.

2.3. Measurement of Iodide, Thyroglobulin, and Thyroid-Stimulating Hormone

Details regarding the iodide measurement in this study population have been published previously and are provided in Appendix A [20]. Briefly, serum samples were thawed at room temperature, vortexed, and transferred to polypropylene tubes. Samples were pretreated, centrifuged, and analyzed by high-performance liquid chromatography (Alliance 2695 HPLC) coupled with electrospray triple-quadrupole mass spectrometry (Micromass, ESI–MS/MS; Waters Corporation, Milford, MA, USA). Identification and quantification of ^{18}O-labeled-perchlorate, ^{13}C-labeled-thiocyante, and iodide was performed using electrospray negative ionization (ESI-) and multiple reaction monitoring. Serum Tg and TSH concentrations were measured using a commercial immunoassay (Siemens AG, Munich, Germany), as they have been shown to be reliable markers of thyroid function in pregnant women [21]. The intra- and inter-assay coefficients of variation for Tg were <8% and <12%, respectively, and for TSH <5% and <5%, respectively.

2.4. Statistical Analysis

Characteristics of the cases and controls were compared using t-tests for continuous variables and χ^2 tests for categorical variables. Equivalent non-parametric tests were used where appropriate. For analyses evaluating continuous exposures, serum iodide, Tg, and TSH values were normalized by log-transformation. Participants were divided into quartiles of iodide and Tg based on the distribution of these biomarkers in the control group. For TSH, we categorized participants as having high TSH (>3.1 and >3.5 mIU/L in the 1st and 2nd trimesters, respectively), normal TSH (0.1–3.1 and 0.2–3.5 in the 1st and 2nd trimesters, respectively), or low TSH (<0.1 and <0.2 mIU/L in the 1st and 2nd trimesters, respectively), according to previously defined reference ranges for this population [22].

Using logistic regression, we estimated unadjusted odds ratios (ORs) and 95% confidence intervals (CIs) for preterm birth and SGA according to each biomarker. We then estimated adjusted ORs and 95% CIs adjusting for maternal age, maternal body mass index (BMI), socioeconomic status, smoking status, parity, and marital status. Covariates were selected for inclusion in multivariable models based on directed acyclic graphs [23]. Individuals with missing data on BMI (N = 7 for preterm birth and N = 3 for SGA) were dropped from multivariable analyses.

We also examined possible non-linear associations of iodide with preterm birth and SGA non-parametrically utilizing restricted cubic spline models. In these models, we specified 3 knots and evaluated the individual spline term contributions to the model fit and overall test for nonlinearity.

In sensitivity analyses, we excluded women with conditions associated with medically-indicated preterm birth (i.e., chronic hypertension, gestational hypertension, gestational diabetes, pre-existing diabetes, thyroid disease) to determine whether these conditions may have influenced the results. All analyses were run using SAS, version 9.4 (SAS Institute Inc., Cary, NC, U.S.).

3. Results

3.1. Descriptive Characteristics

Characteristics of preterm birth and SGA cases and controls at blood draw are presented in Table 1. For preterm birth, cases and controls were similar with regard to maternal age, BMI, smoking status, marital status, parity, gravidity, and socioeconomic status (SES). Preterm birth cases and controls were also similar in terms of gestational age at blood draw (10.9 weeks vs. 10.8 weeks). As expected, cases were more likely to have chronic hypertension (10% vs. 3%), preeclampsia (30% vs. 3%), Type 1 or 2 diabetes (13% vs. 1%), and gestational diabetes (38% vs. 22%), compared to controls. For SGA, cases had lower BMI (24 vs. 25 kg/m^2), gravidity (1.3 vs. 1.4) and parity (0.8 vs. 1.1) than controls, and were also more likely to be smokers (52% vs. 37%). SGA cases were also more likely than controls to have preeclampsia during the pregnancy (16% vs. 4%). The Spearman rank correlation coefficients for each biomarker were as follows: iodide and Tg, $r_s = 0.02$ ($P = 0.54$); iodide and TSH, $r_s = 0.001$ ($P = 0.97$); and Tg and TSH, $r_s = -0.13$ ($P < 0.001$).

Table 1. Maternal characteristics at blood draw according to preterm birth and small for gestational age cases and controls in the Finnish Maternity Cohort and Medical Birth Register, 2012–2013.

Characteristic [1]	Preterm Birth			Small for Gestational Age		
	Controls (n = 242)	Cases (n = 208)	P-value [2]	Controls (n = 241)	Cases (n = 209)	P-value [2]
Maternal age (years)	29.5 (5.3)	29.8 (5.5)	0.49	29.5 (5.3)	29.7 (5.6)	0.70
Body mass index (kg/m^2)	24.6 (4.4)	25.3 (6.0)	0.75	24.8 (4.9)	23.6 (5.1)	<0.001
Gravidity	1.4 (1.8)	1.4 (1.8)	0.80	1.4 (1.8)	1.3 (2.2)	0.03
Parity	1.1 (1.6)	0.9 (1.4)	0.19	1.1 (1.6)	0.8 (1.5)	0.01
Gestational age at screening (weeks)	10.9 (2.9)	10.8 (3.0)	0.89	10.9 (2.9)	11.4 (4.0)	0.12
Gestational age at birth (weeks)	39.7 (1.1)	34.1 (2.7)	<0.01	39.6 (1.5)	38.4 (2.9)	<0.001
Iodide (ng/mL)	28.1 (28.5)	32.8 (31.1)	0.02	28.2 (28.3)	27.7 (28.2)	0.82
Thyroglobulin (ng/mL)	29.6 (29.5)	31.5 (63.3)	0.36	29.9 (29.6)	27.9 (32.9)	0.05
Thyroid stimulating hormone (mIU/L)	1.2 (0.8)	1.3 (2.4)	0.25	1.2 (0.85)	1.4 (2.15)	0.68
Nulliparous	105 (43.4)	108 (51.9)	0.07	103 (42.7)	120 (57.4)	<0.01
Smoking status			0.33			0.03
Nonsmoker	200 (82.6)	164 (78.8)		199 (82.6)	155 (74.2)	
Smoker	37 (15.3)	35 (16.8)		37 (15.4)	52 (24.9)	
Unknown	5 (2.1)	9 (4.3)		5 (2.1)	2 (1.0)	
Socioeconomic status			0.32			0.11
Blue-collar	30 (12.4)	31 (14.9)		31 (12.9)	30 (14.4)	
Lower white-collar	64 (26.4)	60 (28.8)		62 (25.7)	50 (23.9)	
Upper white-collar	28 (11.6)	29 (13.9)		28 (11.6)	34 (16.3)	
Entrepreneur	10 (4.1)	4 (1.9)		10 (4.2)	3 (1.4)	
Student	25 (10.3)	12 (5.8)		24 (10.0)	10 (4.8)	
Other/unknown	85 (35.1)	72 (34.6)		86 (35.7)	82 (39.2)	
Diagnosed thyroid disease	0 (0)	7 (3.4)	<0.01	0 (0)	1 (0.5)	0.28
Chronic hypertension	3 (1.2)	10 (4.8)	0.024	3 (1.2)	4 (1.9)	0.71
Preeclampsia	3 (1.2)	30 (14.4)	<0.01	4 (1.7)	16 (7.7)	<0.01
Gestational hypertension	6 (2.5)	11 (5.3)	0.12	6 (2.5)	11 (5.3)	0.14
Type I or type II diabetes	1 (0.4)	13 (6.3)	<0.01	2 (0.8)	0 (0)	0.50
Gestational diabetes	22 (9.1)	38 (18.3)	0.02	23 (9.5)	23 (11.0)	0.64
Marital status			0.41			0.15
Married or cohabiting	215 (88.8)	176 (84.6)		211 (87.6)	177 (84.7)	
Single or widowed	26 (10.7)	31 (14.9)		30 (12.5)	29 (13.9)	
Unknown	1 (0.4)	1 (0.5)		0 (0)	3 (1.4)	

[1] Values are means (SD) for continuous data and N (%) for categorical data. [2] P-values were estimated using t-tests for continuous data and χ^2 tests for categorical data. Equivalent non-parametric tests were used where appropriate.

3.2. Serum Iodine, Thyroid Hormones, and Preterm Birth

In unadjusted models, each 1 log-unit increase in serum iodide was positively associated with preterm birth (unadjusted OR = 1.22, 95% CI = 1.04–1.42) (Table 2). After adjusting for age, BMI, smoking, and other factors, the positive association persisted (adjusted OR = 1.19, 95% CI = 1.02–1.40), and was robust to the exclusion of women with conditions related to preterm birth (OR = 1.29, 95% CI = 1.06–1.58). In unadjusted models evaluating quartiles of iodide, the OR for preterm birth comparing women with high (quartile 4) versus moderate (quartiles 2+3) serum iodide was 1.32 (95% CI = 0.86–2.04). The OR for preterm birth comparing low (quartile 1) versus moderate (quartiles 2 + 3) serum iodide was 0.75 (95% CI = 0.46–1.22). In adjusted models, the ORs for preterm birth comparing women with high (quartile 4) and low (quartile 1) versus those with moderate (quartiles 2 and 3) serum iodide were 1.22 (95% CI = 0.78–1.93) and 0.76 (95% CI = 0.46–1.26), respectively. In spline analyses, no signifcant departure of linearity was observed for serum iodide and preterm birth (P for non-linearity > 0.05). No associations were observed for Tg and TSH and preterm birth (adjusted OR = 0.87, 95% CI = 0.73–1.05 and OR = 0.97, 95% CI = 0.80–1.19, respectively).

Table 2. Unadjusted and adjusted odds ratios (ORs) and 95% confidence intervals (CIs) for preterm birth according to maternal serum iodide, thyroglobulin, and thyroid stimulating hormone in the Finnish Maternity Cohort and Maternal Birth Register, 2012–2013 [1,2].

Biomarker	Cases: Controls	Median	Unadjusted OR (95% CI)	Adjusted [3] OR (95% CI)
Iodide (ng/mL)				
Quartile (Q)1	38:60	3.4	0.75 (0.46–1.22)	0.76 (0.46–1.26)
Q2 + Q3	102:121	20.3	1 (referent)	1 (referent)
Q4	68:61	59.3	1.32 (0.86–2.04)	1.22 (0.78–1.93)
Log(iodide)	208:242		1.22 (1.04–1.42)	1.19 (1.02–1.40)
Log(iodide) [4]	132:210		1.29 (1.07–1.57)	1.29 (1.06–1.58)
Thyroglobulin (ng/mL)				
Q1	59:59	7.7	1 (referent)	1 (referent)
Q2	55:60	17.4	0.91 (0.55–1.53)	0.83 (0.49–1.41)
Q3	37:60	26.7	0.62 (0.36–1.07)	0.59 (0.34–1.04)
Q4	57:60	52.1	0.95 (0.57–1.58)	0.88 (0.51–1.50)
Log(thyroglobulin)	208:239		0.91 (0.76–1.08)	0.87 (0.73–1.05)
TSH (mIU/L)				
Low	5:11	0.04	0.51 (0.18–1.50)	0.57 (0.19–1.70)
Normal	196:217	1.04	1 (referent)	1 (referent)
High	7:11	3.5	1.14 (0.32–3.95)	1.17 (0.31–4.38)
Log(TSH)	208:239		0.99 (0.82–1.20)	0.97 (0.80–1.19)

[1] ORs and 95% CIs were estimated using logistic regression. [2] Data are missing for 3 controls. [3] Multivariable models are adjusted for maternal age, maternal body mass index, socioeconomic status, smoking status, parity, and marital status. [4] Analyses excluding women with conditions indicated for preterm birth (i.e., preeclampsia, chronic hypertension, gestational hypertension, gestational diabetes, pre-existing diabetes, thyroid disease)

3.3. Serum Iodide, Thyroid Hormones, and Small for Gestational Age

Serum iodide was not associated with odds of having an SGA infant in unadjusted or adjusted models. (Table 3) For example, the unadjusted OR for each log-unit increase in serum iodide was 0.99 (95% CI = 0.85–1.14). Similarly, in unadjusted models, the OR for SGA comparing high (quartile 4) and low (quartile 1) versus moderate (quartiles 2 + 3) serum iodide was 1.15 (95% CI = 0.74–1.80) and 1.05 (95% CI = 0.85–1.14), respectively. Adjustment for age, BMI, and other factors resulted in similar findings (OR per 1 log-unit increase in serum iodide = 1.01, 95% CI = 0.86–1.18). In unadjusted models, log-transformed Tg was inversely associated with SGA (unadjusted OR = 0.84, 95% CI = 0.71-0.99). This inverse association was somewhat stronger after adjustment in multivariable analyses (adjusted OR = 0.78, 95% CI = 0.65–0.94). Likewise, in adjusted models, the OR comparing high (quartile 4) versus low (quartile 1) Tg was 0.45 (95% CI = 0.25–0.79). TSH was not associated with SGA (high versus normal OR = 0.56, 95% CI = 0.14–2.22; low versus normal OR = 1.11, 95% CI = 0.44–2.79). Spline analyses revealed no significant departures of linearity for serum iodide and SGA (P for non-linearity > 0.05).

Table 3. Unadjusted and adjusted odds ratios (ORs) and 95% confidence intervals (CIs) for small for gestational age according to maternal serum iodide, thyroglobulin, and thyroid stimulating hormone in the Finnish Maternity Cohort and Maternal Birth Register, 2012–2013 [1,2].

Biomarker	Cases: Controls	Median	Unadjusted OR (95% CI)	Adjusted [3] OR (95% CI)
Iodide (ng/mL)				
Quartile (Q)1	52:60	3.3	1.05 (0.85–1.14)	1.01 (0.68–1.79)
Q2 + Q3	99:120	19.3	1 (referent)	1 (referent)
Q4	58:61	59.3	1.15 (0.74–1.80)	1.28 (0.79–2.08)
Log(iodide)	209:241		0.99 (0.85–1.14)	1.01 (0.86–1.18)
Log(iodide) [4]	162:206		0.91 (0.77–1.07)	0.91 (0.76–1.09)
Thyroglobulin (ng/mL)				
Q1	75:58	8.3	1 (referent)	1 (referent)
Q2	50:61	17.7	0.63 (0.38–1.05)	0.52 (0.30–0.89)
Q3	36:59	28.2	0.47 (0.27–0.81)	0.41 (0.23–0.72)
Q4	45:60	52.3	0.58 (0.35–0.97)	0.45 (0.25–0.79)
Log(thyroglobulin)	206:238		0.84 (0.71–0.99)	0.78 (0.65–0.94)
TSH (mIU/L)				
Low	10:11	0.04	1.04 (0.43–2.50)	1.11 (0.44–2.79)
Normal	193:221	1.4	1 (referent)	1 (referent)
High	5:6	4.1	0.95 (0.29–3.18)	0.56 (0.14–2.22)
Log(TSH)	208:238		1.05 (0.88–1.26)	1.04 (0.86–1.26)

[1] ORs and 95% CIs were estimated using logistic regression. [2] Data are missing for 3 controls. [3] Multivariable models are adjusted for maternal age, maternal body mass index, socioeconomic status, smoking status, parity, and marital status. [4] Analyses excluding women with conditions indicated for preterm birth (i.e., preeclampsia, chronic hypertension, gestational hypertension, gestational diabetes, pre-existing diabetes, thyroid disease)

4. Discussion

In this population-based, nested case-control study, we found that neither low- nor high-serum iodide was associated with SGA, and some suggestion that higher serum iodide may be associated with increased risk of preterm birth. Levels of TSH, which were largely within the normal range, indicated a mostly euthyroid population. Tg, which is generally higher during periods of both iodine insufficiency and extreme excess [24–26], was inversely associated with risk of having an SGA infant, but was not associated with preterm birth. Levels of TSH were not associated with either outcome, although very few women had values considered to be above or below the normal range in this population. Collectively, our findings suggest that iodine insufficiency, within the range observed among pregnant Finnish women, likely does not play a role in preterm birth or SGA, but that higher serum iodide may be associated with increased risk of preterm birth.

To date, only a handful of studies have evaluated associations of iodine status with preterm birth and SGA, and data are mixed [7–13]. A recent prospective study of pregnant women in the UK reported U-shaped relationships between urinary iodine concentrations and risks of preterm birth and SGA, with elevated risks observed among women with urinary iodine concentration (UIC) <50 and ≥250 µg/L versus those with UIC in the 150–249 µg/L group; however, confidence intervals were wide and included the null value [10]. Another prospective study of pregnant women in the UK with low obstetrical risk reported a borderline significant increased risk of having an SGA infant with increasing UIC, but no association with preterm birth [13]. Similarly, in a largely iodine deficient population of pregnant women in Thailand, insufficient (UIC <150 µg/L) versus sufficient/excess (UIC ≥150 µg/L) iodine status was associated with increased risks of both preterm birth and low birth weight (LBW) infants [9]. Similar associations were observed among pregnant Chinese women, in which UIC

<50 μg/L versus ≥50 μg/L was associated with a non-significant higher risk of LBW and SGA [12]. In another prospective study of Chinese women, both iodine insufficiency and excess were inversely associated with fetal femur length, a measure of fetal growth [11]. Among Spanish women, lower rates of SGA were observed among women with UIC 100–149 μg/L compared to those with <50 μg/L [8], but no associations of UIC with birth weight, SGA, or preterm birth were observed in another study of Spanish women [8]. In our study population of Finnish women, we found that higher serum iodide was positively associated with preterm birth, but neither high nor low serum iodide was associated with SGA.

Only a few previous studies have evaluated associations of Tg and TSH with preterm birth and SGA. In two prospective studies of pregnant Spanish women, high TSH, which is indicative of hypothyroidism, was associated with increased risk of SGA [7,8]. Similarly, in a prospective study of U.S. women, Männistö et al. reported a positive association of hypothyroidism and risk of preterm birth [27], which is consistent with findings of several other studies [28,29]. In our study of Finnish women, we observed an inverse association of Tg and SGA, but no association with preterm birth. TSH was not associated with either outcome, which was somewhat expected given that nearly all women were within the normal range.

While our findings for iodine are somewhat difficult to compare directly with prior studies due to our use of serum versus urine concentrations, the observed elevated risk of preterm birth associated with higher levels of serum iodide in our data are compatible with the possibility of a true U-shaped relationship observed in several previous studies, with both high and low levels of iodine being associated with increased risk of preterm birth. However, because the women who comprised our study population were only mildly iodine insufficient [3], and the prevalence of severe deficiency is low, our results may only capture the right side of this U-shaped relationship. Some data suggest that Tg levels may be sensitive indicators of iodine status among children and pregnant women [24,30], with a U-shaped relationship between Tg and UIC. Thus, the inverse association for SGA observed in analyses comparing high versus low Tg may be explained, at least in part, by mild iodine insufficiency among women with Tg in the lowest quartile. Additional explanations for conflicting findings of previous research and ours may relate to other underlying nutritional deficiencies (e.g., zinc or iron) present in other countries, bioavailable iodine in soil, and genetic factors, as well as differences in the underlying risk of obstetrical complications across study populations [3,31,32].

Potential biological mechanisms to explain our observed positive associations of serum iodide with preterm birth and inverse associations of Tg with SGA are somewhat unclear. During periods of iodine deficiency, TSH, which is secreted from the pituitary gland, increases and stimulates uptake of circulating iodine by thyrocytes in the thyroid [1]. The iodination of Tg produces T_3 and T_4, which are essential for fetal central nervous system and skeletal development. When iodine deficiency is severe (UIC <50 μg/L), the production of T_3 and T_4 is impaired, and circulating levels of the thyroid hormones decrease. Paradoxically, when iodine intake is excessive (defined as UIC >500 μg/L), a transient decrease in T_3 and T_4 also occurs, known as the Wolff–Chaikoff effect [33]. In normal, healthy individuals, this effect lasts only a few days; however, fetuses <36 weeks' gestation cannot escape this effect, resulting in fetal hypothyroidism [34]. Although this phenomenon is not well understood, it is possible that high levels of maternal serum iodide may induce this decrease in fetal thyroid hormones, which in turn, could have implications for fetal skeletal development, placentation, and preterm delivery [33].

Strengths of our study include the population-based, nested case-control design, which ensures minimal impact of selection and recall biases, and improves generalizability to the source population. In addition, our study population included women who were mildly iodine-insufficient, but with relatively low prevalence of other nutritional deficiencies that might otherwise confound the associations between iodine status and preterm birth and SGA [3]. Furthermore, our study is the first to evaluate associations of preterm birth and SGA with serum iodine, a measure of iodine hypothesized to be more stable than urinary iodine concentrations over time. Single spot urinary iodine, which was used to assess iodine status in all previous studies on this subject, exhibits considerable intraindividual variation owing to urine dilution, dietary intake, circadian rhythm, season, and other factors [14–16]. Because of this, UIC is considered an acceptable biomarker of iodine status for whole populations, but not for individuals [35]. Serum iodine on the other hand, is less sensitive to recent dietary intake and may better reflect individual iodine status over longer periods of time [19], possibly reducing misclassification of exposure.

Our study also has limitations. First, we were limited to a single serum iodide measurement, rather than longitudinal iodine measurements over the course of the pregnancy. Serum iodide decreases during pregnancy, and as such, some women may have developed iodine deficiency later in pregnancy. Additionally, serum iodide reference ranges have not been established in this population, making it difficult to compare with prior research and World Health Organization iodine recommendations established for pregnant women. We also cannot rule out potential confounding by unmeasured factors such as dietary patterns, chronic thyroid conditions or iodine supplementation initiated after blood collection. Residual confounding by measured factors such as smoking and socioeconomic status is also possible, but the similarity between unadjusted and adjusted estimates suggest that this is an unlikely source of substantial bias.

5. Conclusions

In conclusion, we found that in a mildly iodine insufficient population of Finnish women, higher-serum iodide was positively associated with risk of preterm birth, but was not associated with risk of having an SGA infant. High levels of Tg were inversely associated with risk of SGA. In light of our findings, it appears that mild iodine insufficiency is unlikely to be a substantial contributor to preterm birth and SGA in Finland. Findings of increased risk of preterm birth associated with high-serum iodide warrant further investigation.

Author Contributions: Conceptualization, J.L.M., T.M.; methodology, J.L.M., A.C.P.-S., K.K., G.A.B., S.L.M., A.L.; software, T.M.; validation, K.K., T.M., U.-J.K.; formal analysis, T.M., A.C.P.-S., G.A.B., A.L.; investigation, E.S., H.-M.S., T.M., M.G.; resources, E.S., H.-M.S., T.M., M.G.; data curation, E.S., H.-M.S., T.M., M.G.; writing—original draft preparation, A.C.P.-S.; writing—review and editing, J.L.M., G.A.B., S.L.M., A.L., E.S., H.-M.S., T.M., M.G., K.K., U.-J.K.; visualization, A.C.P.-S.; supervision, J.L.M.; project administration, J.L.M.; funding acquisition, J.L.M., E.S., H.-M.S., T.M., M.G.

Appendix A

The methods used to measure serum iodide have been described previously by Bell et al. [20]. After samples were thawed at room temperature and vortex mixed for 30 s, 200 μL were transferred to polypropylenes tubes. For sample pretreatment, an internal standard mixture of 40 ng/mL of $Cl^{18}O_4^-$ and 4 μg/mL of $S^{13}CN^-$ was added and mixed. After the standard was thoroughly mixed, 20 μL of acetic acid (HAc, 5% in water) and 10 μL of ascorbic acid solution (AA, 2.5 mg/mL in water) were added, mixed, and incubated for 15 min in an incubator shaker at 37 °C (100 rpm). Following this, 100 μL of tetramethylammonium hydroxide (TMAH) (2.5 weight % solution in water), mixed the solution, and then digested in an oven at 90 °C for 2.5 h. Samples were then cooled to room temperature, after which we added 115 μL of water and 30 μL HAc, and then were mixed and centrifuged for 10 min at 5000 rpm. Finally, 500 μL of the final sample supernatant was transferred to amber vial for high-performance liquid chromatography-triple quadrupole mass spectrometry (HPLC–MS/MS).

An Alliance 2695 high-performance liquid chromatograph (HPLC) coupled with a Micromass Quattro LC tandem mass spectrometer (MS/MS; Waters Corporation, Milford, MA, USA) was used for sample analysis. Micromass MassLynx 3.5 software was used for data acquisition and quantification. The IonPac AS-21 column (guard column; 50 mm × 2 mm, analytical column;

250 mm × 2 mm, Dionex, Sunnyvale, CA, USA) was used to separate iodide. Identification and quantification of ^{18}O-labeled-perchlorate, ^{13}C-labeled-thiocyanate, and iodide was performed using electrospray negative ionization (ESI-) and multiple-reaction monitoring (MRM) mode at 107 ($^{35}Cl^{18}O4$-) > 89 ($^{35}Cl^{18}O3$-); 59 ($S^{13}CN$-) > 59 ($S^{13}CN$-), and 127 (^{127}I-) > 127 (^{127}I-).

A number of quality control checks were performed. A matrix matched calibration standard with a range of concentrations from 0.02 to 100 ng/mL of iodide was used for each 100-sample batch. Calibration curves had regression coefficients of >0.99. Each calibration standard had internal standards ($Cl^{18}O4$- and $S^{13}CN$-) spiked into them at 2 ng/mL and 20 ng/mL. Both internal standards had average recoveries of 70%. Estimated limits of quantification for iodide in blood sera was 0.25 ng/mL. Each 100-sample batch included a procedural blank, a matrix blank, a duplicate, standard reference material, and matrix spike of 25 ng/mL iodide. In analyses, no iodine was detected in procedural blanks, <2 ng/mL of iodide was detected in matrix blanks, 90%–111% of iodine was recovered in standard reference material, and 101%–122% of iodine was recovered in spiked serum matrices. No carry-over was detected from water blanks injected every 20–25 samples. To measure instrumental drift, a mid-point calibration standard was injected in every 10 h as initial calibration verification (ICV) to monitor for drift in instrumental response.

References

1. Zimmermann, M.B.; Jooste, P.L.; Pandav, C.S. Iodine-deficiency disorders. *Lancet* **2008**, *372*, 1251–1262. [CrossRef]
2. Maraka, S.; Ospina, N.M.S.; O'Keeffe, D.T.; Espinosa De Ycaza, A.E.; Gionfriddo, M.R.; Erwin, P.J.; Coddington, C.C., 3rd; Stan, M.N.; Murad, M.H.; Montori, V.M. Subclinical Hypothyroidism in Pregnancy: A Systematic Review and Meta-Analysis. *Thyroid* **2016**, *26*, 580–590. [CrossRef]
3. Nystrom, H.F.; Brantsaeter, A.L.; Erlund, I.; Gunnarsdottir, I.; Hulthen, L.; Laurberg, P.; Mattisson, I.; Rasmussen, L.B.; Virtanen, S.; Meltzer, H.M. Iodine status in the Nordic countries-past and present. *Food Nutr. Res.* **2016**, *60*, 31969. [CrossRef]
4. Leung, A.M.; Pearce, E.N.; Braverman, L.E. Iodine nutrition in pregnancy and lactation. *Endocrin. Metab. Clin.* **2011**, *40*, 765–777. [CrossRef]
5. Mills, J.L.; Ali, M.; Buck Louis, G.M.; Kannan, K.; Weck, J.; Wan, Y.; Maisog, J.; Giannakou, A.; Sundaram, R. Pregnancy Loss and Iodine Status: The LIFE Prospective Cohort Study. *Nutrients* **2019**, *11*, 534. [CrossRef]
6. Granfors, M.; Andersson, M.; Stinca, S.; Åkerud, H.; Skalkidou, A.; Sundström Poromaa, I.; Wikström, A.-K.; Filipsson Nyström, H. Iodine deficiency in a study population of pregnant women in Sweden. *Acta. Obstet. Gynecol. Scand.* **2015**, *94*, 1168–1174. [CrossRef]
7. Alvarez-Pedrerol, M.; Guxens, M.; Mendez, M.; Canet, Y.; Martorell, R.; Espada, M.; Plana, E.; Rebagliato, M.; Sunyer, J. Iodine levels and thyroid hormones in healthy pregnant women and birth weight of their offspring. *Eur. J. Endocrinol.* **2009**, *160*, 423–429. [CrossRef]
8. Leon, G.; Murcia, M.; Rebagliato, M.; Alvarez-Pedrerol, M.; Castilla, A.M.; Basterrechea, M.; Iniguez, C.; Fernandez-Somoano, A.; Blarduni, E.; Foradada, C.M.; et al. Maternal thyroid dysfunction during gestation, preterm delivery, and birthweight. The Infancia y Medio Ambiente Cohort, Spain. *Paediatr. Perinat. Epidemiol.* **2015**, *29*, 113–122. [CrossRef]
9. Charoenratana, C.; Leelapat, P.; Traisrisilp, K.; Tongsong, T. Maternal iodine insufficiency and adverse pregnancy outcomes. *Matern. Child Nutr.* **2016**, *12*, 680–687. [CrossRef]
10. Torlinska, B.; Bath, S.C.; Janjua, A.; Boelaert, K.; Chan, S.Y. Iodine Status during Pregnancy in a Region of Mild-to-Moderate Iodine Deficiency is not Associated with Adverse Obstetric Outcomes; Results from the Avon Longitudinal Study of Parents and Children (ALSPAC). *Nutrients* **2018**, *10*, 291. [CrossRef]
11. Chen, R.; Li, Q.; Cui, W.; Wang, X.; Gao, Q.; Zhong, C.; Sun, G.; Chen, X.; Xiong, G.; Yang, X.; et al. Maternal Iodine Insufficiency and Excess Are Associated with Adverse Effects on Fetal Growth: A Prospective Cohort Study in Wuhan, China. *J. Nutr.* **2018**, *148*, 1814–1820. [CrossRef]
12. Yang, J.; Liu, Y.; Liu, H.; Zheng, H.; Li, X.; Zhu, L.; Wang, Z. Associations of maternal iodine status and thyroid function with adverse pregnancy outcomes in Henan Province of China. *J. Trace Elem. Med. Biol.* **2018**, *47*, 104–110. [CrossRef]

13. Snart, C.J.P.; Keeble, C.; Taylor, E.; Cade, J.E.; Stewart, P.M.; Zimmermann, M.; Reid, S.; Threapleton, D.E.; Poston, L.; Myers, J.E.; et al. Maternal Iodine Status and Associations with Birth Outcomes in Three Major Cities in the United Kingdom. *Nutrients* **2019**, *11*, 411. [CrossRef]

14. Rasmussen, L.B.; Ovesen, L.; Christiansen, E. Day-to-day and within-day variation in urinary iodine excretion. *Eur. J. Clin. Nutr.* **1999**, *53*, 401–407. [CrossRef]

15. Als, C.; Helbling, A.; Peter, K.; Haldimann, M.; Zimmerli, B.; Gerber, H. Urinary iodine concentration follows a circadian rhythm: A study with 3023 spot urine samples in adults and children. *J. Clin. Endocrinol. Metab.* **2000**, *85*, 1367–1369. [CrossRef]

16. Pan, Z.; Cui, T.; Chen, W.; Gao, S.; Pearce, E.N.; Wang, W.; Chen, Y.; Guo, W.; Tan, L.; Shen, J.; et al. Serum iodine concentration in pregnant women and its association with urinary iodine concentration and thyroid function. *Clin. Endocrinol.* **2019**, *90*, 711–718. [CrossRef]

17. Yu, S.; Yin, Y.; Cheng, Q.; Han, J.; Cheng, X.; Guo, Y.; Sun, D.; Xie, S.; Qiu, L. Validation of a simple inductively coupled plasma mass spectrometry method for detecting urine and serum iodine and evaluation of iodine status of pregnant women in Beijing. *Scand. J. Clin. Lab. Inv.* **2018**, *78*, 501–507. [CrossRef]

18. Michalke, B.; Witte, H. Characterization of a rapid and reliable method for iodide biomonitoring in serum and urine based on ion chromatography-ICP-mass spectrometry. *J. Trace Elem. Med. Biol.* **2015**, *29*, 63–68. [CrossRef]

19. Cui, T.; Wang, W.; Chen, W.; Pan, Z.; Gao, S.; Tan, L.; Pearce, E.N.; Zimmermann, M.B.; Shen, J.; Zhang, W. Serum Iodine Is Correlated with Iodine Intake and Thyroid Function in School-Age Children from a Sufficient-to-Excessive Iodine Intake Area. *J. Nutr.* **2019**, *149*, 1012–1018. [CrossRef]

20. Bell, G.A.; Mannisto, T.; Liu, A.; Kannan, K.; Yeung, E.H.; Kim, U.J.; Suvanto, E.; Surcel, H.M.; Gissler, M.; Mills, J.L. The joint role of thyroid function and iodine concentration on gestational diabetes risk in a population-based study. *Acta. Obstet. Gynecol. Scand.* **2019**, *98*, 500–506. [CrossRef]

21. Roti, E.; Gardini, E.; Minelli, R.; Bianconi, L.; Flisi, M. Thyroid function evaluation by different commercially available free thyroid hormone measurement kits in term pregnant women and their newborns. *J. Endocrinol. Invest.* **1991**, *14*, 1–9. [CrossRef]

22. Männistö, T.; Surcel, H.-M.; Ruokonen, A.; Vääräsmäki, M.; Pouta, A.; Bloigu, A.; Järvelin, M.-R.; Hartikainen, A.-L.; Suvanto, E. Early Pregnancy Reference Intervals of Thyroid Hormone Concentrations in a Thyroid Antibody-Negative Pregnant Population. *Thyroid* **2011**, *21*, 291–298. [CrossRef]

23. Shrier, I.; Platt, R.W. Reducing bias through directed acyclic graphs. *BMC. Med. Res. Methodol.* **2008**, *8*, 70. [CrossRef]

24. Stinca, S.; Andersson, M.; Weibel, S.; Herter-Aeberli, I.; Fingerhut, R.; Gowachirapant, S.; Hess, S.Y.; Jaiswal, N.; Jukić, T.; Kusic, Z.; et al. Dried Blood Spot Thyroglobulin as a Biomarker of Iodine Status in Pregnant Women. *J. Clin. Endocrinol. Metab.* **2016**, *102*, 23–32. [CrossRef]

25. Knudsen, N.; Bülow, I.; Jørgensen, T.; Perrild, H.; Ovesen, L.; Laurberg, P. Serum Tg—A Sensitive Marker of Thyroid Abnormalities and Iodine Deficiency in Epidemiological Studies. *J. Clin. Endocrinol. Metab.* **2001**, *86*, 3599–3603. [CrossRef]

26. Vejbjerg, P.; Knudsen, N.; Perrild, H.; Laurberg, P.; Carlé, A.; Pedersen, I.B.; Rasmussen, L.B.; Ovesen, L.; Jørgensen, T. Thyroglobulin as a marker of iodine nutrition status in the general population. *Eur. J. Endocrinol.* **2009**, *161*, 475. [CrossRef]

27. Mannisto, T.; Mendola, P.; Grewal, J.; Xie, Y.; Chen, Z.; Laughon, S.K. Thyroid diseases and adverse pregnancy outcomes in a contemporary US cohort. *J. Clin. Endocrinol. Metab.* **2013**, *98*, 2725–2733. [CrossRef]

28. Casey, B.M.; Dashe, J.S.; Wells, C.E.; McIntire, D.D.; Byrd, W.; Leveno, K.J.; Cunningham, F.G. Subclinical hypothyroidism and pregnancy outcomes. *Obstet. Gynecol.* **2005**, *105*, 239–245. [CrossRef]

29. Casey, B.M.; Thom, E.A.; Peaceman, A.M.; Varner, M.W.; Sorokin, Y.; Hirtz, D.G.; Reddy, U.M.; Wapner, R.J.; Thorp, J.M.; Saade, G.; et al. Treatment of Subclinical Hypothyroidism or Hypothyroxinemia in Pregnancy. *N. Eng. J. Med.* **2017**, *376*, 815–825. [CrossRef]

30. Zimmermann, M.B.; Aeberli, I.; Andersson, M.; Assey, V.; Yorg, J.A.; Jooste, P.; Jukic, T.; Kartono, D.; Kusic, Z.; Pretell, E.; et al. Thyroglobulin is a sensitive measure of both deficient and excess iodine intakes in children and indicates no adverse effects on thyroid function in the UIC range of 100-299 mug/L: A UNICEF/ICCIDD study group report. *J. Clin. Endocrinol. Metab.* **2013**, *98*, 1271–1280. [CrossRef]

31. Ertek, S.; Cicero, A.F.; Caglar, O.; Erdogan, G. Relationship between serum zinc levels, thyroid hormones and thyroid volume following successful iodine supplementation. *Hormones (Athens)* **2010**, *9*, 263–268. [CrossRef]

32. Khatiwada, S.; Lamsal, M.; Gelal, B.; Gautam, S.; Nepal, A.K.; Brodie, D.; Baral, N. Anemia, Iron Deficiency and Iodine Deficiency among Nepalese School Children. *Ind. J. Pediatr.* **2016**, *83*, 617–621. [CrossRef]

33. Pearce, E.N.; Lazarus, J.H.; Moreno-Reyes, R.; Zimmermann, M.B. Consequences of iodine deficiency and excess in pregnant women: An overview of current knowns and unknowns. *Am. J. Clin. Nutr.* **2016**, *104* (Suppl. 3), 918s–923s. [CrossRef]

34. Markou, K.; Georgopoulos, N.; Kyriazopoulou, V.; Vagenakis, A.G. Iodine-Induced hypothyroidism. *Thyroid* **2001**, *11*, 501–510. [CrossRef]

35. Konig, F.; Andersson, M.; Hotz, K.; Aeberli, I.; Zimmermann, M.B. Ten repeat collections for urinary iodine from spot samples or 24-h samples are needed to reliably estimate individual iodine status in women. *J. Nutr.* **2011**, *141*, 2049–2054. [CrossRef]

Nutraceutical Supplements in the Thyroid Setting: Health Benefits beyond Basic Nutrition

Salvatore Benvenga [1,2,3], Ulla Feldt-Rasmussen [4], Daniela Bonofiglio [5] and Ernest Asamoah [6,*]

1   Department of Clinical and Experimental Medicine-Endocrinology, University of Messina,
    via Consolare Valeria-Gazzi, 98125 Messina, Italy; s.benvenga@live.it
2   Master Program on Childhood, Adolescent and Women's Endocrine Health, University of Messina,
    via Consolare Valeria-Gazzi, 98125 Messina, Italy
3   Interdepartmental Program on Molecular and Clinical Endocrinology and Women's Endocrine Health,
    AOU Policlinico G. Martino, via Consolare Valeria-Gazzi, 98125 Messina, Italy
4   Medical Endocrinology and Metabolism PE 2132, Rigshospitalet, Copenhagen University Hospital,
    Blegdamsvej 9, DK-2100 Copenhagen, Denmark; ufeldt@rh.dk
5   Department of Pharmacy, Health and Nutritional Sciences, University of Calabria,
    87036 Arcavacata di Rende (CS), Italy; daniela.bonofiglio@unical.it
6   Community Physicians Network, Diabetes & Endocrinology Care, 8435 Clearvista Place, Suite 101,
    Indianapolis, IN 46256, USA
*   Correspondence: eoasamoah@mac.com

Abstract: In recent years, there has been a growing interest in nutraceuticals, which may be considered as an efficient, preventive, and therapeutic tool in facing different pathological conditions, including thyroid diseases. Although iodine remains the major nutrient required for the functioning of the thyroid gland, other dietary components play important roles in clinical thyroidology—these include selenium, L-carnitine, myo-inositol, melatonin, and resveratrol—some of which have antioxidant properties. The main concern regarding the appropriate and effective use of nutraceuticals in prevention and treatment is due to the lack of clinical data supporting their efficacy. Another limitation is the discrepancy between the concentration claimed by the label and the real concentration. This paper provides a detailed critical review on the health benefits, beyond basic nutrition, of some popular nutraceutical supplements, with a special focus on their effects on thyroid pathophysiology and aims to distinguish between the truths and myths surrounding the clinical use of such nutraceuticals.

Keywords: nutraceuticals; thyroid function; dietary supplements

1. Introduction

1.1. Definition of Nutraceutical

The definition of nutraceuticals is still in the grey area between food, food supplements, and pharmaceuticals. Some definitions [1–5] of nutraceuticals are provided in Table 1. The term "nutraceutical" was coined in 1989 by Stephen De Felice, founder and chairman of the Foundation for Innovation in Medicine, an American organization which encourages medical health research. He defined a nutraceutical as a "food, or parts of a food, that provide medical or health benefits, including the prevention and treatment of disease" [4]. Japan was among the first countries to face the issue of regulating food supplements and foodstuffs. This legislation, originally set in 1991, evolved into the 2003 Health Promotion Law [5]. The current European regulation (Regulation No. 1924/2006 of the European Parliament and of the Council, recently updated by EU Regulation 2015/2283) defines food categories and includes a definition of food supplements, although there is no official mention or recognition the term "nutraceutical" [6]. Accordingly, the European Food Safety Authority (EFSA) does not make any distinction between "food supplements" and "nutraceuticals" for beneficial health claim applications for new products. In a similar way, the Dietary Supplement Health and Education Act (DSHEA, 1994) [7] defined dietary supplements as a category of food, as did the US Food and Drug Administration (FDA) [8]. Indeed, in America "medical foods" and "dietary supplements" are regulatory terms, however "nutraceuticals", "functional foods", and other such terms are determined by consultants and marketers, based on consumer trends. Further information on the dietary supplements given by the Food and Drug Administration (FDA) on its website [9] is summarized in Appendix Table A1.

Table 1. Some definitions of "nutraceutical".

Reference	Definition
[1]	"A foodstuff (such as a fortified food or dietary supplement) that provides health benefits in addition to its basic nutritional value. (First known use: 1990)".
[2]	"A food to which vitamins, minerals, or drugs have been added to make it healthier."
[3]	"Nutraceuticals, which have also been called medical foods, designer foods, phytochemicals, functional foods and nutritional supplements, include such everyday products as "bio" yoghurts and fortified breakfast cereals, as well as vitamins, herbal remedies and even genetically modified foods and supplements. Many different terms and definitions are used in different countries, which can result in confusion."
[4]	"I propose to redefine functional foods and nutraceuticals. When food is being cooked or prepared using "scientific intelligence" with or without knowledge of how or why it is being used, the food is called 'functional food'. Thus, functional food provides the body with the required amount of vitamins, fats, proteins, carbohydrates, etc., needed for its healthy survival. When functional food aids in the prevention and/or treatment of disease(s) and/or disorder(s) other than anemia, it is called a nutraceutical."
[5]	Nutraceutical combines two words the term 'nutrition/nutrients' (a nourishing food component) and 'pharmaceutical' (medicine or a substance used as a medication) applied to food or food component products sometimes with active principle from plants that can provide health and medical benefits, including the prevention and treatment of disease.

1.2. Search of the Literature

A PubMed search, run on 14 July 2017, using the word "nutraceutical" as the entry, yielded 67,344 results. Results fell to 4820 using the entry "nutraceuticals AND hormones" and to 553 using the entry "nutraceuticals AND thyroid". Approximately 18 months later (5 February 2019), the corresponding numbers were 78,919 (+17%), 5538 (+15%) and 642 (+16%), indicating that the interest in the thyroid proceeds with the same pace as that for nutraceuticals in general and hormones in general. Confirmation of these data came from a final search that was run on 9 July 2019 (Table 2).

In the following text, different nutraceuticals possibly influencing human thyroid function and/or immunity will be reviewed and commented upon.

A general effect of the nutraceuticals beyond the thyroid effect is not within the scope of this review, nor is a meticulous review of animal or other experimental studies. We were guided by our clinical practices, particularly those for which patients were most curious. As mentioned in the following section, there is indeed a growing market for such nutraceuticals.

There was relatively scant literature on the topic, and most research focused on thyroid cancer and was experimental in nature, concerning the nutraceuticals illustratively mentioned by the Food and Drug Administration, as shown in Appendix Table A1.

Table 2. Summary of number of articles on given nutraceuticals retrievable on PubMed as of 9 July 2019.

Entry		No. of Items			Proportions		
		Total	Human	Human/Total	Thyroid/Total	Thyroid/Human
1	nutraceuticals	81,422	52,406	64.4%	N/A	N/A
2	nutraceuticals AND hormones	5698	3664	61.4%	N/A	N/A
3	nutraceuticals AND thyroid	656	487	74.2%	0.8%	0.9%
4	carnitine	16,737	7831	46.8%	N/A	N/A
5	carnitine AND thyroid	145	68	46.9%	0.9%	0.9%
6	inositol	44,801	16,700	37.3%	N/A	N/A
7	inositol AND thyroid	295	141	47.8%	0.6%	0.8%
8	melatonin	24,921	10,740	43.1%	N/A	N/A
9	melatonin AND thyroid	514	195	37.9%	2.1%	1.8%
10	resveratrol	11,983	5447	45.4%	N/A	N/A
11	resveratrol AND thyroid	78	47	60.2%	0.6%	0.9%
12	selenium	33,980	13,333	39.2%	N/A	N/A
13	selenium AND thyroid	938	576	61.4%	2.8%	4.3%

Note that the number of items under the keyword "nutraceuticals" underestimates the bulk of the literature. Indeed, by adding items #4, 6, 10, 12, 14 and 16 the sum is 164,513, which is greater than 81,422 for item #1. Similar considerations apply for the corresponding human studies (67,565 vs. 52,406), and for the thyroid studies (total studies = 2305 vs. 656; human studies = 1269 vs. 487).

1.3. Market and Sales

Based on data from a decade ago, annual supplement sales were $23 billion, and about 40,000 supplement products were on the market in the United States [10]. In 2015, the American market for dietary supplements was valued at $37 billion, with the economic impact in the United States for 2016 estimated at $122 billion, including employment wages and taxes [11]. One 2016 analysis estimated the total market for dietary supplements could reach $278 billion worldwide by 2024 [11]. Table 3 summarizes the details for the nutraceuticals reviewed here [12–16].

Table 3. Economic issues for the reviewed nutraceuticals.

Nutraceutical	Market and Sales ^
L-carnitine	L-carnitine market is expected to be worth USD 127 million by 2017, with the United States being the largest market, and the Asia-Pacific region, particularly China, expected to experience a 5.5% annual growth rate through 2017 [12]. No. of items on sale-Amazon: 53; Walgreens: No match; CVS Pharmacy:13.
Myo-inositol	In the consumption market, the global consumption value of inositol increases with the 2.01% average growth rate. Europe and China are the mainly consumption regions [11]. With myo-inositol being the most common form of inositols, over the next five years the inositol market, will register a 6.8% compound annual growth rate in terms of revenue, the global market size will reach US $140 million by 2024, from US $94 million in 2019 [13]. No. of items on sale-Amazon: 3; Walgreens: No match; CVS Pharmacy: No match.
Melatonin	The North America region is the largest supplier of melatonin, with a production market share nearly 54% in 2016, Europe coming next with 27% [14]. The global market size will reach US $2080 million by 2024, from US $700 million in 2019 [14]. No. of items on sale-Amazon: 122; Walgreens: 11; CVS Pharmacy: 91.
Resveratrol	Resveratrol supplements, with annual sales of $30 million in the United States [15] No. of items on sale-Amazon: 45; Walgreens: No match; CVS Pharmacy: 19.
Selenium	Selenium market reached $87 million U.S. in 2017 [16]. No. of items on sale-Amazon: 91; Walgreens: No match; CVS Pharmacy: 84.

^ Numbers in brackets are references. Internet sales by Amazon, Walgreens and CVS Pharmacy are reported. Search was performed for the pure nutraceutical, such as entering "pure melatonin". Search performed on the Amazon website by omitting the word "pure", yielded a greater number of results (973 for L-carnitine, 48 for myo-inositol, 178 for resveratrol, over 1000 for selenium, and over 1000 for biotin). Search on the Walgreens website by omitting the word "pure", yielded a greater number of results (12 for L-carnitine, 1 for myo-inositol, 107 for melatonin, 10 for resveratrol, 21 for selenium, and 71 for biotin).

1.4. The Issue of Purity

"The biggest problem with supplements is that many of them do not actually contain what the label claims. As many as 70% of the supplements on the market either don't have ingredients that match their labels or contain contaminants of some kind" [17]. In his review, Lockwood aimed to investigate the extent of substandard formulated and raw material nutraceuticals [17]. The key findings were that "published evaluations of over 70 formulations of 25 different nutraceuticals revealed variable quality; no nutraceutical showed consistent high quality, but a number revealed consistent low quality, thereby making the case for closer regulation of manufacturers. Whole food sources have also been shown to be widely variable in constituent levels." [17]. Concerning the issue of purity, the illegal presence of thyroid hormones in the majority of dietary health supplements marketed for "thyroid support" potentially exposes patients to the risk of developing iatrogenic thyrotoxicosis [18].

In the following text, we now give some data concerning the nutraceuticals dealt upon in our paper. Concerning carnitine, of 12 over-the-counter carnitine formulations, the actual mean content was only 52% of that indicated on the label [19]. Furthermore, of the same 12 preparations, five had unsatisfactory pharmaceutical dissolution characteristics.

Concerning myo-inositol, one study evaluated label accuracy of four myo-inositol products, designed for polycystic ovary syndrome (PCOS) treatment and available on the Italian market, and performed a cost comparison based on myo-inositol content in milligrams for products analyzed [20]. A significant difference in the myo-inositol content, compared with the labeling was found for the products. Only one product contained more than 95% of the myo-inositol content claimed on the label, and there was a product with less than 75% of the labeling amount. Based on a 2-g myo-inositol per day dose, the cost of a 30-day supply ranged from Euro 20.77 and Euro 71.86, after correction by the actual amount of myo-inositol.

One recent study aimed to determine the dose of melatonin in food supplements marketed in Europe (pharmacies of Spain) and the United States (supermarkets of San Francisco, CA, USA) by validating a liquid chromatography method with diode array detection (LC-DAD) [21]. The authors tentatively identified eight tryptophan-related contaminants in melatonin supplements, with only one supplement declaring its addition on the label. Label melatonin doses varied from 1–1.95 mg/unit and 0.3–5 mg/unit for supplements marketed in Europe (Spain) and the US, respectively. Four out of 17 supplements showed significant deviations from melatonin content declared on the label (from −60% to −20%). Only five out of the eight supplements purchased in Spain actually met the qualifications needed to claim to reduce the time to fall asleep. Another study analyzed the actual melatonin content (and presence of contaminants) in 31 melatonin supplements purchased from groceries and pharmacies in one city in Canada [22]. Melatonin content varied from −83% to +478% of labeled melatonin and approximately three-fourths had melatonin concentration ≤10% of what was claimed. Worse yet, the content of melatonin between lots of the same product varied by as much as 465%. An additional 26% of the 31 melatonin supplements were found to contain serotonin.

Concerning resveratrol, 14 brands of resveratrol-containing nutraceuticals were evaluated [23]. The 14 preparations were purchased directly from online stores during 2010 and were analysed before their expiry dates. Only five out of 14 brands had near label values, compliant with Good Manufacturing Practices (GMP) requirements (95%–105% content of active constituent), four products were slightly out of this range (83%–111%) and three were in the 8%–64% range. Two samples were below the limit of detection. The greater the difference between actual and labeled resveratrol content, the lower the antioxidant and antiproliferative activity strength.

With regard to selenium, one study analysed six different brands of yeast-based selenium food supplements that were obtained from local stores [24]. These supplements were treated with milder extraction and hydrolysis conditions to analyse for the expected selenomethionine content. Only two brands had high levels of selenomethionine, one brand appeared to contain all inorganic selenium, and one brand appeared to contain greater than half inorganic selenium despite label claims of content being only selenomethionine.

2. Carnitine: Compound and Physiology

Carnitine is a quaternary ammonium compound (3-Hydroxy-4-(trimethylazaniumyl) butanoate) that is ubiquitous in tissues and biological fluids of mammals [25]. The natural enantiomer is L-carnitine, which acts as an obligatory cofactor for β-oxidation of fatty acids by facilitating the transport of the long-chain fatty acids across the mitochondrial inner membrane as acyl-carnitine esters. This oxidation liberates energy via the production of ATP in the respiratory chain, thus playing a role in cell's energy metabolism. Particularly, L-carnitine exerted a physiological benefit with a positive impact on cardiac function through reduced oxidative stress, inflammation and necrosis of cardiac myocytes. [26]. Only 25% of the body stores of carnitine come from biosynthesis and 75% comes from the diet. The main source is red meat and dairy products. Muscles are the most prominent carnitine depository since they store about 95% of the 120 mmol total amount contained in the adult human body, and the concentration in skeletal muscle (3.5 mmol/L) is 70-fold greater than that in plasma.

The main interest in carnitine supplementation comes from athletes and other physical exercise performers [27]. Thus, repeated-dose carnitine supplements may increase skeletal muscle content. For instance, long-distance runners given a daily dose of 2 g carnitine for 28 days and subjected to a four-week training period [28] increased skeletal muscle carnitine by approximately 13% as compared to a decrease of about 10% in placebo-treated athletes. In other athletes, supplementation with 1 g/day carnitine for 120 days of training increased carnitine concentrations in skeletal muscle by an average of 9% compared to a decrease of 5% in the placebo-treated athletes [29]. Carnitine is critical for normal skeletal muscle bioenergetics [30–32], and skeletal muscles suffer seriously in states of carnitine deficiency. A relative carnitine deficiency can occur in athletes as a result of increased energy metabolism, unbalanced nutrition, decreased skeletal muscle content and increased renal excretion of carnitine. The important energetic role of carnitine, the relative deficiency associated with sustained physical exercise, and the fact that carnitine is a natural compound, has led healthy subjects aiming to improve their exercise performance to conclude that "more carnitine should be better [30–32], but basically this was proven to be without any beneficial effect.

Carnitine and Thyroid Function

A German group of authors conducted pivotal clinical studies as early as 1959 in a very limited number of patients with Graves' disease, using a mixture of the two isomers (L-and D-carnitine) [33]. The first patient was a 53-year-old bedridden woman with very severe Graves' disease and nervousness, insomnia, weight loss, sweating, tachycardia and Graves' orbitopathy. Basal metabolic rate (BMR) was +82%, and she was administered 1 g/d D,L-carnitine. After 10 days, BMR was unchanged but one week later it fell to +59%. Five weeks after starting D,L-carnitine, BMR was still +50% and the authors switched to the naturally occurring L-carnitine. After only 10 days BMR dropped more rapidly to +8% with associate improvement in general well-being and heart rate. Atrial fibrillation disappeared and heart rate was 80–90 beats/min. To prove that the improvement was due to L-carnitine, it was withdrawn in the 7th week from admission. BMR rose to +39%, but after rechallenge with L-carnitine it fell again to +18% [33].

In the English-language literature, the first three monotherapy carnitine-treated hyperthyroid patients were reported in the mid-1960s [34]. The authors found that patients became clinically euthyroid without any consistent changes in the thyroid function tests, thus supporting the notion that the antithyroid effect of carnitine is one of peripheral antagonism of thyroid hormone, rather than a direct inhibition of thyroid gland function [35]. This was consistent with human tissue culture experiments where L-carnitine inhibited both cell entry and, to a greater extent, nuclear entry of both T3 and T4 [36]. These data are consistent with carnitine being a peripheral antagonist of thyroid hormone action, with a site of inhibition at or before the nuclear envelope [36].

The first controlled clinical trial addressing the value of L-carnitine in antagonizing elevated circulating levels of thyroid hormones was conducted in 50 women under Thyroid stimulating hormone (TSH)-suppressive L-T4 therapy for cytologically benign thyroid nodules who received a simultaneous treatment for six months with placebo ($n = 10$), or for given periods of time with L-carnitine (2g/d or 4 g/d to test dose-dependence) [37]. Evaluation by both extensive clinical and biochemical assessment demonstrated positive effects with the exception of osteocalcin, which increased further during L-carnitine administration and partial exception of total cholesterol (minimal or no increase during L-carnitine administration). Serum FT3, FT4 and TSH remained unchanged throughout the 180 day-duration of the trial. Thus, there was no antagonism from L-carnitine on the negative feedback that thyroid hormones exert on thyrotropin releasing hormone (TRH)/TSH. In addition to the hypothalamic TRH-producing neurons and the pituitary thyrotropin, also osteoblasts were refractory to the thyroid-hormone antagonizing effect of L-carnitine (see above). Thus, L-carnitine synergized with thyroid hormone on the osteoblasts to increase osteocalcin serum concentrations. The favorable effect on the osteoblasts was supported by measuring femur and lumbar bone density by dual-energy-X-ray absorptiometry [37].

More recent cases of severe forms of Graves' disease-related hyperthyroidism, including thyroid storms, were treated successfully with L-carnitine [38–40]. Recently, a pilot study indicated the beneficial effects of a combination of L-carnitine and selenium supplementation in subclinical hyperthyroidism [41]. A rationale for a beneficial effect of L-carnitine supplementation in hyperthyroid patients seems likely because increased levels of thyroid hormones deprive the tissue deposits of L-carnitine itself [42], which is further substantiated by the finding of decreased concentrations of carnitine in the skeletal muscles of hyperthyroid patients. Interestingly, trendwise decreased concentrations of carnitine were found in skeletal muscles of hypothyroid patients [43], which were restored upon regaining euthyroidism. Therefore, decreased concentrations of carnitine in skeletal muscles may contribute to myopathy associated with either hypothyroidism or hyperthyroidism.

Sixty thyroid-hormone adequately replaced hypothyroid Korean patients (age 50.0 ± 9.2 years, 57 females) continued to complain of fatigue [44]. These patients were given L-carnitine (990 mg L-carnitine twice daily; $n = 30$) or placebo ($n = 30$) for 12 weeks. After 12 weeks, although neither the fatigue severity score nor the physical fatigue score changed significantly after 12 weeks, but the mental fatigue score was significantly improved by treatment with L-carnitine compared with placebo ($p < 0.01$). In subgroups, both the physical and mental fatigue scores improved significantly in patients younger than 50 years and those with free T3 ≥ 4.0 pg/mL by treatment with L-carnitine compared with placebo. Other case-based studies have indicated a benefit from L-carnitine on hypothyroid symptoms, but all of them have been case-based [45], while other studies may support benefits in the corticosteroid hormone setting [46].

3. Inositol: Compound and Physiology

Inositol is a water-soluble compound closely associated with the vitamin B group (also known as vitamin B8) [47]. Inositol is a carbohydrate which has a taste half as sweet as that of sucrose. Inositol has long been known for its metabolic effects in humans, where it plays a part in the synthesis of secondary messengers within cells. It is an essential component of the phospholipids that makes up cellular membranes and is found in virtually all cells. The most abundant form of the nutrient is myo-inositol. It assists in the transmission of nerve signals, helps to transport lipids within the body, and is also critical for the proper action of insulin and maintenance of cellular calcium balance. Foods containing the highest concentrations of myo-inositol include fruits, beans, grains and nuts. However, in grains, it is in a non-available form called phytate. The more bioavailable form of inositol comes from lecithin. Inositol is a necessary component of all cellular membranes. It is a member of the B-vitamin family that contributes to muscular and nerve function and participates in the metabolism of fats in the liver. Myo-inositol is the most abundant form of this nutrient, with its highest concentrations being found in the brain and central nervous system. Myo-inositol in particular is a versatile nutrient for the promotion of emotional and mental wellness, healthy eating patterns, and restful sleep through its critical role in neurotransmitter messaging systems. In addition, it is an important nutritional element for the maintenance of ovarian health and normal blood sugar maintenance, especially in women.

Inositol is a non-essential member of the B-complex family with dietary sources from both animal and plant foods. The form of inositol used in this product is myo-inositol, the most abundant form of this nutrient. Inositol is found in all cell membranes, with the highest concentrations in the brain and central nervous system, where it plays an important role in neurotransmitter signaling. Inositol is also critical for the proper action of insulin, lipid metabolism, and for the maintenance of cellular calcium balance. Inositol is a necessary component of all cellular membranes. It is a member of the inositols are marketed as beneficial nutraceutics for improving mood and for the treatment of polycystic ovary syndrome [20]. A significant difference in the myo-inositol content of available products, and there are no regulations to ensure homogenous quality and accuracy [20].

Inositol and Thyroid Function/Autoimmunity

Inositols are essential for the signaling of hormones such as insulin, gonadotropins (follicle stimulating hormone [FSH] and luteinizing hormone [LH]), and TSH. In the thyroid, imbalances in the inositol metabolism can impair thyroidal hormone biosynthesis, storage and secretion [47]. TSH signaling is rather complex involving two different signal cascades. One branch of the signal cascade involves as second messenger cyclic AMP (cAMP), while another branch is inositol-dependent [48]. In a controlled trial, 48 women with autoimmune subclinical hypothyroidism were randomized to treatment with either selenomethionine alone or selenomethionine plus myo-inositol. The authors demonstrated that patients with autoimmune thyroiditis and subclinical hypothyroidism, treated with myo-inositol and selenomethionine, had a reduction of the increased TSH, which selenomethionine supplementation alone was not able to promote. However, the concentration of both thyroperoxidase and thyroglobulin autoantibodies (TPOAb and TgAb) declined in both groups [48]. In a subsequent study of 86 patients with Hashimoto's thyroiditis and subclinical hypothyroidism, the same authors found that the administration of myo-inositol and selenomethionine for six months significantly decreased TSH, TPOAb, and TgAb concentrations, while at the same time enhancing thyroid hormones and personal wellbeing, thereby restoring euthyroidism in patients diagnosed with autoimmune thyroiditis [49]. This was confirmed in a larger study of 168 patients with Hashimoto's thyroiditis and subclinical hypothyroidism (TSH 3–6 mU/L) [50].

The mechanism of this effect might be through immune modulation rather than through thyroid function *per se* [51]. Using the afore-mentioned combined treatment in 22 patients with autoimmune thyroiditis, the initial TSH levels in the high normal range (2.1 < TSH < 4.0) significantly declined, suggesting that the combined treatment can reduce the risk of progression to hypothyroidism in subjects with autoimmune thyroid diseases. Antithyroid autoantibody levels also declined and, moreover, the suspected immune-modulatory effect was confirmed by the finding that the concentration of the chemokine CXCL10 also declined. Studies are, however, awaited to extend the observations in a larger population, to evaluate the effect on the quality of life, and to study the mechanism of the effect on chemokines.

Very recently, thyroid nodular disease also seemed to improve after the combined treatment with myo-inositol and selenomethionine [52], but this also needs confirmation. Final data in this study was analyzed from 34 patients with subclinical hypothyroidism: in 76% of mixed thyroid nodules a significant reduction of their size was observed and 56% of them significantly regressed nodule stiffness following oral supplementation with the combined nutraceutics for six months. The mean number of mixed thyroid nodules shifted from 1.4 ± 0.2 to 1.1 ± 0.2 ($p \leq 0.05$) and the TSH concentrations dropped from 4.2 ± 0.2 mIU/L at baseline to 2.1 ± 0.2 mIU/L post-treatment ($p < 0.001$). In the control group, 38% of the thyroid nodules reduced their diameter but TSH concentrations significantly increased up to the threshold after six months (from 4.0 ± 0.2 mIU/L to 4.3 ± 0.2 mIU/L, $p \leq 0.05$). However, further studies are required, both in vitro and in vivo, in order to investigate the mechanism of this effect on the one hand, and a possible clinical treatment use of myo-inositol plus selenomethionine for the general management of thyroid nodules on the other.

4. Melatonin: Compound and Physiology

The isolation of melatonin was first reported in 1958 [53]. Since the demonstration that pineal melatonin synthesis reflects both daily and seasonal time, melatonin has become a key element of chronobiology research. In mammals, pineal melatonin is essential for transducing day-length information into seasonal physiological responses. Due to its lipophilic nature, melatonin is able to cross the placenta and is believed to regulate multiple aspects of perinatal physiology. The endogenous daily melatonin rhythm is also likely to play a role in the maintenance of synchrony between circadian clocks throughout the adult body. Pharmacological doses of melatonin are effective in resetting circadian rhythms if taken at an appropriate time of day and can acutely regulate factors such as body temperature and alertness, especially when taken during the day. Despite the extensive literature on melatonin physiology, several key questions remain unanswered. Particularly the amplitude of melatonin rhythms has recently been associated with diseases such as type 2 diabetes mellitus but the physiological significance of melatonin rhythm amplitude remains poorly understood.

As a nutraceutical, melatonin is easily available over the counter and is marketed to regulate the sleep pattern and adaptation to time zone differences among numerous other conditions.

Melatonin and Thyroid Function

Melatonin has antioxidant properties, which is one of the reasons why it is assumed to be beneficial for many disease conditions. However, very few human studies exist, and they are primarily of a physiological nature. One such study considers several endocrine and immune interactions in healthy persons at different ages [54] and found statistically significant time-qualified correlations among lymphocyte subset percentages and hormone serum levels in the young and middle aged and one could speculate that the phenomenon of lymphocyte subpopulation redistribution may be more complex, and may involve other hormones such as TRH, TSH, GH (growth hormone), IGF1 (insulin-like growth factor 1), monoamines such as melatonin, cytokines such as IL2 (Interleukin 2), and chemokines. The aging of immune system function may be related to the alteration of circadian rhythmicity, with a loss of interaction among key lymphocyte subsets, immunomodulating hormones, as well as cytokines/chemokines.

Thirty-six perimenopausal and 18 postmenopausal women between 42 and 62 years of age with no pathology or medication were selected for a randomized study of melatonin or placebo at bedtime (22:00–00:00). The melatonin concentration was measured in saliva to divide the participants into low, medium, and high-melatonin subjects [55]. Three- and six-months later, blood was taken for the determination of pituitary (LH and FSH), ovarian, and thyroid hormones (T3 and T4). The results showed that women low in melatonin after treatment with melatonin significantly increased thyroid hormones levels and improved gonadal functions [55]. These results were confirmed by the same authors in another study where peri- and menopausal women ($N = 139$) took a daily dose of 3 mg synthetic melatonin or placebo for 6 months. Melatonin concentrations were determined from five daily saliva samples at fixed times while other hormone levels were determined from blood samples three times over the six-month period [56]. The conclusion was that the six-months treatment with melatonin produced a remarkable and highly significant improvement of thyroid function, positive changes of gonadotropins towards more juvenile levels, and the abrogation of menopause-related depression.

In 40 menopausal women the combination of myo-inositol plus melatonin seemed to positively affect glucose metabolism. Myo-inositol alone seemed to improve thyroid function, while addition of melatonin increased the serum TSH concentration [57]. The reason for this is unknown, but all melatonin products warn against worsening of autoimmune diseases on basis of its potential effect on the immune system. Recently, SNPs related to melatonin receptor gene polymorphism haplotypes were associated with susceptibility to Graves' disease in an ethnic Chinese population and thus support the involvement of the melatonin pathway in the pathogenesis of this autoimmune thyroid disease [58].

In conclusion, there is to date no controlled trials to substantiate a use of melatonin for general thyroid health improvement.

5. Resveratrol: Compound and Physiology

Resveratrol (3,4',5-trihydroxy-trans-stilbene) belongs to the flavonoids family and is a major natural polyphenolic compound found in several fruit and vegetables such as grapes, peanuts, and peanut sprouts. It seems to play an important role as a therapeutic and chemopreventive agent used in the treatment of various illnesses [59,60] and has therefore recently gained much attention among health professionals as well as other nutrition experts. Resveratrol exhibits effects against several cancers [61,62] through different pathways and, furthermore, it has antidiabetic, anti-inflammatory, and antioxidant effects. The cardiovascular protective capacities of resveratrol are believed to be associated with multiple molecular targets such as inflammation, oxidative stress, apoptosis, mitochondrial dysfunction, angiogenesis and platelet aggregation [59].

Similarly, resveratrol is a potent scavenger for free radicals. The high efficiency of resveratrol might be due to the three hydroxyl groups in its structure. Thus, the use of resveratrol as a health-promoting dietary supplement is rapidly increasing in today's market. Many reports have shown that resveratrol offers a wide range of preventive and therapeutic alternatives against various diseases including different types of cancer.

Resveratrol is a member of a family of enzymes, under the general name of stilbene synthase, which makes up part of a larger family of proteins with numerous functions. Notably, its chemical structure resembles that of L-T4, however it is not clear if this has any functional implications [63]. Resveratrol synthase is developed from chalcone synthase via gene duplication and mutations. The absorption in humans is approximately 75% (delayed by food) by trans-epithelial diffusion, while tissue accumulation enhances efficacy at target sites.

Resveratrol and Thyroid Function

Resveratrol may arrest the proliferation of thyroid cancer cells by increasing the abundance and phosphorylation of p53 [64–66]. Moreover, resveratrol mediates the regulation of TSH while, due to its effects on iodine trapping, it shows promise as a prospective anti-thyroid drug. On the other hand, these effects also resulted in a pronounced proliferative action on thyrocytes and resveratrol may therefore be a thyroid disrupting compound [67]. No clinical studies on the compound's effect on the thyroid has been performed in humans, so all available evidence is based on animal and in vitro cellular studies.

Finally, resveratrol as an antioxidant agent is a free radical scavenger and this property can be of interest in thyroid disease states that are accompanied by increased production of hydrogen peroxide and radical oxygen species, such as autoimmune thyroiditis and hyperthyroidism [68]. Proper randomized clinical trials would, however, be required before implementing any use.

Resveratrol supplements can be easily purchased over the counter but they are not regulated by the FDA or any other health authority. Most resveratrol capsules sold in the U.S. contain extracts from an Asian plant called *Polygonum cuspidatum*. Other resveratrol supplements are made from red wine or red grape extracts. The dosages in most resveratrol supplements typically contain 250 to 500 milligrams, which is much lower than the amounts that have been shown beneficial in research (2000 milligrams of resveratrol or more a day).

6. Selenium: Compound and Physiology

Selenium is a non-metal chemical element that is an essential micronutrient. Selenium salts are toxic in large amounts, but trace amounts are necessary for cellular function in many organisms, including all animals. Dietary selenium comes from nuts, cereals, and mushrooms. Brazil nuts are the richest dietary source (though this is soil-dependent since the Brazil nut does not require high levels of the element for its own needs). Selenium is an ingredient in many multivitamins and other dietary supplements. It is a component of the antioxidant enzymes glutathione peroxidase and thioredoxin reductase, which indirectly reduce certain oxidized molecules in animals and some plants. It is also found in three deiodinase enzymes, which convert one thyroid hormone to another. In living systems, selenium is found in the amino acids selenomethionine, selenocysteine, and methylselenocysteine.

The U.S. recommended dietary allowance (RDA) for teenagers and adults is 55 µg/day. Selenium as a dietary supplement is available in many forms, including multi-vitamins/mineral supplements, which typically contain 55 or 70 µg/serving. Selenium-specific supplements typically contain either 100 or 200 µg/serving. In June 2015, the U.S. FDA published its final rule establishing the requirement of minimum and maximum levels of selenium in infant formula. The reference values of EFSA for selenium range from 15 µg/day for children aged one to three years to 70 µg/day for adolescents aged 15–17 years [69]. The selenium content in the human body is believed to be in the range of 13–20 milligram [70].

Selenium food supplements are most efficient as yeast-based selenomethionine, but the contents are not standardized or under any control. For instance, six different brands of yeast-based selenium food supplements were analysed for the expected selenomethionine content [23]. Only two brands had high levels of selenomethionine; one brand appeared to contain only inorganic selenium, and one brand appeared to contain more than half inorganic selenium despite label claims of content being only selenomethionine. Nevertheless, selenium supplementation is increasingly prescribed by endocrinologists as recently documented for Italian endocrinologists [70]. In detail, approximately one in four respondents use selenium often/always, with only one in either use never. Rates were approximately one-fourth of respondents prescribing selenium often/always in Hashimoto's thyroiditis, and one-fifth prescribing selenium in the case presented. In patients with autoimmune thyroiditis (AIT) who are planning pregnancy or are already pregnant, approximately 40% of respondents suggest selenium use [71]. It is worth underlining that the American Thyroid Association (ATA) pregnancy guideline reported that "selenium supplementation is not recommended for the treatment of TPOAb-positive women during pregnancy" [72].

Selenium and Thyroid Function/Autoimmunity

Among all tissues, the thyroid gland has the highest concentration of selenium, of which much is stored in the thyrocytes as the selenoproteins [73,74]: deiodinases (DI1, DI2), glutathion peroxidase (GPx1, GPx3, GPx4), and thioredoxin reductases (TR1, TR2). Both the thyroid gland and all other cells that are dependent of thyroid hormone for proper function use selenium as a cofactor for three of the four known types of thyroid hormone deiodinases, which can both activate and deactivate thyroid hormones and their metabolites—the iodothyronine deiodinases are the subfamily of deiodinase enzymes that use selenium, as does the otherwise rare amino acid selenocysteine. Only iodotyrosine deiodinase does not use selenium.

Adequate selenium intake is required for normal function of thyrocytes and the angiofollicular units in thyroid hormone biosynthesis and storage. Inadequate selenium intake has been associated with increased thyroid volume in females, but not males in one study [75], and in a larger Danish population, this negative correlation between selenium status and thyroid volume was confirmed, and there was, furthermore, a trend toward increased numbers of thyroid nodules with inadequate selenium status [74,76]. Adequate selenium intake, with respect to proper thyroid function, can be monitored by the analysis of serum or plasma selenoproteins such as selenoprotein P or plasma GPx3 [74,77,78]. Intoxication has been reported in several places in China from dietary intake and soil contamination [79,80]. Measurement of these variables is becoming more important in the view of the increased interest in selenium supplementation in various patient groups particularly with autoimmune thyroid diseases (see below) and since there is a risk of overdosing by general too high doses on the one hand and supplementation of selenium sufficient individuals on the other. The U-shaped curve of beneficial effects from selenium concentrations, i.e., exhibiting major advantages in selenium-deficient individuals but specific health risks in those with selenium excess should be seriously considered [81].

Selenium status has been shown to affect immune functions, e.g., T cell differentiation, and selenium deficiency has been associated with Th2 cells/markers, while higher selenium concentrations seem to favor an increased Th1 and Treg response [82]. These observations are thus in keeping with the suggestion of beneficial effects of selenium supplementation in autoimmune diseases of the thyroid [73,83]. Newly diagnosed autoimmune hyperthyroidism, Graves' disease, has been associated with low selenium concentrations [84], an observation which has fuelled several interventional treatment studies of selenium supplementation as adjunctive to antithyroid drugs in Graves' disease [85–88]. A very recent systematic review and meta-analysis of 10 randomized clinical trials could not substantiate a systematic effect of selenium supplementation as an adjunctive treatment in Graves' disease [89]. Generally, the studies were all underpowered, of too short a duration, and with too broad clinical characteristics of the patients, and the issue is therefore yet to be resolved—results from larger ongoing prospective studies are awaited [90].

Concerning the subpopulations of Graves' disease, however, a prospective case-control study demonstrated lower serum selenium concentrations in patients with Graves' orbitopathy compared to Graves' patients without orbitopathy in an Australian study population with marginal selenium status [91]. Against this background, relative selenium deficiency may be an independent risk factor for orbitopathy in patients with Graves' diseases. This has been further substantiated by one major multicentric prospective, placebo and serum-controlled study of Graves' patients with orbitopathy, with demonstration of improved quality of life and disease activity scores [92].

Several placebo-controlled and double-blind studies, both observational and prospective, have been performed to demonstrate the improved quality of life, wellbeing, thyroid hormone status, and disease symptoms of chronic autoimmune thyroiditis of the Hashimoto type with or without hypothyroidism. Although many studies have consistently demonstrated a reduction in thyroid autoantibody concentrations by selenium supplementation, including some compared with control/placebo [93–96], recent meta-analyses found insufficient evidence for the clinical efficacy of selenium supplementation in chronic autoimmune thyroiditis [97,98]. Hopefully, future trials can ultimately provide reliable evidence to help inform clinical decision making. Results were less optimistic than the individual study results, many of which were, however, underpowered, and therefore, in this autoimmune patient group, results are unclear and further ongoing study results are awaited [99].

In women at risk of postpartum thyroiditis, adequate selenium status prevents its development. In a prospective placebo-controlled double-blind prevention study [100], there were fewer cases of postpartum thyroiditis—these results, however, have not been confirmed in other studies [73,101].

Finally, there has been no indication of an increased risk of thyroid cancer in either selenium deficiency or with supplementation of selenium [74].

In conclusion, selenium status has a high impact on normal thyroid development and function, and it is still a potential candidate for improvement of clinical markers and quality of life in some situations of autoimmune thyroid diseases by supplementation, e.g., Graves' orbitopathy and possibly postpartum thyroiditis. However, more solid evidence is awaited until firm conclusions can be made concerning recommendations for global routine clinical use.

7. Perspective and Conclusions

As clinicians, we often see patients who are taking all sorts of supplements with the hope of improving their health and medical conditions, as well as simply feeling better.

Thyroid supplements attract a disproportionately large amount of attention, just as the thyroid gland gets "blamed" for multiple symptoms. There are truths and myths that this review had tried to clarify. Of the numerous nutraceuticals out there for thyroid disease management, we focused on the common or popular ones we encounter in the clinical practice.

Clinicians should acknowledge that over 30% of our patients are using supplements and thus should inquire about them during our office encounters. Apart from improving their general health, patients are using these alleged thyroid supplements to help "improve their metabolism, have more energy, and to lose weight".

It is important that we do not just dismiss these patients, but rather have honest discussions about the claimed benefits and potential risks. Physicians would do well to familiarize themselves with the main supplements being used, and also to know the scientific evidence available to support or refute these claims. More importantly, physicians should understand the potential risks or side effects in order to properly counsel patients about their use.

Based on the literature reviewed in the preceding sections, the evidence for the clinical use and potential benefit of the nutraceuticals addressed in this paper is summarized in Table 4. It is, however, worth noting that very few studies have been randomized clinical trials and generally all the studies have lacked proper power and even attempts to perform power calculations including the few randomized clinical trials. For selenium, two randomized, properly powered, placebo controlled clinical trials are ongoing and results are awaited [89,98]. Similar studies are required also for the most relevant nutraceuticals with a possible influence on the thyroid, in order to provide proper guidance both to patients and clinicians.

Table 4. Summary of evidence for clinical use of the nutraceuticals reviewed here in the thyroid setting *.

Question: Is There Evidence for Clinical Use of ... ?	Answer
Carnitine	Currently available evidence supports the usefulness of L-carnitine in hyperthyroid patients. Carnitine ameliorates a number of symptoms and signs, including cardiac arrhythmia. Case reports have shown benefits even in the setting of thyroid storm. However, no changes in thyroid function tests were reported. One practical setting for the use of L-carnitine (two grams per day) is the control of hyperthyroidism symptomatology when the patients need to take low doses of antithyroid drugs. Only one Korean study is currently available for hypothyroidism, thus precluding conclusions.
Inositols	Only in one study, MI alone (2 g twice a day) or MI plus melatonin (2 g/d MI plus 3 g/d melatonin) were given in two groups of euthyroid postmenopausal women, and serum FT4 and TSH evaluated. MI alone caused an almost 3.5% increase in serum FT4 and a 10% decrease in serum TSH. This contrasted with the opposite changes (3.5% decrease in serum FT4 and almost 10% increase in serum TSH) observed in the group under MI plus melatonin. Few studies have been conducted only in one Western country (Italy), and with the combination of MI plus selenium or MI plus carnitine. Supplementation with the first combination has been used in the setting of patients with Hashimoto's thyroiditis related SCHypo, and it decreased both serum thyroid autoantibodies and TSH. The combination of MI plus carnitine was only investigated in one study of patients with SCHyper, thus precluding conclusions.
Melatonin	There has been interest in melatonin and autoimmunity and the thyroid gland has been implicated in the discussion. It is thought that melatonin may have a paracrine role and in thyroid disease under a condition of oxidative stress may reduce the processes involved in thyroid antoimmunity. However, there are no controlled trials or definite data to show conclusively that melatonin can be beneficial in thyroid disease.
Resveratrol	No answer can be given, simply for lack of studies.
Selenium	Benefits have been demonstrated for mild forms of Graves' ophthalmopathy. Benefits for the clinical course of GD itself are controversial. In the setting of HT, a benefit has been shown more on serum thyroid autoantibodies than on thyroid function. There is only one study on the benefit given by selenium supplementation, both in terms of serum thyroid autoantibodies and thyroid dysfunction, in the setting of PPT. For the combinations of selenium with MI see above.

Abbreviations, in alphabetical order: GD = Graves' disease; HT = Hashimotos' thyroiditis; MI = myo-inositol; PPT = postpartum thyroiditis. SCHyper = subclinical hyperthyroidism; SCHypo = subclinical hypothyroidism.

Author Contributions: S.B., U.F.-R. and E.A. conceptualized, searched literature and wrote the first versions of the manuscript. D.B. took care of the final update, revision and editing.

Acknowledgments: UF-R's research salary is sponsored by an unrestricted research grant from the NovoNordisk Foundation. This paper received no administrative or technical support.

Appendix A

Table A1. Information on the dietary supplements provided by the Food and Drug Administration *.

Questions	Answers
What is a dietary supplement? §	Congress defined the term "dietary supplement" in the Dietary Supplement Health and Education Act (DSHEA) of 1994. A dietary supplement is a product taken by mouth that contains a "dietary ingredient" intended to supplement the diet. The "dietary ingredients" in these products may include vitamins, minerals, herbs or other botanicals, amino acids, and substances such as enzymes, organ tissues, glandulars, and metabolites. Dietary supplements can also be extracts or concentrates and may be found in many forms such as tablets, capsules, softgels, gelcaps, liquids, or powders. They can also be in other forms, such as a bar, but if they are, information on their label must not represent the product as a conventional food or a sole item of a meal or diet. Whatever their form may be, DSHEA places dietary supplements in a special category under the general umbrella of "foods", not drugs, and requires that every supplement be labeled a dietary supplement.
What is a "new dietary ingredient" in a dietary supplement? §	The Dietary Supplement Health and Education Act (DSHEA) of 1994 defined both of the terms "dietary ingredient" and "new dietary ingredient" as components of dietary supplements. In order for an ingredient of a dietary supplement to be a "dietary ingredient," it must be one or any combination of the following substances: a vitamin, a mineral, an herb or other botanical, an amino acid, a dietary substance for use by man to supplement the diet by increasing the total dietary intake (e.g., enzymes or tissues from organs or glands), or a concentrate, metabolite, constituent or extract. A "new dietary ingredient" is one that meets the above definition for a "dietary ingredient" and was not sold in the U.S. in a dietary supplement before 15 October 1994.
What are the benefits of dietary supplements?	Some supplements can help assure that you get enough of the vital substances the body needs to function; others may help reduce the risk of disease. But supplements should not replace complete meals which are necessary for a healthful diet–so, be sure you eat a variety of foods as well. Unlike drugs, supplements are not permitted to be marketed for the purpose of treating, diagnosing, preventing, or curing diseases. That means supplements should not make disease claims, such as "lowers high cholesterol" or "treats heart disease." Claims like these cannot be legitimately made for dietary supplements.
Are there any risks in taking supplements?	Yes. Many supplements contain active ingredients that have strong biological effects in the body. This could make them unsafe in some situations and hurt or complicate your health. For example, the following actions could lead to harmful–even life-threatening–consequences. Combining supplements Using supplements with medicines (whether prescription or over the counter) Substituting supplements for prescription medicines Taking too much of some supplements, such as vitamin A, vitamin D, or iron Some supplements can also have unwanted effects before, during, and after surgery. So, be sure to inform your healthcare provider, including your pharmacist about any supplements you are taking.

Table A1. *Cont.*

Questions	Answers
Some Common Dietary Supplements	Calcium Echinacea Fish Oil Glucosamine and/or Chondroitin Sulphate Garlic Vitamin D St. John's Wort Saw Palmetto Ginkgo Green Tea Note: These examples do not represent either an endorsement or approval by FDA.
How can I find out more about the dietary supplement I'm taking?	Dietary supplement labels must include name and location information for the manufacturer or distributor. If you want to know more about the product that you are taking, check with the manufacturer or distributor about: Information to support the claims of the product. Information on the safety and effectiveness of the ingredients in the product.
Report Problems to FDA	Notify the FDA if the use of a dietary supplement caused you or a family member to have a serious reaction or illness (even if you are not certain that the product was the cause, or you did not visit a doctor or clinic). Follow these steps: • Stop using the product. • Contact your healthcare provider to find out how to take care of the problem. • Report problems to FDA in either of these ways: • Contact the Consumer Complaint Coordinator in your area. • File a safety report online through the Safety Reporting Portal.

§ Source is [7]. * Source is [8].

References

1. Merriam-Webster Dictionary. Available online: https://www.merriam-webster.com/dictionary/nutraceutical (accessed on 3 September 2019).
2. Cambridge Dictionary. Available online: http://dictionary.cambridge.org/dictionary/english/nutraceutical (accessed on 3 September 2019).
3. Bull, E.; Rapport, L.; Lockwood, B. What is a nutraceutical? *Pharm. J.* **2000**, *265*, 57–58. Available online: https://www.pharmaceutical-journal.com/download?ac=1064856 (accessed on 3 September 2019).
4. Kalra, E.K. Nutraceutical-definition and introduction. *AAPS Pharm. Sci.* **2003**, *5*, E25. [CrossRef] [PubMed]
5. Available online: https://www.eu-japan.eu/sites/default/files/publications/docs/2016-03-nutraceuticals-japan-min.pdf (accessed on 3 September 2019).
6. European Parliament. Regulation EU 2015/2283 of the European Parliament and of the Council of 25 November 2015 on novel foods, amending Regulation (EU) No 1169/2011 of the European Parliament and of the Council and repealing Regulation (EC) No 258/97 of the European Parliament and of the Council and Commission Regulation (EC) No 1852/2001. Available online: https://eur-lex.europa.eu/legal-content/en/TXT/?uri=CELEX%3A32015R2283 (accessed on 3 September 2019).
7. DSHEA 1994. United States Food and Drug Administration (FDA). Dietary Supplement Health and Education Act (DSHEA). U.S. Department of Health and Human Services. United States. Public Law 103–417. Available online: https://ods.od.nih.gov/About/DSHEA_Wording.aspx (accessed on 3 September 2019).
8. Dietary Supplements: What You Need to Know. Available online: https://www.fda.gov/Food/DietarySupplements/UsingDietarySupplements/ucm109760.htm (accessed on 3 September 2019).
9. Questions and Answers on Dietary Supplements. Available online: https://www.fda.gov/Food/DietarySupplements/UsingDietarySupplements/ucm480069.htm#what_is (accessed on 3 September 2019).
10. Wootan, G.D.; Brittain, P.M. *Detox Diets for Dummies*; Wiley Publishing, Inc.: Hoboken, NJ, USA, 2010; p. 88.
11. Available online: https://en.wikipedia.org/wiki/Dietary_supplement (accessed on 3 September 2019).

12. Daniells, S. L-carnitin market to hit $ 130 million by 2017, predicts report. 2011. Available online: https://www.nutraingredients-usa.com/Article/2011/04/22/L-carnitine-market-to-hit-130-million-by-2017-predicts-report (accessed on 3 September 2019).

13. Inositol Market Worth 140 Million USD Industry Making 6.8% of CAGR by 2024. Inositol Market Report. 2019. Available online: https://pmrpressrelease.com/inositol-market-worth-140-million-usd-industry-making-6-8-of-cagr-by-2024/ (accessed on 3 September 2019).

14. Global Melatonin Market Growth 2019–2024. 2019. Available online: https://www.lpinformationdata.com/reports/154866/global-melatonin-market (accessed on 3 September 2019).

15. Yoshino, J.; Conte, C.; Fontana, L.; Mittendorfer, B.; Imai, S.; Schechtman, K.B.; Gu, C.; Kunz, I.; Rossi Fanelli, F.; Patterson, B.W.; et al. Resveratrol supplementation does not improve metabolic function in nonobese women with normal glucose tolerance. *Cell Metab.* **2012**, *16*, 658–664. [CrossRef] [PubMed]

16. National Business Journal Reports: $87 Million U.S. Selenium Sales by Channel in 2017. Supplement Business Report 2018 Informa. Available online: https://www.nutritionbusinessjournal.com/reports/2018-nbj-supplement-business-report/ (accessed on 3 September 2019).

17. Lockwood, G.B. The quality of commercially available nutraceutical supplements and food sources. *J. Pharm. Pharmacol.* **2011**, *63*, 3–10. [CrossRef] [PubMed]

18. Kang, G.Y.; Parks, J.R.; Fileta, B.; Chang, A.; Abdel-Rahim, M.M.; Burch, H.B.; Bernet, V.J. Thyroxine and triiodothyronine content in commercially available thyroid health supplements. *Thyroid* **2013**, *23*, 1233–1237. [CrossRef] [PubMed]

19. Millington, D.S.; Dubag, G. Dietary supplement L-carnitine: Analysis of different brands to determine bioavailability and content. *Clin. Res. Reg. Affairs* **1993**, *10*, 71–80.

20. Papaleo, V.; Molgora, M.; Quaranta, L.; Pellegrino, M.; De Michele, F. Myo-inositol products in polycystic ovary syndrome (PCOS) treatment: Quality, labeling accuracy, and cost comparison. *Eur. Rev. Med. Pharmacol. Sci.* **2011**, *15*, 165–174. [PubMed]

21. Cerezo, A.B.; Leal, A.; Alvarez-Fernandez, M.A.; Hornedo-Ortega, R.; Troncoso, A.M.; Garcia-Parrilla, M.C. Quality control and determination of melatonin in food supplements. *J. Food Compos. Anal.* **2016**, *45*, 80–86. [CrossRef]

22. Erland, L.A.; Sazena, P.K. Melatonin Natural Health Products and Supplements: Presence of Serotonin and Significant Variability of Melatonin Content. *J. Clin. Sleep. Med.* **2017**, *13*, 275–281. [CrossRef]

23. Rossi, D.; Guerrini, A.; Bruni, R.; Brognara, E.; Borgatti, M.; Gambari, R.; Maietti, S.; Sacchetti, G. trans-Resveratrol in nutraceuticals: Issues in retail quality and effectiveness. *Molecules* **2012**, *17*, 12393–12405. [CrossRef]

24. B'Hymer, C.; Caruso, J.A. Evaluation of yeast-based selenium food supplements using high-performance liquid chromatography and inductively coupled plasma mass spectrometry. *J. Anal. At. Spectrom.* **2000**, *15*, 1531–1539. [CrossRef]

25. Hoppel, C. The physiologic role of carnitine. In *L-Carnitine and its Role in Medicine: From Function to Therapy*; Ferrari, R., Di Mauro, S., Sherwood, G., Eds.; Academic Press: San Diego, CA, USA, 1990; pp. 5–19.

26. Wang, Z.Y.; Liu, Y.Y.; Liu, G.H.; Lu, H.B.; Mao, C.Y. L-Carnitine and heart disease. *Life Sci.* **2018**, *194*, 88–97. [CrossRef] [PubMed]

27. Benvenga, S. Effects of L-carnitine on thyroid hormone metabolism and on physical exercise tolerance. *Horm. Metab. Res.* **2005**, *37*, 566–571. [CrossRef] [PubMed]

28. Arenas, J.; Huertas, R.; Campos, Y.; Diaz, A.E.; Villalon, J.M.; Vilas, E. Effects of L-carnitine on the pyruvate dehydrogenase complex and carnitine palmitoyl transferase in muscle athletes. *FEBS Lett.* **1994**, *341*, 91–93. [CrossRef]

29. Arenas, J.; Ricoy, J.R.; Encinas, A.R.; Pola, P.; D'Iddio, S.; Zeviani, M.; Di Donato, S.; Corsi, M. Carnitine in muscle, serum and urine of non-professional athletes; effects of physical exercise, training, and L-carnitine administration. *Muscle Nerve* **1991**, *14*, 598–604. [CrossRef]

30. Brass, E.P.; Hiatt, W.R. The role of carnitine and carnitine supplementation during excercise in man and in individuals with special needs. *J. Am. Coll. Nutr.* **1998**, *17*, 207–215. [CrossRef]

31. Brass, E.P. Supplemental carnitine and exercise. *Am. J. Clin. Nutr.* **2000**, *72*, 618S–623S. [CrossRef]

32. Brass, E.P. Carnitine and sports medicine: Use or abuse? *Ann. NY Acad. Sci.* **2004**, *1033*, 67–78. [CrossRef]

33. Strack, E.; Wortz, G.; Rotzsch, W. Wirkungen von Carnitin bei Uberfunktion der Schildruse (Effects of Carnitine in cases of Thyroid Hyperfunction). *Endocrinologie* **1959**, *38*, 218–225.

34. Gilgore, S.G.; De Felice, S.L. Evaluation of carnitine—An antagonist of thyroid hormone. *J. N. Drugs* **1966**, *6*, 349–350. [CrossRef]

35. De Felice, S.L.; Gilgore, S.G. The antagonistic effect of carnitine in hyperthyroidism. Preliminary report. *J. N. Drugs* **1966**, *6*, 351–353. [CrossRef]

36. Benvenga, S.; Lakshmanan, M.; Trimarchi, F. Carnitine is a naturally occurring inhibitor of thyroid hormone nuclear uptake. *Thyroid* **2000**, *12*, 1043–1050. [CrossRef] [PubMed]

37. Benvenga, S.; Ruggeri, R.M.; Russo, A.; Lapa, D.; Campenni, A.; Trimarchi, F. Usefulness of L-carnitine, a naturally occurring peripheral antagonist of thyroid hormone action, in iatrogenic hyperthyroidism: A randomized, double-blind, placebo-controlled clinical trial. *J. Clin. Endocrinol. Metab.* **2001**, *86*, 3579–3594. [CrossRef] [PubMed]

38. Benvenga, S.; Lapa, D.; Cannavò, S.; Trimarchi, F. Successive thyroid storms treated with L-carnitine and low doses of methimazole. *Am. J. Med.* **2003**, *115*, 417–418. [CrossRef]

39. Chee, R.; Agah, R.; Vita, R.; Benvenga, S. Severe hyperthyroidism treated with L-carnitine, propranolol, and finally with thyroidectomy in a seriously ill cancer patient. *Hormones* **2014**, *13*, 407–412. [PubMed]

40. Kimmoun, A.; Munagamage, G.; Dessalles, N.; Gerard, A.; Feillet, F.; Levy, B. Unexpected awakening from comatose thyroid storm after a single intravenous injection of L-carnitine. *Intensive Care Med.* **2011**, *37*, 1716–1717. [CrossRef] [PubMed]

41. Nordio, M. A novel treatment for subclinical hyperthyroidism: A pilot study on the beneficial effects of L-carnitine and selenium. *Eur. Rev. Med. Pharmacol. Sci.* **2017**, *21*, 2268–2273.

42. Maebashi, M.; Kawamura, N.; Sato, N.; Imamura, A.; Yoshinaga, K. Urinary excretion of carnitine in patients with hyperthyroidism and hypothyroidism: Augmentation by thyroid hormone. *Metabolism* **1977**, *26*, 351–356. [CrossRef]

43. Sinclair, C.; Gilchrist, J.M.; Hennessey, J.V.; Kandula, M. Muscle carnitine in hypo- and hyperthyroidism. *Muscle Nerve* **2005**, *32*, 357–359. [CrossRef]

44. An, J.H.; Kim, Y.J.; Kim, K.J.; Kim, S.H.; Kim, N.H.; Kim, H.Y.; Kim, N.H.; Choi, K.M.; Baik, S.H.; Choi, D.S.; et al. L-carnitine supplementation for the management of fatigue in patients with hypothyroidism on levothyroxine treatment: A randomized, double-blind, placebo-controlled trial. *Endocr. J.* **2016**, *63*, 885–895. [CrossRef]

45. Benvenga, S.; Sindoni, A. L-carnitine supplementation for the management of fatigue in patients with hypothyroidism on levothyroxine treatment. *Endocr. J.* **2016**, *63*, 937–938. [CrossRef] [PubMed]

46. Alesci, S.; De Martino, M.U.; Mirani, M.; Benvenga, S.; Trimarchi, F.; Kino, T.; Chrousos, G.P. L carnitine: A nutritional modulator of glucocorticoid receptor functions. *FASEB J.* **2003**, *17*, 1553–1555. [CrossRef] [PubMed]

47. Benvenga, S.; Antonelli, A. Inositol(s) in thyroid function, growth and autoimmunity. *Rev. Endocr. Metab. Disord.* **2016**, *17*, 471–484. [CrossRef] [PubMed]

48. Nordio, M.; Pajalich, R. Combined treatment with Myo-inositol and selenium ensures euthyroidism in subclinical hypothyroidism patients with autoimmune thyroiditis. *J. Thyroid Res.* **2013**, *2013*, 424163. [CrossRef] [PubMed]

49. Nordio, M.; Basciani, S. Treatment with Myo-Inositol and Selenium Ensures Euthyroidism in Patients with Autoimmune Thyroiditis. *Int. J. Endocrinol.* **2017**. [CrossRef]

50. Nordio, M.; Basciani, S. Myo-inositol plus selenium supplementation restores euthyroid state in Hashimoto's patients with subclinical hypothyroidism. *Eur. Rev. Med. Pharmacol. Sci.* **2017**, *21* (Suppl. 2), 51–59.

51. Ferrari, S.M.; Fallahi, P.; Di Bari, F.; Vita, R.; Benvenga, S.; Antonelli, A. Myo-inositol and selenium reduce the risk of developing overt hypothyroidism in patients with autoimmune thyroiditis. *Eur. Rev. Med. Pharmacol. Sci.* **2017**, *21* (Suppl. 2), 36–42.

52. Nordio, M.; Basciani, S. Evaluation of thyroid nodule characteristics in subclinical hypothyroid patients under a myo-inositol plus selenium treatment. *Eur. Rev. Med. Pharmacol. Sci.* **2018**, *22*, 2153–2159.

53. Johnston, J.D. 60 Years of neuroendocrinology: Regulation of mammalian neuroendocrine physiology and rhythms by melatonin. *J. Endocrinol.* **2015**, *226*, T187–T198. [CrossRef]

54. Mazzoccoli, G.; De Cata, A.; Carughi, S.; Greco, A.; Inglese, M.; Perfetto, F.; Tarquini, R. A possible mechanism for altered immune response in the elderly. *In Vivo* **2010**, *24*, 471–487.

55. Bellipanni, G.; Bianchi, P.; Pierpaoli, W.; Bulian, D.; Ilyia, E. Effects of melatonin in perimenopausal and menopausal women: A randomized and placebo controlled study. *Exp. Gerontol.* **2001**, *36*, 297–310. [CrossRef]

56. Bellipanni, G.; Di Marzo, F.; Blasi, F.; Di Marzo, A. Effects of melatonin in perimenopausal and menopausal women: Our personal experience. *Ann. N. Y. Acad. Sci.* **2005**, *1057*, 393–402. [CrossRef] [PubMed]

57. D'Anna, R.; Santamaria, A.; Giorgianni, G.; Vaiarelli, A.; Gullo, G.; Di Bari, F.; Benvenga, S. Myo-inositol and melatonin in the menopausal transition. *Gynecol. Endocrinol.* **2017**, *33*, 279–282. [CrossRef] [PubMed]

58. Lin, J.D.; Yang, S.F.; Wang, Y.H.; Fang, W.F.; Lin, Y.C.; Liou, B.C.; Lin, Y.F.; Tang, K.T.; Cheng, C.W. Association of melatonin receptor gene polymorphisms with Graves' disease. *PLoS ONE* **2017**, *12*, e0185529. [CrossRef]

59. Rauf, A.; Imran, M.; Suleria, H.A.R.; Ahmad, B.; Peters, D.G.; Mubarak, M.S. A comprehensive review of the health perspectives of resveratrol. *Food Funct.* **2017**, *8*, 4284–4305. [CrossRef] [PubMed]

60. Limmongkon, A.; Janhom, P.; Amthong, A.; Kawpanuk, M.; Nopprang, P.; Poohadsuan, J.; Somboon, T.; Saijeen, S.; Surangkul, D.; Metawee, S.; et al. Antioxidant activity, total phenolic, and resveratrol content in five cultivars of peanut sprouts. *Asian Pac. J. Trop. Biomed.* **2017**, *7*, 332–338. [CrossRef]

61. Rauf, A.; Imran, M.; Butt, M.S.; Nadeem, M.; Peters, D.G.; Mubarak, M.S. Resveratrol as an anti-cancer agent: A review. *Crit. Rev. Food Sci. Nutr.* **2016**. [CrossRef]

62. Aggarwal, B.B.; Bhardwaj, A.; Aggarwal, R.S.; Seeram, N.P.; Shishodia, S.; Takada, Y. Role of resveratrol in prevention and therapy of cancer: Preclinical and clinical studies. *Anticancer Res.* **2004**, *24*, 2783–2840.

63. Duntas, L.H. Resveratrol and its impact on aging and thyroid function. *J. Endocrinol. Investig.* **2011**, *34*, 788–792.

64. Yu, X.M.; Jaskula-Sztul, R.; Ahmed, K.; Harrison, A.D.; Kunnimalaiyaan, M.; Chen, H. differentiation markers expression in anaplastic thyroid carcinoma via activation of Notch1 signaling and suppresses cell growth. *Mol. Cancer Ther.* **2013**, *12*, 1276–1287. [CrossRef]

65. Shih, A.; Davis, F.B.; Lin, H.Y.; Davis, P.J. Resveratrol induces apoptosis in thyroid cancer cell lines via a MAPK- and p53-dependent mechanism. *J. Clin. Endocrinol. Metab.* **2002**, *87*, 1223–1232. [CrossRef] [PubMed]

66. Truong, M.; Cook, M.R.; Pinchot, S.N.; Kunnimalaiyaan, M.; Chen, H. Resveratrol induces Notch2-mediated apoptosis and suppression of neuroendocrine markers in medullary thyroid cancer. *Ann. Surg. Oncol.* **2011**, *18*, 1506–1511. [CrossRef] [PubMed]

67. Giuliani, C.; Iezzi, M.; Ciolli, L.; Hysi, A.; Bucci, I.; Di Santo, S.; Rossi, C.; Zucchelli, M.; Napolitano, G. Resveratrol has anti-thyroid effects both in vitro and in vivo. *Food Chem. Toxicol.* **2017**, *107*, 237–247. [CrossRef] [PubMed]

68. Sebai, H.; Hovsepian, S.; Ristorcelli, E.; Aouani, E.; Lombardo, D.; Fayet, G. Resveratrol increases iodide trapping in the rat thyroid cell line FRTL-5. *Thyroid* **2010**, *20*, 195–203. [CrossRef] [PubMed]

69. Available online: https://efsa.onlinelibrary.wiley.com/doi/epdf/10.2903/j.efsa.2014.3846 (accessed on 3 September 2019).

70. GB Health Watch. Available online: https://www.gbhealthwatch.com/Nutrient-Selenium-Overview.php (accessed on 3 September 2019).

71. Negro, R.; Attanasio, R.; Grimaldi, F.; Marcocci, C.; Guglielmi, R.; Papini, E. A 2016 Italian Survey about the Clinical Use of Selenium in Thyroid Disease. *Eur. Thyr. J.* **2016**, *5*, 164–170. [CrossRef] [PubMed]

72. Alexander, E.K.; Pearce, E.N.; Brent, G.A.; Brown, R.S.; Chen, H.; Dosiou, C.; Grobman, W.A.; Laurberg, P.; Lazarus, J.H.; Mandel, S.J.; et al. 2017 Guidelines of the American Thyroid Association for the Diagnosis and Management of Thyroid Disease During Pregnancy and the Postpartum. *Thyroid* **2017**, *27*, 315–389. [CrossRef] [PubMed]

73. Drutel, A.; Archambeaud, F.; Caron, P. Selenium and the thyroid gland: More good news for clinicians. *Clin. Endocrinol. (Oxf)* **2013**, *78*, 155–164. [CrossRef] [PubMed]

74. Köhrle, J. Selenium and the thyroid. *Curr. Opin. Endocrinol. Diabetes Obes.* **2013**, *20*, 441–448. [CrossRef]

75. Derumeaux, H.; Valeix, P.; Castetbon, K.; Bensimon, M.; Boutron-Ruault, M.C.; Arnaud, J.; Hercberg, S. Association of selenium with thyroid volume and echostructure in 35- to 60-year-old French adults. *Eur. J. Endocrinol.* **2003**, *148*, 309–315. [CrossRef]

76. Rasmussen, L.B.; Schomburg, L.; Köhrle, J.; Pedersen, I.B.; Hollenbach, B.; Hög, A.; Ovesen, L.; Perrild, H.; Laurberg, P. Selenium status, thyroid volume, and multiple nodule formation in an area with mild iodine deficiency. *Eur. J. Endocrinol.* **2011**, *164*, 585–590. [CrossRef]

77. Burk, R.F.; Hill, K.E. Selenoprotein P: An extracellular protein with unique physical characteristics and a role in selenium homeostasis. *Ann. Rev. Nutr.* **2005**, *25*, 215–235. [CrossRef] [PubMed]

78. Burk, R.F.; Norsworthy, B.K.; Hill, K.E.; Motley, A.K.; Byrne, D.W. Effects of chemical form of selenium on plasma biomarkers in a high-dose human supplementation trial. *Cancer Epidemiol. Biomarkers Prev.* **2006**, *15*, 804–810. [CrossRef] [PubMed]

79. Cui, Z.; Huang, J.; Peng, Q.; Yu, D.; Wang, S.; Liang, D. Risk assessment for human health in a seleniferous area, Shuang'an, China. *Environ. Sci. Pollut. Res. Int.* **2017**, *24*, 17701–17710. [CrossRef] [PubMed]

80. Dinh, Q.T.; Cui, Z.; Huang, J.; Tran, T.A.T.; Wang, D.; Yang, W.; Zhou, F.; Wang, M.; Yu, D.; Liang, D. Selenium distribution in the Chinese environment and its relationship with human health: A review. *Environ. Int.* **2018**, *112*, 294–309. [CrossRef] [PubMed]

81. Duntas, L.; Benvenga, S. Selenium: An element for life. *Endocrine* **2015**, *48*, 756–775. [CrossRef] [PubMed]

82. Huang, Z.; Rose, A.H.; Hoffmann, P.R. The role of selenium in inflammation and immunity: From molecular mechanisms to therapeutic opportunities. *Antioxid. Redox Signal.* **2012**, *16*, 705–743. [CrossRef] [PubMed]

83. Toulis, K.A.; Anastasilakis, A.D.; Tzellos, T.G.; Goulis, D.G.; Kouvelas, D. Selenium supplementation in the treatment of Hashimoto's thyroiditis: A systematic review and a metaanalysis. *Thyroid* **2010**, *20*, 1163–1173. [CrossRef]

84. Bülow Pedersen, I.; Knudsen, N.; Carlé, A.; Schomburg, L.; Köhrle, J.; Jørgensen, T.; Rasmussen, L.B.; Ovesen, L.; Laurberg, P. Serum selenium is low in newly diagnosed Graves' disease: A population-based study. *Clin. Endocrinol. (Oxf)* **2013**, *79*, 584–590. [CrossRef]

85. Leo, M.; Bartalena, L.; Rotondo Dottore, G.; Piantanida, E.; Premoli, P.; Ionni, I.; Di Cera, M.; Masiello, E.; Sassi, L.; Tanda, M.L. Effects of selenium on short-term control of hyperthyroidism due to Graves' disease treated with methimazole: Results of a randomized clinical trial. *J. Endocrinol. Investig.* **2017**, *40*, 281–287. [CrossRef]

86. Calissendorff, J.; Mikulski, E.; Larsen, E.H.; Möller, M. A Prospective Investigation of Graves' Disease and Selenium: Thyroid Hormones, Autoantibodies and Self-Rated Symptoms. *Eur. Thyroid J.* **2015**, *4*, 93–98. [CrossRef]

87. Wang, L.; Wang, B.; Chen, S.R.; Hou, X.; Wang, X.F.; Zhao, S.H.; Song, J.Q.; Wang, Y.G. Effect of Selenium Supplementation on Recurrent Hyperthyroidism Caused by Graves' Disease: A Prospective Pilot Study. *Horm. Metab. Res.* **2016**, *48*, 559–564. [CrossRef]

88. Kahaly, G.J.; Riedl, M.; König, J.; Diana, T.; Schomburg, L. Double-blind, placebo-controlled, randomized trial of selenium in graves hyperthyroidism. *J. Clin. Endocrinol. Metab.* **2017**, *102*, 4333–4341. [CrossRef] [PubMed]

89. Zheng, H.; Wei, J.; Wang, L.; Wang, Q.; Zhao, J.; Chen, S.; Wei, F. Effects of Selenium Supplementation on Graves' disease: A Systematic Review and Meta-Analysis. *Evid. Based Complement. Alternat. Med.* **2018**, *2018*, 3763565. [CrossRef] [PubMed]

90. Watt, T.; Cramon, P.; Bjorner, J.B.; Bonnema, S.J.; Feldt-Rasmussen, U.; Gluud, C.; Gram, J.; Hansen, J.L.; Hegedüs, L.; Knudsen, N. Selenium supplementation for patients with Graves' hyperthyroidism (the GRASS trial): Study protocol for a randomized controlled trial. *Trials* **2013**, *14*, 119. [CrossRef] [PubMed]

91. Khong, J.J.; Goldstein, R.F.; Sanders, K.M.; Schneider, H.; Pope, J.; Burdon, K.P.; Craig, J.E.; Ebeling, P.R. Serum selenium status in Graves' disease with and without orbitopathy: A case-control study. *Clin. Endocrinol. (Oxf)* **2014**, *80*, 905–910. [CrossRef] [PubMed]

92. Marcocci, C.; Kahaly, G.J.; Krassas, G.E.; Bartalena, L.; Prummel, M.; Stahl, M.; Altea, M.A.; Nardi, M.; Pitz, S.; Boboridis, K. European Group on Graves' Orbitopathy. Selenium and the course of mild Graves' orbitopathy. *N. Engl. J. Med.* **2011**, *364*, 1920–1931. [CrossRef] [PubMed]

93. Gärtner, R.; Gasnier, B.C.H.; Dietrich, J.W.; Krebs, B.; Angstwurm, M.W. Selenium supplementation in patients with autoimmune thyroiditis decreases thyroid peroxidase antibodies concentrations. *J. Clin. Endocrinol. Metab.* **2002**, *87*, 1687–1691. [CrossRef] [PubMed]

94. Duntas, L.H.; Mantzou, E.; Koutras, D.A. Effects of a six month treatment with selenomethionine in patients with autoimmune thyroiditis. *Eur. J. Endocrinol.* **2003**, *148*, 389–393. [CrossRef]

95. Turker, O.; Kumanlioglu, K.; Karapolat, I.; Dogan, I. Selenium treatment in autoimmune thyroiditis: 9-month follow-up with variable doses. *J. Endocrinol.* **2006**, *190*, 151–156. [CrossRef]

96. Winther, K.H.; Bonnema, S.J.; Cold, F.; Debrabant, B.; Nybo, M.; Cold, S.; Hegedüs, L. Does selenium supplementation affect thyroid function? Results from a randomized, controlled, double-blinded trial in a Danish population. *Eur. J. Endocrinol.* **2015**, *172*, 657–667. [CrossRef]

97. Van Zuuren, E.J.; Albusta, A.Y.; Fedorowicz, Z.; Carter, B.; Pijl, H. Selenium supplementation for Hashimoto's thyroiditis. *Cochrane Database Syst. Rev.* **2013**, *6*, CD010223. [CrossRef] [PubMed]

98. Winther, K.H.; Wichman, J.E.; Bonnema, S.J.; Hegedüs, L. Insufficient documentation for clinical efficacy of selenium supplementation in chronic autoimmune thyroiditis, based on a systematic review and meta-analysis. *Endocrine* **2017**, *55*, 376–385. [CrossRef] [PubMed]

99. Winther, K.H.; Watt, T.; Bjørner, J.B.; Cramon, P.; Feldt-Rasmussen, U.; Gluud, C.; Gram, J.; Groenvold, M.; Hegedüs, L.; Knudsen, N. The chronic autoimmune thyroiditis quality of life selenium trial (CATALYST): Study protocol for a randomized controlled trial. *Trials* **2014**, *15*. [CrossRef] [PubMed]

100. Negro, R.; Greco, G.; Mangieri, T.; Pezzarossa, A.; Dazzi, D.; Hassan, H. The influence of selenium supplementation on postpartum thyroid status in pregnant women with thyroid peroxidase autoantibodies. *J. Clin. Endocrinol. Metab.* **2007**, *92*, 1263–1268. [CrossRef] [PubMed]

101. Mao, J.; Pop, V.J.; Bath, S.C.; Vader, H.L.; Redman, C.W.; Rayman, M.P. Effect of low-dose selenium on thyroid autoimmunity and thyroid function in UK pregnant women with mild-to-moderate iodine deficiency. *Eur. J. Nutr.* **2016**, *55*, 55–61. [CrossRef] [PubMed]

Endemic Goiter and Iodine Prophylaxis in Calabria, a Region of Southern Italy: Past and Present

Cinzia Giordano [1,2], **Ines Barone** [1], **Stefania Marsico** [1,2], **Rosalinda Bruno** [1,2], **Daniela Bonofiglio** [1,2,*], **Stefania Catalano** [1,2,*] and **Sebastiano Andò** [1,2,*]

[1] Department of Pharmacy, Health and Nutritional Sciences, University of Calabria, 87036 Rende (CS), Italy; cinzia.giordano@unical.it (C.G.); ines.barone@unical.it (I.B.); stefania.marsico@unical.it (S.M.); rosalinda.bruno@unical.it (R.B.)

[2] Centro Sanitario, University of Calabria, 87036 Rende (CS), Italy

[*] Correspondence: daniela.bonofiglio@unical.it (D.B.); stefcatalano@libero.it (S.C.); sebastiano.ando@unical.it (S.A.)

Abstract: Iodine, a micronutrient that plays a pivotal role in thyroid hormone synthesis, is essential for proper health at all life stages. Indeed, an insufficient iodine intake may determine a thyroid dysfunction also with goiter, or it may be associated to clinical features such as stunted growth and mental retardation, referred as iodine deficiency disorders (IDDs). Iodine deficiency still remains an important public health problem in many countries, including Italy. The effective strategy for the prevention and control of IDDs is universal salt iodization, which was implemented in Italy in 2005 as a nationwide program adopted after the approval of an Italian law. Despite an improvement in the iodine intake, many regions in Italy are still characterized by mild iodine deficiency. In this review, we provide an overview of the historical evolution of the iodine status in the Calabria region, located in the South of Italy, during the past three decades. In particular, we have retraced an itinerary from the first epidemiological surveys at the end of the 1980s to the establishment of the Regional Observatory of Endemic Goiter and Iodine Prophylaxis, which represents an efficient model for the surveillance of IDDs and monitoring the efficacy of iodine prophylaxis.

Keywords: iodine deficiency; iodine prophylaxis; goiter; urinary iodine concentration

1. Introduction

Iodine deficiency and related disorders are still a public health problem that affects most countries, including industrialized and developing regions [1,2]. At the end of 2018, a global survey on iodine status, covering more than 97% of the world's population, indicated that 21 countries remain vulnerable to iodine deficiency. Specifically, nationally-representative surveys revealed insufficient iodine intake in 14 countries (Burkina Faso, Burundi, Finland, Haiti, Israel, Iraq, the Democratic People's Republic of Korea, Lebanon, Mali, Madagascar, Mozambique, Samoa, Vanuatu, and Vietnam). Moreover, in sub-national surveys, seven other countries, including Angola, Italy, Morocco, Norway, Russia, South Sudan, and Sudan were reported as being iodine insufficient [3].

Iodine deficiency impairs thyroid hormone production and has many adverse effects during the course of life, which are collectively termed the iodine deficiency disorders (IDDs). The frequency and severity of IDD manifestations are related to the degree of iodine deficiency and the age of the affected subjects. Although thyroid enlargement (goiter) is the classic sign of iodine deficiency, and can take place at any age, the most serious adverse effects of iodine deficiency occur during pregnancy, including impaired fetal growth and brain development [4–6]. The iodine status of the population can be assessed by using four methods: urinary iodine (UI) concentration, the goiter rate, serum thyroid stimulating hormone (TSH), and serum thyroglobulin (Tg) levels [7–10]. UI is the most sensitive indicator of current iodine intake because >90% of dietary iodine is excreted in the urine [11]. UI concentration can be measured in spot urine samples and the median UI values were used to assess iodine nutrition among school-age children, as recommended by World Health Organization (WHO), United Nations International Children's Emergency Fund (UNICEF), and the Iodine Global Network (IGN) [7]. The cut-off values for urinary iodine levels were used to define iodine deficiency (<100 µg/L) were classified as mild (50–99 µg/L), moderate (20–49 µg/L), or severe (<20 µg/L). Daily iodine intake for population can be extrapolated from UI concentration using the following formula: urinary iodine (µg/L) × 0.0235 × body weight (Kg) = daily intake (µg) [12].

This allows us to assume that a median UI concentration of 100 µg/L corresponds roughly to an average daily iodine intake of 150 µg.

An important indicator of IDDs is represented by the goiter rate measured by ultrasound in school-age children. However, a standardized approach should be adopted worldwide to improve the reliability of thyroid volume in the context of IDD monitoring [8]. Supplementary indicators of iodine deficiency include blood-spot TSH measurement only in neonates [13], while Tg measured in a dried blood spot has been reported to be a good marker of iodine intake in infancy [14].

Universal salt iodization is the most cost-effective strategy for IDDs and the WHO, UNICEF, and IGN recommend that iodine is added at a concentration of 20–40 mg per kg salt, dependent on local salt intake [15].

Over the last decades, intensive efforts have been made by the governments of IDD-affected countries to implement and control salt iodization program [9,16–19]. India was one of the first countries in the world to initiate and maintain a sustained increase in the coverage of adequately iodized salt, achieving the goal of universal salt iodization levels of greater than 90% in urban areas of the Central, North, and North-East zones of its territory in 2015 [20–22]. Following the introduction of mandatory salt iodization in 1995, Madagascar showed a swift growth in iodized salt coverage, however a recent national survey reported that iodine deficiency remains a serious public health problem there [23]. This implies that to maintain an effective program on salt iodization over the long term, it is necessary to set up a system that coordinates and monitors the sale trend of iodized salt and communicates the health benefits of consuming iodized salt. A good example of national progress is represented by Ethiopia in which the national coverage of iodized salt increased from 4.2% in 2005 to 95% in 2014. These results stem from multi-level and multi-sector efforts involving public-private partnerships that focused on enforcing iodization legislation [24,25]. Also in Italy, a nationwide salt iodization program was implemented in 2005 with the approval of the law n. 55/2005 that requires the addition of potassium iodate to table salt at 30 mg/kg and the mandatory availability of iodized salt in food shops and supermarkets. The law also permits the use of iodized salt in the food and catering industries. To the aim of evaluating the efficiency and effectiveness of the nationwide program of iodine prophylaxis, in 2009 the Italian National Observatory for Monitoring Iodine Prophylaxis (OSNAMI) was established at the Italian National Institute of Health [26]. Although a significant improvement of iodine nutrition has been observed over the years, some regions in Italy still remain at risk of deficiency.

In this review we provide an overview of the iodine status in Calabria, a region of Southern Italy, over the past three decades. Particularly, we report data obtained from the first epidemiological surveys up to the establishment of the Regional Observatory of Endemic Goiter and Iodine Prophylaxis (Figure 1), that represents an efficient model for the surveillance of IDDs and monitoring the efficacy of iodine prophylaxis.

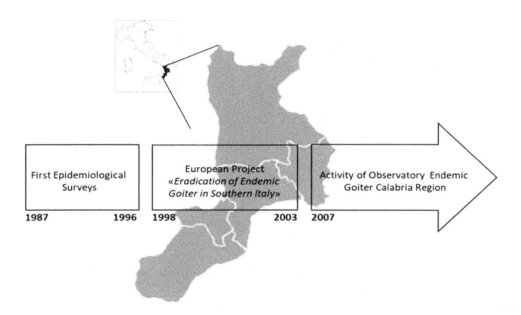

Figure 1. Schematic representation of the key steps of epidemiological surveys conducted from the late 1980s to the present for assessing and monitoring iodine status in the Calabria region.

2. History of Goiter and Iodine Deficiency in Calabria: Epidemiological Surveys during the 1980–2000 Period

The Calabria region located in the Southern of Italy is a peninsula of irregular shape, referred to as the "toe" of the Italian "boot", with a coastline of 738 km on the Ionian and Tyrrhenian coasts of the Mediterranean Basin. The regional orography highlights mountainous features: 42% of the land is mountainous, 49% is hilly, and only 8% is completely flat with an average elevation of 597 m [27]. This region, comprising five provinces with a total population of about 2 million inhabitants, has been historically exposed to iodine deficiency.

Data obtained from epidemiological surveys carried out between 1987–1996 allowed us to draw a first map of iodine deficiency and endemic goiter in Calabria by evaluating the mean of UI excretion and the size of thyroid gland. Since ultrasonography was not easy to perform in a large scale of epidemiological screening and the reference values for ultrasound thyroid volume measurement in children living in iodine-sufficient areas were not well established, the goiter rate was assessed using WHO's 1960 palpation system [28].

The first study was conducted by our research group [29] in 1987–1989 on 34 villages of extraurban areas of Catanzaro (A) and Cosenza (B) provinces. In this survey, 4468 and 2721 schoolchildren (aged between 6–12 years) of area A and area B, respectively, were examined. The prevalence of endemic goiter was 53% in the population living in Catanzaro's province with the highest percentage found in Zagarise (67%), while the rate in schoolchildren from Cosenza's province was 44% with the highest percentage found in Laino Castello (69%). Interestingly, in both areas the goiter prevalence was independent from area altitude as well as the distance of the villages from the main town, and was significantly higher than that observed among the 1170 age-matched schoolchildren living in the urban area of the Calabria region (7.7%). Mean UI concentration was 49.7 ± 5.3 µg/L and 70.7 ± 3.1 µg/L in area A and B, respectively, indicating the presence of a mild iodine deficiency respect to the UI values of urban area that reflect an iodine sufficiency (104 ± 6.6 µg/L).

After two years of voluntary iodine prophylaxis (1991–1992) 855 schoolchildren from five small villages (Laino Borgo, Laino Castello, San Basile, Saracena and Mormanno) of Cosenza province were examined. These five villages were chosen since their drug-stores carried iodized salt and the population was advised to use it. As shown in Figure 2, an increase of UI concentration along with a reduced goiter prevalence were found, suggesting that an effective program of iodine prophylaxis is urgently needed in this region [29].

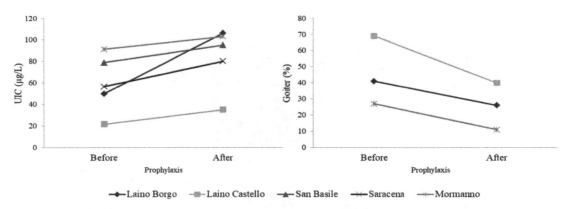

Figure 2. Urinary iodine concentration (UIC) and goiter prevalence before and after iodine prophylaxis in schoolchildren of the Cosenza province.

Another epidemiological study, which are useful to better define the map of endemic goiter and to characterize iodine deficiency in the whole Calabrian territory, was performed during the years 1990–1996 by Costante et al. [30]. A total of 13,984 schoolchildren, aged 6–14 years, was examined for the goiter prevalence, while UI excretion was evaluated in 284 samples that were randomly collected. Goiter prevalence ranged from 19% to 64% and from 5.3% to 25.7% in the inland territory and at the coastal area, respectively, while the mean of UI excretion was 53.8 ± 43.4 µg/L in the inland territory and 89.6 ± 59.8 µg/L at sea level, confirming that moderate levels along with pockets of severe iodine deficiency was present in the inland region, while iodine supply varied from sufficient to marginally low in the coastal areas. Moreover, the presence of mild to moderate iodine deficiency was also established by the results of neonatal TSH levels from the congenital hypothyroidism regional screening program. Indeed, the authors reported 14.8% frequency of TSH levels >5 µU/mL in newborns from the inland territory and 14.1% frequency from coastal areas [30].

Overall, these first epidemiological surveys clearly indicate that at the end of the 1990s, the whole Calabria region was a mild to moderate iodine deficient area. Interestingly, the data obtained in the Calabria region were in line with a series of surveys carried out from 1978 to 1991 in different regions of Italy, in which a total number of 72,112 schoolchildren was examined, including 5046 controls living in urban areas and 66,066 subjects residing in rural endemic areas. Surveys were carried out throughout Italy in predominantly hilly and mountainous areas. Globally, the goiter prevalence ranged from 14% to 73%, which inversely correlated with urinary iodine excretion (10–122 µg/g creatinine) and was more prevalent in Central and Southern Italy (reference [31] and references therein).

At the end of the 1990s, as part of a European project entitled "Eradication of endemic goiter and of disorders of iodine deficiency in Southern Italy" with cooperation between the National Research Council and the Ministry of Health, and financed by the European Union, a survey to assess the iodine nutrition was conducted in eight regions of Southern Italy, including Calabria [32]. The grade of iodine deficiency was assessed through the measurement of UI excretion in 23,103 samples randomly collected from the schoolchildren population aged 11–14 years living in urban and rural areas and in different geographic locations. Median UI excretion in the all studied population was 74 µg/L, showing significantly higher values in urban areas compared to rural areas (81 µg/L vs. 73 µg/L, $p < 0.0001$). Besides, median UI excretion was significantly lower in inland mountainous/hilly areas respect to coastal mountainous/hilly areas (68 µg/L vs. 79 µg/L, $p < 0.0001$). The results of this extensive survey indicated that in Southern Italy, mild to moderate iodine deficiency still persisted [32]. Particularly in the Calabria region, data obtained from a total of 2693 spot urinary samples expressed as median as well as mean (±SD) displayed insufficient iodine intake in all five provinces of the Calabria region (Table 1, data unpublished).

Table 1. Mean (±DS) and median urinary iodine concentration (UIC) in schoolchildren in the Calabria region.

Provinces	Samples (n)	UIC Mean (±SD) µg/L	UIC Median µg/L
Catanzaro	1024	85 ± 71	65
Cosenza	701	91 ± 71	73
Crotone	257	84 ± 78	54
Reggio Calabria	346	91 ± 69	75
Vibo Valentia	365	83 ± 64	67

Similar results were obtained in Campania, another region of Southern Italy, in which UI excretion from 10,552 schoolchildren were determined. The analysis of frequency distribution showed values below 50 and 100 µg/L of UI in 32% and 61% of children, respectively, highlighting the Campania region as a mild iodine deficiency area [33].

As a part of the same European project, another important challenge was to implement the use of iodized salt through interactive meetings with schoolchildren. In the Calabria region, we have interviewed 49,840 subjects in their classrooms, providing detailed information on the beneficial effects of iodine salt prophylaxis along with informative materials consisting of leaflets and table-games about iodine deficiency disorders. A final goal of this project was to establish an Observatory for Monitoring Iodine Prophylaxis in each Italian region.

3. Status of Iodine Intake Over the Last Two Decades in the Calabria Region: The Epidemiological Observatory for Endemic Goiter and Iodine Prophylaxis

Based on our extensive studies carried out in the entire regional territory and taking into account the final goal of the European project, the Epidemiological Observatory and Promotion of Health of the Calabria Region, Section "Goiter Endemic and Iodine Prophylaxis" (OERC) was established by the Calabria region (regional law n. 755/2003) at the Health Center of the University of Calabria. The OERC represents the epidemiological structure through which the regional-scale surveillance of the iodine prophylaxis program is carried out using: (i) epidemiological surveys to periodically evaluate the iodine intake and the prevalence of goiter in the adolescent and to verify the prevalence of thyroid diseases in the adult population; (ii) a promotional campaign on the advantages of iodine prophylaxis; (iii) the sale trend of iodized salt.

3.1. Epidemiological Surveys

The first survey was carried out in the years 2007–2009 on 11–14 year old children recruited from long standing iodine sufficient urban areas (U) and from rural areas (R) in which an iodine insufficiency was previously documented [29,30]. In agreement with the guidelines of WHO, UNICEF, and International Council for Control of Iodine Deficiency Disorders (ICCIDD) [9], monitoring was based on both the percentage of goiter and the median value of UI concentration in schoolchildren. A total of 2733 subjects (1686 U and 1047 R) from the five provinces of Calabria were examined to evaluate thyroid volume by ultrasonography, while 1358 (794 U and 565 R) spot-urine samples were collected to determine adequacy of iodine intake. The prevalence of goiter, calculated on the basis of the reference values proposed by WHO [8], and the median values of ioduria are shown in Figure 3 (data unpublished).

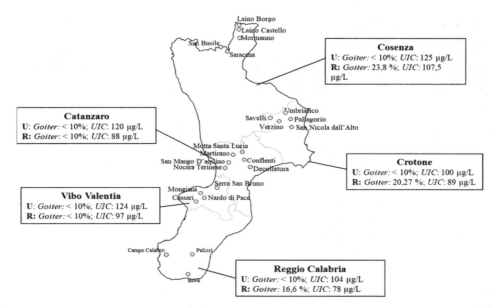

Figure 3. Goiter prevalence and median urinary iodine concentration in schoolchildren population from iodine sufficient urban areas (U) and rural areas (R) of the Calabria region.

Our data indicated that a mild iodine deficiency was still present in the rural areas of the provinces of Cosenza, Reggio Calabria, and Crotone, whereas all the areas in which the prevalence of goiter was less than 10% showed an adequate iodine status.

On the basis of these findings, we focused our attention on a vast territory of mild to-moderate endemic area of Cosenza province, including four villages (Laino, San Basile, Saracena, and Mormanno). In particular, we assessed both goiter prevalence and UI concentration in children aged 11–14 years. Using WHO criteria, the goiter prevalence was 7.1% and 10.95% normalized for body surface area (BSA) and age, respectively, while median UI excretion was 113 μg/L. Moreover, we also evaluated the efficacy of the iodine prophylaxis in an adult population living in Laino. We observed reduced goiter prevalence in the studied population that was subjected for two decades to a program of salt iodization. More interestingly, the beneficial effects of iodine prophylaxis were also observed in the youngest adult population investigated (ranged 18–27 years), which showed almost an absence of thyroid enlargement, whereas the older adult population (>58 years), which have mostly lived in a severe iodine deficient area before beginning iodine supplementation, were less responsive in reducing goiter prevalence [34].

The epidemiological studies on iodine status by OERC continued until 2012 in the context of the activities carried out by OSNAMI. Median UI concentration and goiter prevalence in 729 schoolchildren recruited in Calabria region were 87 μg/L and 7.5%, respectively, which showed that further efforts were still required to encourage the use of iodized salt [35].

Despite the clear benefits of iodine prophylaxis, continuous surveillance of adverse effects induced by iodine intake needs to be carefully maintained. Thus, the frequency of thyroid disorders along with the levels of antithyroid antibodies (TgAb and TPOAb) in 560 adult subjects from Laino and from the urban area of Cosenza were evaluated [36]. As expected, the prevalence of subjects affected by goiter was significantly higher in the rural area than in the urban area, but interestingly it was significantly lower compared with that reported in the adult population living in the same rural area in 2007 (42.6% rural area in 2007 vs. 13.8% rural area in 2015, $p < 0.0001$). Moreover, we have observed a significant increase of TgAb levels in subjects living in a long-standing iodine sufficient area that may be an epiphenomenon with no pathogenic significance [37]. Interestingly, no changes were detected for concentrations of TPOAbs, the levels of which are typically high in thyroid autoimmune disease [38].

More recently, preliminary data from the national program of iodine deficiency monitoring activities of OSNAMI have reported an increased UI concentration in rural areas as well as urban areas together with a reduction in goiter prevalence in schoolchildren population of most Italian regions, including Calabria [39].

3.2. Promotional Campaign

An intense and widespread iodine prophylaxis campaign was carried out during 2007–2009. At the end of the promotional survey, the OERC medical team visited 1012 primary schools involving more than 100,000 children in all provinces of Calabria, outlining the health benefits of iodine through the distribution of information materials, pamphlets, gadgets, and posters. Besides, other strategies to increase consumer awareness towards iodized salt and its beneficial health effects have been developed and are currently ongoing. These include a promotional campaign using mass media (newspaper, TV), billboards on buses, and a website [40] that offers a useful platform containing national and international links to other reliable sources of information about iodine nutrition.

3.3. Sale Trend of Iodized Salt

The activities of the OERC also include an assessment of the iodine content in salt on the market. Salt samples, taken from the subjects screened (131 subjects from the rural area and 235 subjects from the urban area) during our epidemiological surveys, were found to be compliant with the iodine content permitted by Italian law (30 mg/kg) [36]. The data on sale trends of iodized salt in Calabria, supplied by the Italian Salt Company, one of the most important sales producers/distributors in the region, showed an increasing trend over the last few decades, reaching a coverage rate of approximately 65% [36]. These data are in line with those obtained from the national salt producers and collected by the Italian National Institute of Health that specifically reported an increase in the percentage of sold iodized salt from 34% in 2006 to 65% in 2017 [39]. However, since a usage rate of iodized salt of at least 90% is recommended by WHO, UNICEF, and the ICCIDD [3] for effective prevention of IDDs, further efforts should be made to better inform the population on the benefits of using iodized salt.

4. Conclusions

The IDD control program in Calabria is one of the success stories of public health in Italy. The epidemiological data over the last three decades clearly indicate the improvement of iodine status in the Calabria region also due to the commitment of the Regional Observatory of Endemic Goiter and Iodine Prophylaxis. Although substantial progress has been made, efforts should focus on ensuring there is adequate iodine intake in the entire population to achieve and maintain the IDD control goal.

Author Contributions: D.B., S.C. and S.A. conceptualized, C.G., searched literature, I.B., S.M., R.B. searched literature and data curation, C.G., D.B., S.C. wrote the first versions of the manuscript. D.B., S.C. and S.A. took care of the final update, revision and editing. All authors approved the final version.

Acknowledgments: Authors thank the school-children, teachers and the authorities of the schools for their participation and collaboration.

References

1.   Li, M.; Eastman, C.J. The changing epidemiology of iodine deficiency. *Nat. Rev. Endocrinol.* **2012**, *8*, 434–440. [CrossRef] [PubMed]
2.   Mohammadi, M.; Azizi, F.; Hedayati, M. Iodine deficiency status in the WHO Eastern Mediterranean Region: A systematic review. *Environ. Geochem. Health* **2018**, *40*, 87–97. [CrossRef] [PubMed]
3.   The Iodine Global Network: 2018 Annual Report. Available online: https://www.ign.org/cm_data/IGN_2018_Annual_Report_5_web.pdf (accessed on 5 September 2019).

4.   Zimmermann, M.B. The role of iodine in human growth and development. *Semin Cell Dev. Biol.* **2011**, *22*, 645–652. [CrossRef] [PubMed]

5.   Eastman, C.J.; Zimmermann, M.B. The iodine deficiency disorders. In *Endotext*; Feingold, K.R., Anawalt, B., Boyce, A., Chrousos, G., Dungan, K., Grossman, A., Hershman, J.M., Kaltsas, G., Koch, C., Kopp, P., et al., Eds.; MDText.com, Inc.: South Dartmouth, MA, USA, 2000. Available online: https://www.ncbi.nlm.nih.gov/books/NBK285556/ (accessed on 5 September 2019).

6.   Morreale de Escobar, G.; Obregon, M.J.; Escobar del Rey, F. Role of thyroid hormone during early brain development. *Eur. J. Endocrinol.* **2004**, *151* (Suppl. 3), U25–U37. [CrossRef]

7.   World Health Organization. Urinary iodine concentrations for determining iodine status in populations. Available online: https://apps.who.int/iris/bitstream/handle/10665/85972/WHO_NMH_NHD_EPG_13.1_eng.pdf (accessed on 5 September 2019).

8.   Zimmermann, M.B.; Hess, S.Y.; Molinari, L.; De Benoist, B.; Delange, F.; Braverman, L.E.; Fujieda, K.; Ito, Y.; Jooste, P.L.; Moosa, K.; et al. New reference values for thyroid volumen by ultrasound in iodine-sufficient school children: A World Health Organization/Nutrition for Health and Development Iodine Deficiency Study Group Report. *Am. J. Nutr.* **2004**, *79*, 231–237. [CrossRef] [PubMed]

9.   World Health Organization/International Council for the Control of the Iodine Deficiency Disorders/United Nations Children's Fund (WHO/ICCIDD/UNICEF). *Assessment of the Iodine Deficiency Disorders and Monitoring Their Elimination*; World Health Organization: Geneva, Switzerland, 2007.

10.   Zimmermann, M.B.; de Benoist, B.; Corigliano, S.; Jooste, P.L.; Molinari, L.; Moosa, K.; Pretell, E.A.; Al-Dallal, Z.S.; Wei, Y.; Zu-Pei, C.; et al. Assessment of iodine status using dried blood spot thyroglobulin: Development of reference material and establishment of an international reference range in iodine-sufficient children. *J. Clin. Endocrinol. Metab.* **2006**, *91*, 4881–4887. [CrossRef] [PubMed]

11.   *Principles of Nutritional Assessment*; Gibson, R. (Ed.) Oxford University Press: Oxford, UK, 2005.

12.   Institute of Medicine. *Academy of Sciences 2001 Dietary Reference Intakes for Vitamin A, Vitamin K, Arsenic, Boron, Chromium, Copper, Iodine, Iron, Manganese, Molybdenum, Nickel, Silicon, Vanadium, and Zinc*; National Academy Press: Washington, DC, USA, 2001.

13.   Eastman, C.J. Screening for thyroid disease and iodine deficiency. *Pathology* **2012**, *44*, 153–159. [CrossRef] [PubMed]

14.   Farebrother, J.; Zimmermann, M.B.; Assey, V.; Castro, M.C.; Cherkaoui, M.; Fingerhut, R.; Jia, Q.; Jukic, T.; Makokha, A.; San Luis, T.O.; et al. Thyroglobulin is markedly elevated in 6- to 24-month-old infants at both low and high iodine intakes and suggests a narrow optimal iodine intake range. *Thyroid* **2019**, *29*, 268–277. [CrossRef]

15.   World Health Organization/International Council for the Control of the Iodine Deficiency Disorders/United Nations Children's Fund (WHO/ICCIDD/UNICEF). *Assessment of the Iodine Deficiency Disorders and Monitoring Their Elimination*; WHO/NHD/01.1; World Health Organization: Geneva, Switzerland, 2001.

16.   World Health Organization. *Guideline: Fortification of Food-Grade Salt with Iodine for the Prevention and Control of Iodine Deficiency Disorders*; World Health Organization: Geneva, Switzerland, 2014; Available online: https://apps.who.int/iris/handle/10665/136908 (accessed on 5 September 2019).

17.   Rasmussen, L.B.; Carlé, A.; Jørgensen, T.; Knudsen, N.; Laurberg, P.; Pedersen, I.B.; Perrild, H.; Vejbjerg, P.; Ovesen, L. Iodine intake before and after mandatory iodization in Denmark: Results from the Danish Investigation of Iodine Intake and Thyroid Diseases (DanThyr) study. *Br. J. Nutr.* **2008**, *100*, 166–173. [CrossRef]

18.   Charlton, K.E.; Yeatman, H.; Brock, E.; Lucas, C.; Gemming, L.; Goodfellow, A.; Ma, G. Improvement in iodine status of pregnant Australian women 3 years after introduction of a mandatory iodine fortification programme. *Prev. Med.* **2013**, *57*, 26–30. [CrossRef]

19.   Zimmermann, M.B.; Aeberli, I.; Torresani, T.; Bürgi, H. Increasing the iodine concentration in the Swiss iodized salt program markedly improved iodine status in pregnant women and children: A 5-y prospective national study. *Am. J. Clin. Nutr.* **2005**, *82*, 388–392. [CrossRef] [PubMed]

20.   Ministry of Health and Family Welfare. Government of India & International Institute of Population Sciences (2007) National Family Health Survey-3 National Report (2005–06). Available online: http://rchiips.org/nfhs/nfhs3_national_report.shtml (accessed on 2 October 2019).

21.   Pandav, C.S.; Yadav, K.; Srivastava, R.; Pandav, R.; Karmarkar, M.G. Iodine deficiency disorders (IDD) control in India. *Indian J. Med. Res.* **2013**, *138*, 418–433. [PubMed]

22. Pandav, C.S.; Yadav, K.; Salve, H.R.; Kumar, R.; Goel, A.D.; Chakrabarty, A. High national and sub-national coverage of iodised salt in India: Evidence from the first National Iodine and Salt Intake Survey (NISI) 2014–2015. *Public Health Nutr.* **2018**, *21*, 3027–3036. [CrossRef] [PubMed]

23. Randremanana, R.V.; Bastaraud, A.; Rabarijaona, L.P.; Piola, P.; Rakotonirina, D.; Razafinimanana, J.O.; Ramangakoto, M.H.; Andriantsarafara, L.; Randriamasiarijaona, H.; Tucker-Brown, A.; et al. First national iodine survey in Madagascar demonstrates iodine deficiency. *Matern. Child. Nutr.* **2019**, *15*, e12717. [CrossRef] [PubMed]

24. Chuko, T.; Bagriansky, J.; Brown, A.T. Ethiopia's long road to USI. *IDD Newsl.* **2015**, *43*. Available online: https://www.ign.org/cm_data/IDD_may15_1.pdf (accessed on 2 October 2019).

25. IFPRI. *Global Nutrition Report 2016: From Promise to Impact: Ending Malnutrition by 2030*; International Food Policy Research Institute: Washington, DC, USA, 2016; p. 182. Available online: http://www.ifpri.org/publication/global-nutrition-report-2016-promise-impact-ending-malnutrition-2030 (accessed on 2 October 2019).

26. OSNAMI—Istituto Superiore di Sanità. Osservatorio Nazionale per il Monitoraggio della Iodoprofilassi in Italia. Available online: http://old.iss.it/osnami/index.php?lang=1 (accessed on 5 September 2019).

27. Pellicone, G.; Caloiero, T.; Coletta, V.; Veltri, A. Phytoclimatic map of Calabria (Southern Italy). *J. Maps* **2014**, *10*, 109–113. [CrossRef]

28. Stanbury, J.B.; Ermans, A.M.; Hetzel, B.S.; Pretell, E.A.; Querido, A. Endemic goitre and cretinism: Public health significance and prevention. *WHO Chron.* **1974**, *28*, 220–228.

29. Andò, S.; Maggiolini, M.; Di Carlo, A.; Diodato, A.; Bloise, A.; De Luca, G.P.; Pezzi, V.; Sisci, D.; Mariano, A.; Macchia, V. Endemic goiter in Calabria: Etiopathogenesis and thyroid function. *J. Endocrinol. Investig.* **1994**, *17*, 329–333. [CrossRef]

30. Costante, G.; Grasso, L.; Schifino, E.; Marasco, M.F.; Crocetti, U.; Capula, C.; Chiarella, R.; Ludovico, O.; Nocera, M.; Parlato, G.; et al. Iodine deficiency in Calabria: Characterization of endemic goiter and analysis of different indicators of iodine status region-wide. *J. Endocrinol. Investig.* **2002**, *25*, 201–207. [CrossRef]

31. Aghini-Lombardi, F.; Antonangeli, L.; Vitti, P.; Pinchera, A. Status of iodine nutrition in Italy. In *Iodine Deficiency in Europe*; Delange, F., Dunn, J.T., Glinoer, D., Eds.; A continuing concern; Plenum Press: New York, NY, USA, 1993; pp. 403–408.

32. Aghini-Lombardi, F.; Vitti, P.; Antonangeli, L.; Fiore, E.; Piaggi, P.; Pallara, A.; Consiglio, E.; Pinchera, A. Southern Italy Study Group for Iodine Deficiency Disorders. The size of the community rather than its geographical location better defines the risk of iodine deficiency: Results of an extensive survey in Southern Italy. *J. Endocrinol. Investig.* **2013**, *36*, 282–286. [CrossRef]

33. Mazzarella, C.; Terracciano, D.; Di Carlo, A.; Macchia, P.E.; Consiglio, E.; Macchia, V.; Mariano, A. Iodine status assessment in Campania (Italy) as determined by urinary iodine excretion. *Nutrition* **2009**, *25*, 926–929. [CrossRef] [PubMed]

34. Bonofiglio, D.; Catalano, S.; Perri, A.; Baldini, M.P.; Marsico, S.; Tagarelli, A.; Conforti, D.; Guido, R.; Andò, S. Beneficial effects of iodized salt prophylaxis on thyroid volume in an iodine deficient area of southern Italy. *Clin. Endocrinol.* **2009**, *71*, 124–129. [CrossRef] [PubMed]

35. Olivieri, A.; Di Cosmo, C.; De Angelis, S.; Da Cas, R.; Stacchini, P.; Pastorelli, A.; Vitti, P. Regional Observatories for Goiter Prevention. The way forward in Italy for iodine. *Minerva. Med.* **2017**, *108*, 159–168. [PubMed]

36. Bonofiglio, D.; Catalano, S.; Perri, A.; Santoro, M.; Siciliano, L.; Lofaro, D.; Gallo, M.; Marsico, S.; Bruno, R.; Giordano, C.; et al. Monitoring the effects of iodine prophylaxis in the adult population of southern Italy with deficient and sufficient iodine intake levels: A cross-sectional, epidemiological study. *Br. J. Nutr.* **2017**, *117*, 170–175. [CrossRef] [PubMed]

37. Tomer, Y. Anti-thyroglobulin autoantibodies in autoimmune thyroid disease: Cross-reactive or pathogenic? *Clin. Immunol. Immunopathol.* **1997**, *82*, 3–11. [CrossRef] [PubMed]

38. Chen, C.R.; Hamidi, S.; Braley-Mullen, H.; Nagayama, Y.; Bresee, C.; Aliesky, H.A.; Rapoport, B.; McLachlan, S.M. Antibodies to thyroid peroxidase arise spontaneously with age in NOD. H-2h4 mice and appear after thyroglobulin antibodies. *Endocrinology* **2010**, *151*, 4583–4593. [CrossRef] [PubMed]

39. Olivieri, A.; De Angelis, S.; Rotondi, D.; Pastorelli, A.; Stacchini, P.; Da Cas, R.; Medda, E. The Regional Observatories for Goiter Prevention. Attività di monitoraggio del programma nazionale per la prevenzione dei disordini da carenza iodica: La situazione italiana a 14 anni dall'approvazione della Legge 55/2005. *L'Endocrinologo.* **2019**, *20*, 245–248. [CrossRef]

Sodium, Potassium and Iodine Intake, in a National Adult Population Sample of the Republic of Moldova

Lanfranco D'Elia [1,2], Galina Obreja [3], Angela Ciobanu [4,5], Joao Breda [6], Jo Jewell [5,7], Francesco P. Cappuccio [1,8,*]

[1] World Health Organization Collaborating Centre for Nutrition, University of Warwick, Coventry CV4 7AL, UK; lanfranco.delia@unina.it
[2] Department of Clinical Medicine and Surgery, "Federico II" University of Naples, 80131 Naples, Italy
[3] Department of Social Medicine and Health Management, State University of Medicine and Pharmacy Nicolae Testemitanu, 2004 Chişinău, Moldova; galina.obreja@gmail.com
[4] World Health Organization Country Office, 2012 Chişinău, Moldova; ciobanua@who.int
[5] World Health Organization European Office for Prevention and Control of Noncommunicable Diseases, 2100 Copenhagen, Denmark; jewellj@who.int
[6] World Health Organization European Office for Prevention and Control of Noncommunicable Diseases, 229994 Moscow, Russia; rodriguesdasilvabred@who.int
[7] United Nations Children's Fund, UNICEF, New York, NY 10017, USA
[8] Division of Health Sciences, Warwick Medical School, University of Warwick, Coventry CV4 7AL, UK
*   Correspondence: f.p.cappuccio@warwick.ac.uk
†   Membership of the Salt Consumption Survey in the Republic of Moldova Study Group is provided in the Acknowledgments.

Abstract: In the Republic of Moldova, more than half of all deaths due to noncommunicable diseases (NCDs) are caused by cardiovascular disease (CVD). Excess salt (sodium) and inadequate potassium intakes are associated with high CVD. Moreover, salt iodisation is the preferred policy to prevent iodine deficiency and associated disorders. However, there is no survey that has directly measured sodium, potassium and iodine consumption in adults in the Republic of Moldova. A national random sample of adults attended a screening including demographic, anthropometric and physical measurements. Sodium, potassium and iodine intakes were assessed by 24 h urinary sodium (UNa), potassium (UK) and iodine (UI) excretions. Knowledge, attidues and behaviours were collected by questionnaire. Eight-hundred and fifty-eight participants (326 men and 532 women, 18–69 years) were included in the analysis (response rate 66%). Mean age was 48.5 years (SD 13.8). Mean UNa was 172.7 (79.3) mmoL/day, equivalent to 10.8 g of salt/day and potassium excretion 72.7 (31.5) mmoL/day, equivalent to 3.26 g/day. Only 11.3% met the World Health Organization (WHO) recommended salt targets of 5 g/day and 39% met potassium targets (>90 mmoL/day). Whilst 81.7% declared limiting their consumption of processed food and over 70% not adding salt at the table, only 8.8% looked at sodium content of food, 31% still added salt when cooking and less than 1% took other measures to control salt consumption. Measures of awareness were significantly more common in urban compared to rural areas. Mean urinary iodine was 225 (SD: 152; median 196) mcg/24 h, with no difference between sexes. According to WHO criteria, 41.0% had adequate iodine intake. Iodine content of salt table was 21.0 (SD: 18.6) mg/kg, lower in rural than urban areas (16.7, SD = 18.6 vs. 28.1, SD = 16.5 mg/kg, $p < 0.001$). In most cases participants were not using iodised salt as their main source of salt, more so in rural areas. In the Republic of Moldova, salt consumption is unequivocally high, potassium consumption is lower than recommended, both in men and in women, whilst iodine intake is still inadequate in one in three people, although severe iodine deficiency is rare. Salt consumed is often not iodised.

Keywords: Republic of Moldova; salt; sodium; potassium; iodine; population

1. Introduction

Non-communicable diseases (NCDs) are the leading causes of death globally [1] and their reduction is a health priority [2], with reduction in population salt consumption a cost-effective policy option ('best buys') [3]. In the Republic of Moldova, NCDs are the leading causes of death, and cardiovascular disease (CVD) represents the main cause of population morbidity and mortality, accounting for every second death in 2016 [4]. High blood pressure (BP) and unhealthy diets are major causes CVD in the world and account for most of the disease burden in the Republic of Moldova [5]. High salt in the diet (i.e., sodium chloride, 1 g = 17.1 mmoL of sodium) causes high BP, a high risk of vascular diseases [6–10] and other adverse health effects [11–13]. A lower salt intake reduces BP [7,8], cardiovascular events and overall mortality [9,10].

The World Health Organization (WHO) currently recommends for adults a consumption not higher than 5 g of salt daily [14]. However, in most countries in the world this recommendation is unmet [15–17]. Salt enters our diet not only as added salt to food and cooking by the consumer, but, in the Western diet, more often from processed food, food prepared in restaurants and other food outlets [18,19]. There is no direct estimate of population dietary salt intake in Republic of Moldova. However, it is likely to be high, as in neighbouring countries like Serbia (9.85 g/day) [20], Slovenia (11.3 g/day) [21] and Montenegro (11.6 g/day) [22]. In the Republic of Moldova it is a common habit to add salt to food at the table and when cooking, as well as eating processed food that have high salt content. In 2013 a national survey indicated that 24.3% of those surveyed always or often added salt to food, and 32.4% always or often ate processed foods that are high in salt [5]. Salt reduction strategies in the European region, including the Republic of Moldova, include monitoring and evaluation actions as one of their pillars [23].

In contrast to sodium, dietary potassium has beneficial effects on BP and cardiovascular health [24–26]. The Republic of Moldova lacks data on actual potassium consumption. The WHO currently recommends that adults should consume not less than 90 mmoL of potassium daily [27]. Finally, in the Republic of Moldova the prevention of iodine deficiency disorders recommends universal salt iodization [28]. Starting in 2009, the Ministry of Health authorised the production and placing on the market of iodized bottled water additionally to iodized salt. Since more than 90% of iodine consumed is excreted in the urine within 24–48 hours [29,30], 24 h urinary iodine excretion is a good marker of recent iodine intake and an ideal biomarker for estimating iodine status [31] in the entire adult population.

The aim of the present study was to establish current baseline average consumption of sodium, potassium and iodine by 24h urine collection, in a national random sample of men and women. The study also aimed to explore knowledge, attitudes and behaviour towards dietary salt.

2. Materials and Methods

2.1. Participants and Recruitment

A total of 1307 randomly selected men and women participated in the survey. They were all aged 18–69 years. They comprised residents of all Districts and Administrative Territorial Units 'Gagauz-Yeri', along with Chişinău and Bălti Municipalities. The survey did not cover the Districts from the left bank of the Nistru River and the Municipality of Bender (Figure 1). A probabilistic master sample from the National Bureau of Statistics' Household Budget Survey was used to select the sample for the survey which was extracted in three phases: 150 Primary Sampling Units (PSU—communes, cities or sectors within cities) were selected; list of households from PSU were drawn; eligible individuals from households were identified. Random sampling proportional to size were stratified by sex, geography (north, centre, south and Chişinău), urban/rural, size of cities.

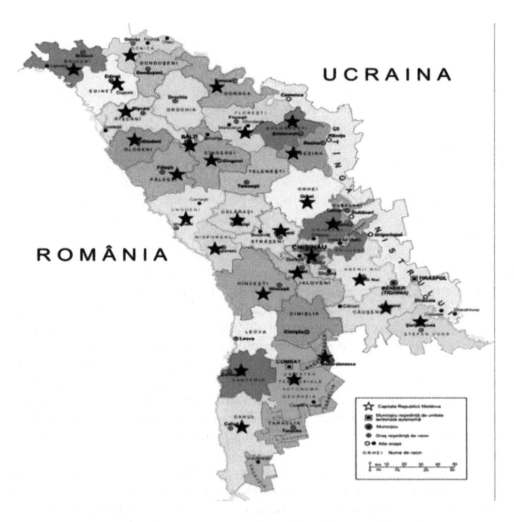

Figure 1. Geographical sampling from the Republic of Moldova. National proportional random sampling from 28 (marked with a star) of 37 Districts and Administrative Territorial Units 'Gagauz-Yeri', along with Chişinău and Bălti Municipalities. The sampling was as follows: Anenii Noi (1.3%), Balti (0.8%), Basarabeasca (1.4%), Briceni (4.7%), Cahul (3.5%), Călăraşi (2.4%), Cantemir (2.4%), Căuşeni (0.8%), Chişinău (30.7%), Comrat/ATU 'Gagauz-Yeri' (4.4%), Criuleni (4.3%), Edineţ (3.1%), Făleşti (2.4%), Floreşti (2.2%), Glodeni (1.2%), Hînceşti (0.7%), Ialoveni (4.4%), Nisporeni (3.0%), Ocniţa (2.7%), Orhei (4.8%), Rezina (1.7%), Rîşcani (0.6%), Sîngerei (1.9%), Şoldaneşti (2.6%), Soroca (2.2%), Ştefan Vodă (0.6%), Străşeni (2.7%) and Ungheni (6.3%).

From the sampling frame and according to PAHO/WHO and EMRO-WHO Protocols [32,33], we excluded the following groups: pregnant women, individuals with heart failure, severe kidney disease, stroke, liver disease, people who had started diuretic therapy in the last two weeks, any other conditions that would compromise the collection of 24 h urine samples or a reliable informed consent.

The survey took place between 21st July and 5th September 2016. From the 1307 participants interviewed, 858 (66%) provided data for inclusion in the analysis. Thirteen had missing data, 263 admitted missing more than one void, 77 provided either under-collections (<23 h) or over-collections (>25 h) and 37 had urinary creatinine excretion outside two standard deviations (SDs) of the sex-specific distribution of urinary creatinine in the sample (Figure 2).

The survey was carried out in accordance with the Declaration of Helsinki and Good Clinical Practice [34]. Ethical approval for the survey was obtained from the Committee of Research Ethics of the National Agency for Public Health of the Republic of Moldova and participants provided written informed consent to take part.

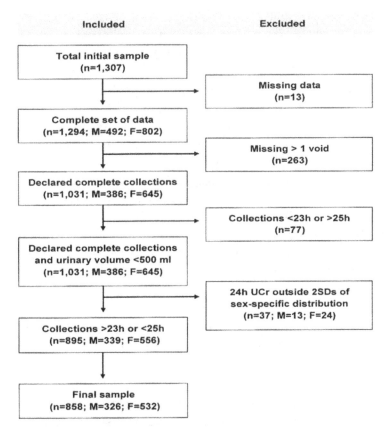

Figure 2. Stepwise procedure for the selection of valid participants according to protocol adherence, quality control and completeness of 24 hour urine collections.

2.2. Data Collection

The full methodology is reported in the supplementary material (Text S1). In brief, there were three stages: (a) questionnaire, (b) physical measurements and (c) 24 h urine collections.

The questionnaire (adapted version of the WHO STEPS Instrument for NCD Risk Factor Surveillance) [35] obtained demographic and socio-economic status, frequency of salty food, fruit and vegetable consumptions, knowledge attitudes and behaviour on dietary salt.

Anthropometry, blood pressure (BP) and heart rate were measured in all participants with standardized protocols and validated equipment, as also described elsewhere [22,32,33]. Hypertension is defined as systolic and/or diastolic BP ≥ 140/90 mmHg or regular antihypertensive treatment [36].

After detailed and careful instructions (Text S1), participants provided a 24 h urine collection [32,33]. Sodium, potassium and creatinine determinations were carried out immediately [37,38]. Sodium and potassium concentration in the urine samples were determined using a Ion Selective Electrode with a Beckman Coulter Synchron CX5PRO system (High Wycombe, UK) and expressed in mmoL/L [37]. Creatinine concentration was determined through the Creatinine (urinary) Jaffé kinetic method and expressed in mg/dL [38]. These determinations were carried out at the ICS Medical Laboratory Synevo SRL in Chişinău. Urinary iodine was measured separately at the National Agency for Public Health of the Republic of Moldova using the ammonium persulfate digestion method with spectrophotometric detection by Sandell–Kolthoff reaction, expressed as mcg/L [39]. Iodine determinations in table salt were carried out by the titration method [40].

2.3. Statistical Analysis

With a standard deviation of 75 mmoL/24 h (alpha = 0.05, power = 0.80) in urinary sodium excretion, the study was designed to detect a reduction in salt consumption over time of around 1 g per day (~20 mmoL sodium/24 h). Considering an attrition rate of 50%, we aimed to select

240 participants per age and sex group [32,33]. The population was stratified in groups by sex (men and women), age (18–29 years, 30–44 years, 45–59 years, 60–69 years) and urban/rural areas. Therefore, 1920 individuals were originally needed to be selected (total $n = 120 \times 8$ groups/0.5 attrition = 1920). T-test for unpaired samples or analysis of variance (ANOVA) was used to test differences between groups. The chi-square test was used for categorical variables. To convert urinary output into dietary intake, the urinary excretion of sodium (UNa) or potassium (UK) in mmoL/day were first converted to mg/day (for sodium 1 mmol = 23 mg of sodium, for potassium 1 mmol = 39 mg). The conversion from dietary sodium (Na) intake to salt (NaCl) intake was made by multiplying the sodium value by 2.542. Then, sodium values were multiplied by 1.05 (assuming that aproximately 95% of sodium ingested is excreted) [41]. For potassium dietary intake was calculated assuming 80% of the potassium ingested is excreted in the urine [42]. Urinary iodine was expressed in mcg/day. We used the cut-off targets for iodine consumption set by WHO (based on urinary iodine concentrations in mcg/L derived from 24h collections) [31]. Statistical analyses were carried out using SPSS, version 20 (SPSS Inc., Chicago, IL, USA). The results were reported as mean (SD and/or 95% CI) or as percentages, as appropriate. Two-sided p below 0.05 were considered statistically significant.

3. Results

The final population sample included 858 participants between 18 and 69 years old ($n = 326$ or 38% men and $n = 532$ or 62% women), recruited nationally (Figure 1).

3.1. Characteristics of the Participants

Mean age was similar in men and women, but men were taller and heavier than women and had a higher systolic BP (Table 1). The point prevalence of hypertension was 45.5% (385/858), comparable in men (148/326 or 45.8%) and women (237/532 or 45.2%; $p > 0.05$).

Table 1. Characteristics of the participants.

Variable	All ($n = 858$)	Men ($n = 326$)	Women ($n = 532$)
Age (years)	48.5 (13.8)	47.3 (13.6)	49.2 (13.9)
Height (cm)	166.7 (8.8)	172.8 (8.1)	162.9 (7.0) [†]
Weight (kg)	78.2 (15.8)	82.0 (15.8)	75.8 (15.3) [†]
B.M.I. (kg/m^2)	28.1 (5.4)	27.4 (4.9)	28.6 (5.7) [‡]
Waist circumference (cm)	–	93.8 (15.5)	91.8 (15.1)
Hip circumference (cm)	–	100.5 (12.3)	106.5 (14.0)
Systolic BP (mmHg)	134.3 (21.2)	136.1 (18.5)	133.1 (22.6) *
Diastolic BP (mmHg)	86.8 (11.9)	87.1 (10.8)	86.6 (12.6)
Pulse rate (b/min)	76.2 (9.5)	78.0 (10.3)	75.2 (8.8)
Hypertension [#] n (%)	385 (45.5)	148 (45.8)	237 (45.2)

Results are mean (SD) or as percentage; [†] $p < 0.001$; [‡] $p = 0.002$; * $p = 0.04$ vs. men. [#] SBP ≥ 140 mmHg and/or DBP ≥ 90 mmHg or on anti-hypertensive medications.

3.2. Daily Urinary Excretions of Volume, Sodium, Potassium and Creatinine and Salt and Potassium Intake

Urinary volume excretion was, on average, 1441 mL per day, higher in men than women, and higher in urban than rural areas (Table 2). Urinary creatinine excretion was 11.7 mmol per day, higher in men than women, but lower in urban than rural areas (Table 2). Mean urinary sodium was 172.7 (SD 79.3, median 161.9) mmoL/24h (Table 2), equivalent to a mean consumption of 10.8 (4.9) g of salt per day (Table 2). Men excreted more sodium than women (mean difference 18.1 mmoL/24h, $p < 0.001$), equivalent to ~1.1 g of higher salt consumption than women. WHO recommended levels of 5 g or less were met by just 97 participants (11.3%), with no difference between sex and area of residence. Mean urinary potassium was 72.7 (SD 31.5, median 68.8) (Table 2), equivalent to a mean consumption of 3.40 (1.47) g of potassium per day (Table 2).

Table 2. Daily urinary excretions of volume, sodium, potassium and creatinine and estimates of salt and potassium intake.

Variables	All (n = 858)	Men (n = 326)	Women (n = 532)	Rural (n = 531)	Urban (n = 327)
Volume (mL/24 h)	1441 (529)	1505 (536)	1401 (521) ^	1333 (427)	1616 (624) #
Sodium (mmoL/24 h)	172.7 (79.3)	183.9 (86.0)	165.8 (74.1) †	180.4 (80.2)	160.1 (76.2) #
Salt intake (g/day)	10.8 (4.9)	11.5 (5.4)	10.3 (4.6) #	11.3 (5.0)	10.0 (4.8) #
Potassium (mmoL/24 h)	72.7 (31.5)	76.0 (33.4)	70.7 (30.1) *	73.8 (31.6)	71.0 (31.2)
Potassium intake (g/day)	3.40 (1.47)	3.55 (1.56)	3.31 (1.41) *	3.45 (1.47)	3.32 (1.46)
Creatinine (mmol/24h)	11.7 (5.0)	13.3 (5.6)	10.7 (4.2) #	12.3 (4.8)	11.4 (5.0) †

Results are mean (SD). $^{\#}$ $p < 0.001$; $^{\wedge}$ $p < 0.005$; † $p < 0.01$; * $p < 0.02$ vs. men or vs. rural

Men excreted more potassium than women. Thirty-nine per cent of participants met the levels of potassium excretion of 90 mmoL/day or more recommended by the WHO, with no difference between sexes and areas of residence.

3.3. Daily Intake of Iodine and Use of Iodised Salt

Urinay iodine excretion (as measure of intake) was adequate in 40.9% of participants, irrespective of sex or area of residence (Table 3). Iodine consumption was above requirement or excessive in 30.3% of the participants, irrespective of sex or area of residence. Of the 28.6% who fell into the category indicating insufficient consumption (equally distributed by sex or area of residence), only 2.3% had severe deficiency (Table 3).

Table 3. Proportions of participants meeting WHO targets for iodine consumption (based on urinary iodine concentrations in mcg/L derived from 24 h collections).

Group (mcg/L)	All (n = 858)	Men (n = 326)	Women (n = 532)	Rural (n = 531)	Urban (n = 327)
	n (%)	n (%)	n (%)	n (%)	n (%)
Insufficient (<100)	245 (28.6)	95 (29.1)	150 (28.2)	104 (31.8)	141 (26.6)
Severe (<20)	20 (2.3)	6 (1.8)	14 (2.6)	4 (1.2)	16 (3.0)
Moderate (20–49)	60 (7.0)	24 (7.4)	36 (6.8)	28 (8.6)	32 (6.0)
Mild (50–99)	165 (19.2)	65 (19.9)	100 (18.8)	72 (22.0)	93 (17.5)
Adequate (100–199)	351 (40.9)	132 (40.5)	219 (41.2)	131 (40.1)	220 (41.4)
Above requirement (200–299)	152 (17.7)	59 (18.1)	93 (17.5)	58 (17.7)	94 (17.7)
Excessive (≥300)	108 (12.6)	40 (12.3)	68 (12.8)	34 (10.4)	74 (13.9)

Results are number (%).

Average urinary iodine excretion was 225 (SD: 152, median 196) mcg per day (Table 4), with no difference between sexes or areas of residence. Iodine salt content was, on average 21.0 (18.6) mg/kg, with no difference between men and women. However, participants in rural areas consumed table salt with significantly less iodine concentrations than those samples consumed in urban areas ($p < 0.001$; Table 4).

Table 4. Daily urinary excretions of iodine and iodine content of household salt samples.

Variables	All (n = 858)	Men (n = 326)	Women (n = 532)	Rural (n = 531)	Urban (n = 327)
Iodine (mcg/24 h)	225 (152)	232 (154)	221 (150)	225 (145)	224 (128)
Iodine in table salt (mg/kg)	21.0 (18.6)	22.1 (18.2)	20.3 (18.9)	16.7 (18.6)	28.1 (16.5) #

Results are mean (SD). $^{\#}$ $p < 0.001$ vs. rural.

There were weak correlations between the amount of sodium excreted in the urine and the amount of excreted iodine in men and women or rural and urban settings (Figure 3).

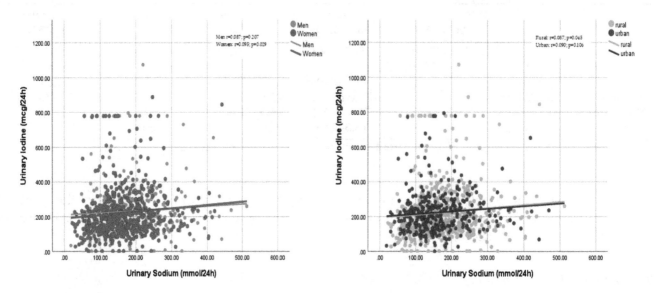

Figure 3. Correlations between urinary sodium and urinary iodine excretions by sex (left) and areas of residence (right). Left: men r = 0.087, p = 0.207, women r = 0.095, p = 0.029; right: rural r = 0.087, p = 0.045, urban r = 0.090, p = 0.106.

There were also weak correlations between the amount of urinary iodine excreted in a day and the amount of iodine present in the table salt sampled from the households of individual participants (Figure 4).

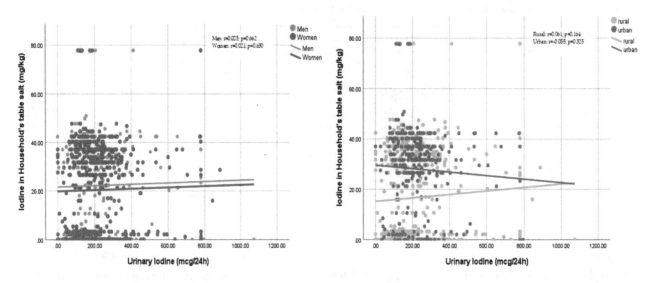

Figure 4. Correlations between urinary iodine excretions and iodine content of household's table salt by sex (left) and areas of residence (right). Left: men r = 0.025, p = 0.662, women r = 0.021, p = 0.630; right: rural r = 0.061, p = 0.164, urban r = −0.055, p = 0.325.

3.4. Knowledge, Attitude and Behaviours Towards Salt Intake

Knowledge, attitude and behaviours toward the consumption of salt was assessed by asking participants about the frequency, quantity and type of salt used in the household, as well as their cooking habits and their attitudes towards dietary salt. A total of 35.4% of respondents mentioned that they added salt always or often before or while eating. The percentage of men who added salt always or often to their meal was significantly higher than that of women (47.8% vs. 27.7%; p < 0.001). A total of 61.3% of respondents reported that they always or often added salt when cooking or preparing food at home; this was the case more often in rural than in urban areas (69.8% vs. 47.5%; $p < 0.001$). More than half of the respondents (64.4%) mentioned that they used iodised salt when cooking or preparing food at home. Consumption of iodised salt, however, was higher in urban than in rural areas (86.1% vs. 52.9%; $p < 0.001$). About a quarter (26.7%) felt they consumed too much or far too much salt, women being more likely (32.1% vs. 23.3%; $p < 0.01$). More than half (67.2%) acknowledged that consuming too much salt could cause serious health problems; however, only 28.2% considered lowering salt intake in the diet to be very important. More than a quarter of respondents (27.8%) mentioned that they consumed processed foods high in salt, with more men than women doing so (34.9% vs. 23.5%; $p < 0.001$), and more often in urban than rural settings (39.2% vs. 20.8%; $p < 0.001$).

Participants were asked about actions they take to control salt intake on a regular basis. A total of 81.7% limited their consumption of processed food high in salt (Table 5). A total of 22.3% would use spices rather than salt, one in three would not add salt when cooking. Only 8% looked at salt/sodium content on food labels and 14.3% bought alternatives to salt. One in three avoided eating food prepared outside home and 0.8% took any other measure to reduce salt intake.

Table 5. Knowledge, attitudes and behaviour towards the consumption of salt.

Participants Who:	All ($n = 858$)	Men ($n = 326$)	Women ($n = 532$)	Rural ($n = 531$)	Urban ($n = 327$)
Limit their consumption of processed food	81.7	79.7	82.4	80.4	83.9
Look at salt/sodium content in foods	8.8	10.1	8.2	3.8	17.2 *
Buy low salt/sodium alternatives	14.3	17.4	13.2	3.8	24.7 *
Do not add salt at the table	77.3	69.6	80.2	75.9	79.6
Do not add salt when cooking	31.1	24.6	33.5	13.3	61.3 *
Use spices instead of salt when cooking	22.3	15.9	24.7	25.3	17.2
Avoid eating food prepared outside a home	33.1	27.5	35.2	43.7	15.1 *
Take other measures to control salt intake	0.8	1.4	0.5	1.3	0

Results are expressed as % of column total. * $p \leq 0.001$ vs. rural by Fisher's exact test.

4. Discussion

This is the first national survey on sodium, potassium and iodine consumption ever carried out in adults in the Republic of Moldova, using the gold standard measure of 24 h urinary sodium, potassium and iodine excretions as biomarkers of intake. The results show unequivocally that salt consumption is high, potassium consumption is lower than recommended, both in men and in women. Furthermore, iodine intake is still inadequate in one in three people, although severe iodine deficiency is rare. However, universal salt iodization cover is still inadequate in many households both in urban and rural areas, where the use of iodized salt is still limited in the Moldovan diet.

4.1. Salt Consumption

Average salt intake was nearly 11 g per day, over two-fold of the WHO recommended maximum population target of 5 g per day [14]. Only 11.3% of the participants met the WHO salt targets. Men excreted more sodium than women, and in rural areas salt consumption was higher than in urban areas. Discretionary use of salt is common in the Republic of Moldova, with a third of participants adding salt regularly to food and half also using it regularly when cooking. The majority of participants knew that high salt causes serious health problems. However, only less than half thought it would be useful to reduce its consumption, and even fewer felt their own intake was not excessive and were doing anything to reduce it. The answers to these questions reveal an insufficient level of knowledge of the problem associated with high salt consumption amongst the participants and the unreadiness to transfer this knowledge to behavioural changes in using discretionary salt.

4.2. Potassium Consumption

Average population potassium intake was estimated at around 3.26 g per day, still lower than the WHO recommended minimum population target of 3.51 g per day (equivalent to 90 mmol per day [27]. Between 31% and 50% met WHO potassium targets. Men ate more potassium than women, likely due to the larger body size and volume of food eaten, rather than the quality of it. Salt and potassium are expressed as total quantities rather than consumption per calorie intake, hence the gender difference is mainly explained by the larger body size of men compared to women and the corresponding total food consumption compared to women. No difference in potassium intake was detected between rural and urban areas.

4.3. Iodine Consumption

Average daily iodine consumption was 225 mcg per day, with no difference between sexes or areas of residence. Severe iodine deficiency (<20 mcg/L according to WHO criteria [31]) was rare. However, more than a quarter had levels below 100 mcg/L (insufficient), and a quarter had levels either above requirement or excessive (above 300 mcg/L). The Republic of Moldova has adopted for a long time a policy of universal salt iodization for the control of iodine deficiency disorders [28]. It should be mentioned that as from 2009 the production and placing on the market of iodized bottled water was authorised by the government, which may have contributed to the increasing iodine supply, especially among more affluent population groups. By measuring the iodine content of the table salt used in the households visited for the screening, we were able to detect a significant lower iodine content in rural compared to urban areas (16.7 vs. 28.1 mg/kg). Moreover, the percentage of households with no iodized salt was greater in rural than urban areas (30.9% vs. 9.8%; $p < 0.001$). These results seem to suggest a variety of barriers, including possibly deterioration of iodized salt before reaching the users, reduced access, lower use, lack of awareness, costs, lack of use of iodized salt in food preparation by local producers, street vendors and the food industry. Another finding in our study was the lack of strong relationships between urinary sodium and iodine excretions and between urinary iodine excretion and iodine content in households' table salt. These findings may, in part, indicate that some salt in diet derives from non-iodized sources. Assuming that the food eaten in the households is prepared with iodized salt (since the country has a national policy of universal salt iodization), a major component of the salt consumed may derive from food eaten outside the household prepared with non-iodized salt. It is also possible that the use of iodized bottled water has become an important source of iodine, not captured in the correaltions with iodized salt.

4.4. Comparison with Other European Countries

Our main findings show that the salt intake in the Republic of Moldova is as high or higher than that reported in many other European and neighbouring countries, both in men and women. In the recent MINISAL study in Italy, the daily salt intake of Italians was 10.9 g for men and 8.5 g for women [43], with large variations by region and socio-economic status [44]. In Northern Greece average intakes were 11.1 and 9.1 g per day for men and women, respectively [45]. In the national survey of salt consumption in Slovenia men ate 13.0 g and women 9.9 g per day [21]. Recently, in the city of Podgorica, in Montenegro, salt consumption was measured at 13.9 g in men and 9.9 g per day in women [22]. In the SALTURK II survey in Turkey, men consumed 15.7 g of salt per day and women 14.0 g per day, with higher salt consumption in rural compared to urban areas [46]. Finally, in Portugal a national survey as estimated the consumption of salt at 10.7 g per day in men and 10.2 g per day in women [47]. Potassium intake in the Republic of Moldova was lower than in Portugal [47] and higher than that measured in Italy [43], Greece [45], and Montenegro [22]. Men eat more potassium than women.

4.5. Strengths and Limitations

Our study included a large random sample of men and women representative of the Republic of Moldova. Salt and potassium intake were measured using the gold-standard method of 24 h urine collections [33]. We applied a rigorous quality control and used a highly standardized protocol to ensure completeness of urine collections, and a strict protocol of inclusion only of those fulfilling the quality control criteria, such as length of collection time and urinary creatinine excretion, markers of the accuracy of the collection. Our study is one of few studies having carried out at the same time a population based evaluation of daily iodine excretion in an adult population using 24 h urinary iodine excretion as a biomarker (rathe than spot urine samples), to assess the iodine status of a group of individuals who, whilst being supplemented with the universal salt iodization program, is not usually included in the population monitoring and surveillance on the effects of such policy.

Selection bias remains a possibility that we cannot rule out. We excluded a third of the participants as a result of the robust quality control for completeness of urine collections. Participants not delivering complete urines had lower weight, BMI, waist and hip circumferences and lower diastolic BP than those complying. No other differences were seen in their general characteristics (Table S1). Urinary sodium and potassium excretions were only assessed once. Whilst we cannot characterise an individual's intake [48], there is less likelihood that group estimates be biased. Finally, the absence of measurements of thyroid hormones does not allow a full assessment of the impact of both insufficient and excessive iodine intake on the adult population.

4.6. Impact and Policy Implications

The population of the Republic of Moldova is of just over 4 million, of whom approximately 75% over the age of 25 years. According to national health statistics from 2016, the mortality rate from diseases of the cardiovascular system is 617.3 per 100,000 population [49]. To meet the 30% reduction in population salt consumption set by WHO, the Republic of Moldova should aim at a 3.24 g per day reduction nationally. This reduction would be expected to avert 7.9% CVD events and 10.7% strokes every year, approximately 1460 CVD deaths per year.

The Republic of Moldova adopted the National Strategy on Prevention and Control of Noncommunicable Diseases 2012–2020 and its Action Plan [50]. Part of this pledge is to continue on the awareness campaigns already in place and to establish a comprehensive strategy involving legal measures, mandatory reformulation, nutritional labelling, efficient enforcement and good leadership [28]. Furthermore, a feasibility study of implementation and evaluation of essential interventions for the prevention of CVD in primary healthcare is currently under way in the Republic of Moldova, with a view towards a national scale-up [51].

The evidence of the level of sodium and potassium intake in the Republic of Moldova provides robust evidence to support action and to facilitate evaluation. Awareness, attitudes and behaviours about salt and its implication for health suggest that there is an intensification of public awareness campaigns and health promotion to improve the take up of preventive strategies aiming at reducing salt consumption, whilst at the same time increasing potassium intake by encouraging higher consumption of potassium-rich food. Awareness about hidden salt in processed food should be highlighted. The national program for reducing salt intake in the Republic of Moldova needs a multisectoral collaborative approach including not only public awareness and behaviour-change communication (including via health care professionals), but, more importantly, structured programs for reformulation that set the framework for the food industry to reduce salt in bread and bakery products and processed foods, major source of salt intake.

4.7. Conclusions

The present study provides valuable insights into ways to improve and adapt the universal salt iodization program. From one hand our results suggest that there are improvements to be made for a comprehensive take up of the policy nationally. On the other hand it confirms that both iodization and salt reduction policies are fully compatible, as agreed in a WHO Consensus Statement [31] and more recently confirmed in case studies in Italy [52] and China [53] where a moderate salt reduction in unlikely to compromise iodine status. Our data provides a useful baseline against which to monitor the impact of future initiatives.

Author Contributions: F.P.C. developed the protocol, trained local teams, co-ordinated quality control and data analysis and drafted the manuscript. L.D. carried out quality control and statistical analysis. G.O. and A.C. developed the research protocol, trained local teams, coordinated the study, carried out the fieldwork and liaised with the local laboratory. J.J. and J.B. contributed to the design and interpretation of the findings. All authors contributed significantly to the final version of the manuscript.

Acknowledgments: The following are members of Salt Consumption Survey in the Republic of Moldova Study Group (in alphabetical order): Igor Berbec, Iurie Bobu, Valentina Bors, Joao Breda, DumitruCalincu, Francesco P Cappuccio, Veaceslav Carp, Angela Ciobanu, Nicolae David, Lanfranco D'Elia, Tatiana Eremciuc, Lilian Galer, Ala Gheorghiev, Mariana Gincu, Lilia Gurin, Jo Jewell, Alexandra Mandric, Vasile Moraru, Galina Obreja, Vasile Odobescu, Sveatoslav Ovcinicov, Vitalie Puris, Elena Revenco, Ecaterina Salaru, Ion Salaru, Stefan Savin, Raisa Scurtu, Natalia Silitrari, Alexandra Silnic, Nelea Tabuncic. The present analysis was carried out under the terms of reference of the WHO Collaborating Centre for Nutrition at the University of Warwick. The WHO Office for Europe and the authors would like to express gratitude to Svetlana Cebotari, Minister of Health, Labour and Social Protection, Aliona Serbulenco, State Secretary of the Ministry of Health, Labour and Social Protection and Haris Hajrulahovic, WHO Representative to the Republic of Moldova, for their keen interest, encouragement, support and endorsement. Special thanks go to the team of the National Agency for Public Health involved in the preparation of the survey and data collection. The authors alone are responsible for the content and views expressed in this publication and they do not necessarily represent the decisions, policy or views of the World Health Organization.

References

1. GBD 2015 Mortality and Causes of Death Collaborators. Global, regional, and national life expectancy, all-cause mortality, and cause-specific mortality for 249 causes of death, 1980–2015: A systematic analysis for the Global Burden of Disease Study 2015. *Lancet* **2016**, *388*, 1459–1544.

2. World Health Organization. *Global Action Plan. for the Prevention and Control of NCDs 2013–2020*; World Health Organization: Geneva, Switzerland, 2013; pp. 1–103.

3. World Health Organization. Tackling NCDs: "Best buys" and Other Recommended Interventions for the Prevention and Control of Noncommunicable Diseases. 2017. Available online: http://www.who.int/ncds/management/best-buys/en/ (accessed on 27 October 2019).

4. National Center for Health Management. Health Yearbook: Public Health in Moldova. 2015. Available online: http://www.cnms.md/ro/rapoarteo (accessed on 27 October 2019).

5. World Health Organization. *Prevalence of Noncommunicable Disease Risk Factors in the Republic of Moldova (STEPS 2013)*; Regional Office for Europe, World Health Organization: Copenhagen, Denmark, 2014; pp. 1–221.

6. European Heart Network. *Transforming European Food and Drink Policies for Cardiovascular Health*; European Heart Network: Brussels, Belgium, 2017; pp. 1–137.

7. Aburto, N.J.; Ziolkovska, A.; Hooper, L.; Elliott, P.; Cappuccio, F.P.; Meerpohl, J. Effect of lower sodium intake on health: Systematic review and meta-analysis. *Br. Med. J.* **2013**, *346*, f1326. [CrossRef] [PubMed]

8. He, F.J.; Li, J.; MacGregor, G.A. Effect of longer-term modest salt reduction on blood pressure: Cochrane systematic review and meta-analysis of randomised trials. *Br. Med. J.* **2013**, *346*, f1325. [CrossRef] [PubMed]

9. Strazzullo, P.; D'Elia, L.; Kandala, N.-B.; Cappuccio, F.P. Salt intake, stroke, and cardiovascular disease: Meta-Analysis of prospective studies. *Br. Med. J.* **2009**, *339*, b4567. [CrossRef] [PubMed]

10. Cook, N.R.; Cutler, J.A.; Obarzanek, E.; Buring, J.E.; Rexrode, K.M.; Kumanyika, S.K.; Appel, L.J.; Whelton, P.K. Long term effects of dietary sodium reduction on cardiovascular disease outcomes: Observational follow-up of the Trials of Hypertension Prevention (TOHP). *Br. Med. J.* **2007**, *334*, 885–888. [CrossRef]

11. Cappuccio, F.P. Cardiovascular and other effects of salt consumption. *Kidney Int.* **2013**, *3*, 312–315. [CrossRef]

12. D'Elia, L.; Rossi, G.; Schiano di Cola, M.; Savino, I.; Galletti, F.; Strazzullo, P. Meta-Analysis of the effect of dietary sodium restriction with or without concomitant renin–angiotensin–aldosterone system-inhibiting treatment on albuminuria. *Clin. J. Am. Soc. Nephrol.* **2015**, *10*, 1542–1552. [CrossRef]

13. D'Elia, L.; Galletti, F.; La Fata, E.; Sabino, P.; Strazzullo, P. Effect of dietary sodium restriction on arterial stiffness: Systematic review and meta-analysis of the randomized controlled trials. *J. Hypertens.* **2018**, *36*, 734–743. [CrossRef]

14. World Health Organization. *Guideline: Sodium Intake for Adults and Children*; World Health Organization (WHO): Geneva, Switzerland, 2012.

15. Brown, I.J.; Tzoulaki, I.; Candeias, V.; Elliott, P. Salt intakes around the world: Implications for public health. *Int. J. Epidemiol.* **2009**, *38*, 791–813. [CrossRef]

16. Cappuccio, F.P.; Capewell, S. Facts, issues, and controversies in salt reduction for the prevention of cardiovascular disease. *Funct. Food Rev.* **2015**, *7*, 41–61.

17. WHO Regional Office for Europe. *Mapping Salt Reduction Initiatives in the WHO European Region*; WHO Regional Office for Europe: Copenhagen, Denmark, 2013.

18. Mattes, R.D.; Donnelly, D. Relative contributions of dietary sources. *J. Am. Coll. Nutr.* **1991**, *10*, 383–393. [CrossRef] [PubMed]

19. Sanchez-Castillo, C.P.; Warrender, S.; Whitehead, T.P.; James, W.P. An assessment of the sources of dietary salt in a British population. *Clin. Sci.* **1987**, *72*, 95–102. [CrossRef] [PubMed]

20. Jovicic-Bata, J.; Grujicic, M.; Raden, S.; Novakovic, B. Sodium intake and dietary sources of sodium in a sample of undergraduate students from Novi Sad, Serbia. *Vojnosanit. Pregl.* **2016**, *73*, 1044–1049. [CrossRef] [PubMed]

21. Ribič, C.H.; Zakotnik, J.M.; Vertnik, L.; Vegnuti, M.; Cappuccio, F.P. Salt intake of the Slovene population assessed by 24-hour urinary sodium excretion. *Public Health Nutr.* **2010**, *13*, 1803–1809. [CrossRef]

22. D'Elia, L.; Brajovic, M.; Klisic, A.; Breda, J.; Jewell, J.; Cadjenovic, V.; Cappuccio, F.P.; on behalf of Salt Consumption Survey in Montenegro Study Group. Sodium and potassium intake, knowledge attitudes and behaviour towards salt consumption, amongst adults in Podgorica, Montenegro. *Nutrients* **2019**, *11*, 160. [CrossRef]

23. Cappuccio, F.P.; Capewell, S.; Lincoln, P.; McPherson, K. Policy options to reduce population salt intake. *Br. Med. J.* **2011**, *343*, 402–405. [CrossRef]

24. Aburto, N.J.; Hanson, S.; Gutierrez, H.; Hooper, L.; Elliott, P.; Cappuccio, F.P. Effect of increased potassium intake on cardiovascular risk factors and disease: Systematic review and meta-analyses. *Br. Med. J.* **2013**, *346*, f1378. [CrossRef]

25. D'Elia, L.; Barba, G.; Cappuccio, F.P.; Strazzullo, P. Potassium Intake, Stroke, and Cardiovascular Disease: A meta-analysis of Prospective Studies. *J. Am. Coll. Cardiol.* **2011**, *57*, 1210–1219. [CrossRef]

26. D'Elia, L.; Iannotta, C.; Sabino, P.; Ippolito, R. Potassium rich-diet and risk of stroke: Updated meta-analysis. *Nutr. Metab. Cardiovasc. Dis.* **2014**, *24*, 585–587. [CrossRef]

27. World Health Organization. *Guideline: Potassium Intake for Adults and Children*; World Health Organization (WHO): Geneva, Switzerland, 2012; pp. 1–52.

28. Obreja, G.; Raevschi, E.; Penina, O. Informing national salt reduction strategy. *Mold. Med. J.* **2018**, *61*, 9–16.

29. Nath, S.K.; Moinier, B.; Thullier, F.; Rongier, M.; Desjeux, J.F. Urinary excretion of iodide and fluoride from supplemented food grade salt. *Int. J. Vitam. Nutr. Res.* **1992**, *62*, 66–72. [PubMed]

30. Jahreis, G.; Hausmann, W.; Kiessling, G.; Franke, K.; Leiterer, M. Bioavailability of iodine from normal diets rich in dairy products: Results of balance studies in women. *Exp. Clin. Endocrinol. Diabetes* **2001**, *109*, 163–167. [CrossRef] [PubMed]

31. World Health Organization. *Guideline: Fortification of Food-Grade Salt with Iodine for the Prevention and Control of Iodine Deficiency Disorders*; World Health Organization: Geneva, Switzerland, 2014; pp. 1–54.

32. Pan American Health Organization/World Health Organization. *Salt-Smart Americas: A Guide for Country-Level Action*; PAHO: Washington, DC, USA, 2013; pp. 1–159.

33. World Health Organization. *How to Obtain Measures of Population-Level Sodium Intake in 24-Hour Urine Samples*; WHO-EM/NUT/279/E; World Health Organization/Regional Office of the Eastern Mediterranean: Cairo, Egypt, 2018; pp. 1–51.

34. World Medical Association. Declaration of Helsinki: Recommendations guiding doctors in clinical research. *Bull. World Health Org.* **2008**, *86*, 650–651.

35. World Health Organization. *The WHO STEPwise Approach to Chronic Disease Risk Factor Surveillance (STEPS)*; World Health Organization: Geneva, Switzerland, 2014; Available online: https://www.who.int/ncds/surveillance/steps/STEPS_Instrument_v2.1.pdf (accessed on 27 October 2019).

36. Mancia, G.; Fagard, R.; Narkiewicz, K.; Redón, J.; Zanchetti, A.; Böhm, M.; Christiaens, T.; Cifkova, R.; De Backer, G.; Dominiczak, A.; et al. 2013 ESH/ESC Guidelines for the management of arterial hypertension: The Task Force for the management of arterial hypertension of the European Society of Hypertension (ESH) and of the European Society of Cardiology (ESC). *J. Hypertens.* **2013**, *31*, 1281–1357. [CrossRef] [PubMed]

37. Oesch, U.; Ammann, D.; Simon, W. Ion-Selective membrane electrodes for clinical use. *Clin. Chem.* **1986**, *32*, 1448–1459. [PubMed]

38. Junge, W.; Wilke, B.; Halabi, A.; Klein, G. Determination of reference intervals for serum creatinine, creatinine excretion and creatinine clearance with an enzymatic and a modified Jaffé method. *Clin. Chim. Acta* **2004**, *344*, 137–148. [CrossRef] [PubMed]

39. Ohashi, T.; Yamaki, M.; Pandav, C.S.; Karmarkar, M.G.; Irie, M. Simple microplate method for determination of urinary iodine. *Clin. Chem.* **2000**, *46*, 529–536.

40. Jooste, P.L.; Strydom, E. Methods for determination of iodine in urine and salt. *Best Pract. Res. Clin. Endocrinol. Metab.* **2010**, *24*, 77–88. [CrossRef]

41. Lucko, A.M.; Doktorchik, C.; Woodward, M.; Cogswell, M.; Neal, B.; Rabi, D.; Anderson, C.; He, F.J.; MacGregor, G.A.; L'Abbe, M.; et al. Percentage of ingested sodium excreted in 24-hour urine collections: A systematic review and meta-analysis. *J. Clin. Hypertens.* **2018**, *20*, 1220–1229. [CrossRef]

42. Stamler, J.; Elliott, P.; Chan, Q.; for the INTERMAP Research group. INTERMAP Appendix tables. *J. Hum. Hypertens.* **2003**, *17*, 665–758. [CrossRef]

43. Donfrancesco, C.; Ippolito, R.; Lo Noce, C.; Palmieri, L.; Iacone, R.; Russo, O.; Vanuzzo, D.; Galletti, F.; Galeone, D.; Giampaoli, S.; et al. Excess dietary sodium and inadequate potassium intake in Italy: Results of the MINISAL study. *Nutr. Metab. Cardiovasc. Dis.* **2013**, *23*, 850–856. [CrossRef]

44. Cappuccio, F.P.; Ji, C.; Donfrancesco, C.; Palmieri, L.; Ippolito, R.; Vanuzzo, D.; Giampaoli, S.; Strazzullo, P. Geographic and socio-economic variation of sodium and potassium intake in Italy. Results from the MINISAL-GIRCSI programme. *BMJ Open* **2015**, *5*, e007467. [CrossRef] [PubMed]

45. Vasara, E.; Marakis, G.; Breda, J.; Skepastianos, P.; Hassapidou, M.; Kafatos, A.; Rodopaios, N.; Koulouri, A.; Cappuccio, F.P. Sodium and Potassium Intake in Healthy Adults in Thessaloniki Greater Metropolitan Area-The Salt Intake in Northern Greece (SING) Study. *Nutrients* **2017**, *22*, 417. [CrossRef] [PubMed]

46. Erdem, Y.; Akpolat, T.; Derici, Ü.; Şengül, Ş.; Ertürk, Ş.; Ulusoy, Ş.; Altun, B.; Arici, M. Dietary sources of high sodium intake in Turkey: SALTURK II. *Nutrients* **2017**, *9*, 933. [CrossRef] [PubMed]

47. Polonia, J.; Martins, L.; Pinto, F.; Nazare, J. Prevalence, awareness, treatment and control of hypertension and salt intake in Portugal: Changes over a decade. The PHYSA study. *J. Hypertens.* **2014**, *32*, 1211–1221. [CrossRef]

48. Lerchl, K.; Rakova, N.; Dahlmann, A.; Rauh, M.; Goller, U.; Basner, M.; Dinges, D.F.; Beck, L.; Agureev, A.; Larina, I.; et al. Agreement between 24-hour salt ingestion and sodium excretion in a controlled environment. *Hypertension* **2015**, *66*, 850–857. [CrossRef]

49. National Centre for Health Management. *Statistical Yearbook of the Republic of Moldova*; Ministry of Health, Labour and Social Protection of the Republic of Moldova: Chişinău, Moldova, 2017.

50. Government of the Republic of Moldova. Decision no. 403 of 6 April 2016 on the approval of the National Action Plan for 2016–2020 on the implementation of the National Strategy on Prevention and Control of Noncommunicable Diseases. *Monitorul Oficial Republicii Moldova* **2016**, *100*, 464. (In Romanian)

51. Collins, D.; Ciobanu, A.; Laatikainen, T.; Curocichin, G.; Salaru, V.; Zatic, T.; Anisei, A.; Farrington, J. Protocol for the evaluation of a pilot implementation of essential interventions for the prevention of cardiovascular diseases in primary healthcare in the Republic of Moldova. *BMJ Open* **2019**, *9*, e025705. [CrossRef]

52. Pastorelli, A.A.; Stacchini, P.; Olivieri, A. Daily iodine intake and the impact of salt reduction on iodine prophylaxis in the Italian population. *Eur. J. Clin. Nutr.* **2015** *69*, 211–215. [CrossRef]

Association between Iodine Nutrition Status and Thyroid Disease-Related Hormone in Korean Adults: Korean National Health and Nutrition Examination Survey VI (2013–2015)

Sohye Kim [1,2], Yong Seok Kwon [3], Ju Young Kim [4], Kyung Hee Hong [5] and Yoo Kyoung Park [1,*]

[1] Department of Medical Nutrition, Graduate School of East-West Medical Science, Kyung Hee University, Yongin 17104, Korea; sohye76@daum.net

[2] Nutrition Care Services, Seoul National University of Bundang Hospital, Seongnam 13620, Korea

[3] F&D Communication, Gyeonggi 10433, Korea; shafrang@naver.com

[4] Department of Family Medicine, Seoul National University of Bundang Hospital, Seongnam 13620, Korea; kkamburi@gmail.com

[5] Department of Food Science and Nutrition, Dongseo University, Pusan 47011, Korea; hkhee@gdsu.dongseo.ac.kr

* Correspondence: ypark@khu.ac.kr

Abstract: This study aimed to observe the relationship between iodine nutrition status (dietary iodine intake and estimated iodine intake based on urinary iodine concentration (UIC)) and thyroid disease-related hormones. This study involved 6090 subjects >19 years old with valid UIC, assessed between 2013 and 2015 by the Korean National Health and Nutrition Examination Survey, using a stratified, multistage, clustered probability-sampling design. The estimated iodine intake in participants was measured using UIC and urine creatinine. To examine the effect of iodine intake on thyroid disease, the iodine intake was divided into Korean Dietary Reference Intakes groups, and logistic regression analysis was performed via the surveylogistic procedure to obtain odds ratios (ORs) and 95% confidence intervals (CIs). The estimated iodine intake showed a significant positive correlation with dietary iodine intake (r = 0.021, $p < 0.001$), UIC (r = 0.918, $p < 0.001$), and thyroid-stimulating hormone (TSH) (r = 0.043, $p < 0.001$), but a significant negative correlation with free thyroxine (FT4) (r = −0.037, $p < 0.001$). Additionally, as the estimated iodine intake increased, age, TSH, and UIC increased, but FT4 decreased (p for trend < 0.0001). The risk of thyroid disease was higher in the "≥tolerable upper intake level (UL ≥ 2400 µg/day)" group than in the "<estimated average requirement (EAR < 150 µg/day)" group in females (OR: 2.418; 95% CI: 1.010–5.787). Also, as iodine intake increased, the risk of thyroid disease increased (p for trend < 0.038).

Keywords: iodine nutrition status; thyroid disease; thyrotropin; urine iodine; epidemiologic studies; Korean

1. Introduction

Korea is geographically rich in iodine and one of the iodine-rich countries with a high intake of seaweeds [1]. According to a recent study, the mean dietary iodine intake was 763.5 µg for Korean female subjects and 953.1 µg for males [2]. In a study involving the trend analysis of iodine intake, the iodine intake for males was 326.2–817.0 µg and for females 257.0–802.4 µg [3]. It seems that a majority of the studies indicate that most of the Koreans' iodine intake is within the upper limit (UL) (2400 µg) intake, but over two times higher than the recommended nutrient intake (RNI) (150 µg) [4–8]. Iodine controls the speed of, and is therefore an essential element in, thyroid hormone synthesis. When the iodine intake is insufficient, the hypothalamus hormones, thyrotropin-releasing hormone (TRH) is secreted, and thyroid-stimulating hormone (TSH) further increases the secretion of the thyroid to increase the synthesis and secretion of the thyroid hormone. When blood levels of triiodothyronine (T3) and thyroxine (T4) decrease, and in response the thyroid activity is increased to compensate for iodine deficiency, a sudden excessive intake can increase the risk of hyperthyroidism. Additionally, excessive iodine intake can change the thyroid function, and according to several studies, the prevalence of hypothyroidism, hyperthyroidism, and autoimmune thyroiditis has increased [9–13]. Many studies have reported that deficiency and excess of iodine are associated with thyroid dysfunction [7,10,14,15]. Therefore, it is important to find out effects on thyroid hormones made by level of iodine nutrition status. The iodine nutrition status of the population is measured based on dietary iodine intake or urinary iodine concentration (UIC), which is a well-accepted, cost-effective, and readily available indicator. Furthermore, according to the iodine nutritional epidemiology standard of the World Health Organization (WHO), UIC is a recommended barometer for iodine intake that assesses the iodine status of the population and is a sensitive indicator [16,17].

TSH, T4, T3, and thyroid autoantibodies (TPOAb) measurements are biochemical tests in the diagnosis and control of thyroid disease [18]. Serum TSH is the most sensitive marker for assessing the status of thyroid function and measurement of serum TSH level is used as a screening test for patients with thyroid dysfunction [19]. TSH is known to be affected by factors such as age, sex, race, iodine intake, smoking, presence of antibodies, and body mass index (BMI) [15,20].

The purpose of this study is to investigate the relationship between iodine nutrition status (dietary iodine intake and estimated iodine intake based on UIC) and thyroid disease-related hormones, such as serum TSH and free thyroxine (FT4). Also, we investigated the association of the iodine nutrition status and the thyroid disease incidence among Korean adults.

This is the nationwide study to observe the relationship between thyroid disease-related functions, such as serum TSH and FT4 level, and UIC, which was first introduced by the Korean National Health and Nutrition Examination Survey (KNHANES) VI (2013–2015), and also examined the relationship between iodine nutrition status including iodine intake in people's diet and estimated iodine intake.

2. Methods and Materials

2.1. Study Population

The KNHANES is conducted to obtain national estimates of the health and nutrition status of Koreans by the Korea Centers for Disease Control and Prevention (KCDC) that uses a stratified, multistage clustered probability-sampling design [21]. KNHANES is a nationwide, population-based, cross-sectional study to assess the health and nutrition status of the Korean civilian, noninstitutionalized population. Each survey consists of three sections: health interview, health examinations, and nutritional survey.

We selected from the total population ($n = 22,938$) after the exclusion of <19 years ($n = 4914$), subjects with thyroid cancer ($n = 135$), pregnant and lactating women ($n = 239$), subjects reporting unrealistic daily total energy intakes (<500 kcal, >5000 kcal) ($n = 2251$), subjects who did not test UIC ($n = 9312$), and subjects with missing weight variables ($n = 2$). As a result, a total of 6095 subjects were included in the final analysis (men=2852, women=3243). This subsample of KNHANES VI (2013–2015) consisted of 6095 participants who underwent the thyroid function test (serum TSH and FT4) and UIC stratified subsampling with consideration of sex and age.

This study protocol was approved by the Institutional Review Board of the KCDC and the KNHANES (2013-07CON-03-4C, 2013-12EXP-03-5C, and 2015-01-02-6C). All participants gave written informed consent.

2.2. Measurement of TSH, FT4, and UIC

Serum TSH and FT4 levels analyzed via electrochemiluminescence immunoassay were used. Serum TSH (reference range 0.35–5.50 mU/L) and FT4 (reference range 0.89–1.76 ng/dL) levels were analyzed using E-TSH kit (Roche Diagnostics, Mannheim, Germany) and E-Free T4 kit (Roche Diagnostics, Mannheim, Germany), respectively. UIC, analyzed through inductively coupled plasma mass spectrometry (ICPMS; PerkinElmer, Waltham, MA, USA) using iodine standard (Inorganic Venture, Christiansburg, VA, USA), was used [22].

2.3. Estimated Iodine Intake

The estimated iodine intake in populations was calculated by measuring the UIC and urine creatinine (Ucr) level and the following equation (1) [6,23,24]:

$$\text{Estimated of iodine intake (μg/day)} = \text{UIC (μg/L)} \times \{879.89 + (\text{weight (kg)} \times 12.51) - [(6.19 \times \text{age}) + (34.51 \text{ if black}) - (379.42 \text{ if female})]\} / (\text{Ucr} \times 0.92 \times 10). \tag{1}$$

2.4. Establishment of Iodine Database of Commercial Foods in Korea

The iodine content of foods was based on the values shown in the Food Values of the Korean Nutrition Society [25], Food Composition Tables, 9th revision by the Korean National Institute of Agricultural Science, Rural Development Administration [26], a thesis that established the iodine database for common Korean foods [2], and the Standard tables of food composition in Japan (7th revised version) of the Ministry of Education, Culture, Sport, Science, and Technology, Tokyo, 2015 [27].

The value was selected if the food source existed on the database; however, if there was no matching food, it was replaced by something a similar food item from the database. If there were variations in terms of the processing method for certain foods, such as drying methods, we calculated the iodine values based on the values of the existing source of the foods. Moreover, if there were multiple values from different sources of data for one specific food, the mean value for the specific food was used. The total number of food items was 837, and the number of foods with iodine content was 559, which provided 66.8% coverage.

2.5. Measurement of Dietary Iodine Intake Using 24-hr-Dietary Recall

The nutrition survey data were collected using the 24-h dietary recall method and face-to-face health interviews by trained dietitians and health examination [28]. The daily intake of energy was calculated using the Korean Foods and Nutrients Database of the Rural Development Administration [26]. To calculate the dietary iodine intake, we established an iodine database by merging the data on food items from the 24 h diet recall in the KNHANES database (2013–2015) with the established iodine value for each food item.

2.6. Statistics

As the KNHANES data is based on stratified multistage probability extraction rather than simple random extraction data, this study analyzed the weight (2013, KNHANES; Wt_hmnt, 2014, 2015 KNHANES; Wt_trnt), the stratification variable (KSTRATA) and the primary sampling unit (PSU). To test for significant differences, the t-test was used when calibration was not performed using the surveyreg procedure, and the general linear model was used when calibration was performed using the surveyreg procedure. Additionally, the age and total daily energy intake were used as calibration variables. In addition, the correlation between each of the iodine intake and thyroid function tests was analyzed using Pearson correlation. Using the paired t-test, associations were determined with weighted measures among the estimated iodine intake, dietary iodine intake, and UIC. Lastly, to examine the effect of iodine intake on thyroid disease, this study divided iodine intake into Korean Dietary Reference Intakes (KDRI) groups [4], and logistic regression analysis was performed via the surveylogistic procedure to obtain odds ratios (OR) and 95% confidence intervals (CI). All statistical analyses were performed using SAS Ver. 9.4 (SAS Institute, Cary, NC, USA).

3. Results

3.1. Iodine Nutrition Status

The mean estimated iodine intake for all subjects was 790.1 µg, which was higher than the mean dietary iodine intake (551.0 µg). These results were identical for both the male and female groups (Figure 1).

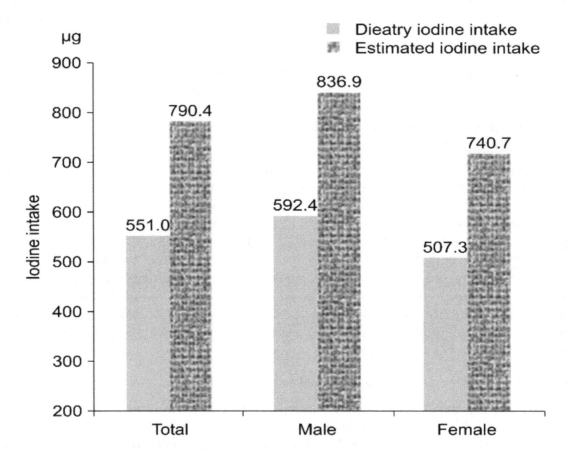

Figure 1. Mean of dietary iodine intake vs. estimated iodine intake.

The results of the analysis of the iodine nutrition status of the subjects are shown in Table 1. The thyroid disease group was higher in the total subjects' energy than in the non-thyroid disease group (unadjusted $p < 0.0001$, adjusted for age $p = 0.001$). In total subjects, the mean dietary iodine intake of the non-thyroid disease group was 554.0 ± 35.8 µg, which was higher than that of the thyroid disease group of 458.8 ± 93.6 µg. However, the mean of estimated iodine intake of the non-thyroid disease group was 780.0 ± 56.1 µg, which was lower than that of the thyroid disease group of 1108.1 ± 195.8 µg. In total subjects, the mean UIC of the non-thyroid disease group was 883.2 ± 92.1 µg, which was lower than that of the thyroid disease group of 1085.9 ± 183.9 µg, but there was no significant difference. Additionally, the same result was obtained in the female group (non-thyroid disease 849.8 µg, thyroid disease group 1145.5 µg), but the result of the male group was the opposite (non-thyroid disease 913.5 µg, thyroid disease group 745.1 µg), and there were no significant differences between these groups. Moreover, there were no significant differences in all groups with UIC, dietary iodine intake, and estimated iodine intake.

Table 1. Iodine nutrition status of the subjects.

	Total (n = 6095)				Male (n = 2852)				Female (n = 3243)			
	Non-Thyroid Disease (n = 5908)	Thyroid Disease (n = 187)	Unadjusted p-Value [a]	Adjusted p-Value [a,b]	Non-Thyroid Disease (n = 2827)	Thyroid Disease (n = 25)	Unadjusted p-Value	Adjusted p-Value	Non-Thyroid Disease (n = 3081)	Thyroid Disease (n = 162)	Unadjusted p-Value	Adjusted p-Value
	Mean ± SE	Mean ± SE			Mean ± SE	Mean ± SE			Mean ± SE	Mean ± SE		
Dietary Iodine (µg/day)	554.0 ± 35.8	458.8 ± 93.6	0.348	0.483	592.9 ± 60.0	533.2 ± 190.8	0.766	0.715	510.9 ± 34.3	445.8 ± 101.5	0.547	0.502
Estimated Iodine (µg/day)	780.0 ± 56.1	1108.1 ± 195.8	0.107	0.162	837.5 ± 97.8	775.7 ± 241.2	0.813	0.624	716.4 ± 39.0	1166.3 ± 226.2	0.051	0.067
UIC [c] (µg/L)	883.2 ± 92.1	1085.9 ± 183.9	0.322	0.400	913.5 ± 164.5	745.1 ± 235.8	0.558	0.462	849.8 ± 52.5	1145.5 ± 211.5	0.172	0.195

[a] p-value was calculated via the surveyreg procedure of SAS; [b] Adjusted for age and energy intake (energy intake was adjusted for age); [c] UIC = Urinary iodine concentration.

3.2. TSH and FT4 of the Subjects

The TSH and FT4 levels of the non-thyroid disease group vs. the thyroid disease group are shown in Figure 2. The mean TSH of the non-thyroid disease group was 2.8 ± 0.1 mIU/L, which was lower than that of the thyroid disease group (3.7 ± 0.4 mIU/L) (adjusted for age and energy intake $p = 0.029$). As a result, TSH in the total subjects was significantly higher in the thyroid disease group than in the non-thyroid disease group. Male and female groups showed similar results, but there were no significant differences. Additionally, the mean FT4 of the non-thyroid disease group was lower than that of the thyroid disease group, but there was no significant difference.

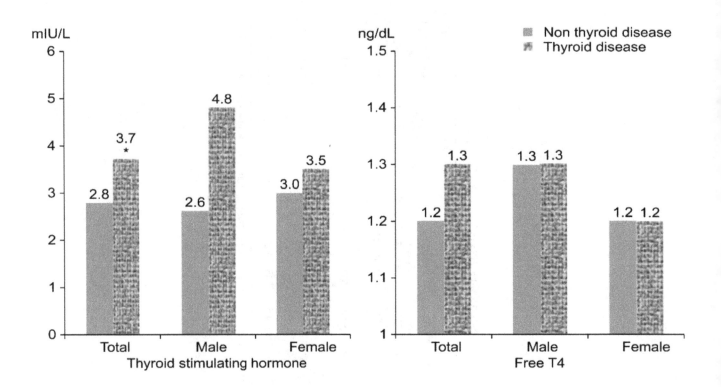

Figure 2. TSH and FT4 of thyroid disease status by sex.

3.3. UIC, TSH, and FT4 According to KDRI of the Estimated Iodine Intake

The estimated iodine intake was divided into KDRI groups, and the results of UIC, TSH, and FT4 tests for each group are presented in Table 2.

The KDRI groups were as follows: "<EAR (estimated average requirement)", <95 µg/day; "≥EAR, <RNI (recommended nutrient intake)," ≥95 µg/day, <150 µg/day; "≥RNI, <UL (tolerable upper intake)," ≥150 µg/day, 2400 µg/day; and "≥UL," ≥2400 µg/day by KDRI [4]. The mean and median values of the UL group were dramatically higher than those of the other groups (Figure 3). In total subjects, both unadjusted and adjusted for age and energy intake, as iodine intake increased, age (p for trend < 0.0001), TSH (p for trend = 0.009) (Figure 3), and UIC (p for trend < 0.0001) tended to increase, but FT4 showed a tendency to decrease (p for trend < 0.0001) (Figure 4). In addition, in both male and female groups, as iodine intake increased, age, TSH, and UIC tended to increase, but FT4 showed a tendency to decrease. All results are significant except for TSH in the female group.

Table 2. UIC, TSH, free T4, and KDRI of the estimated iodine intake by sex.

Estimated Iodine Intake (μg/day)	Korean Dietary Reference Intakes (KDRI)				Unadjusted p for Trend [d]	Adjusted p for Trend [d,e]
	<EAR [a] (<95) (n = 850) Mean ± SE	≥EAR, <RNI [b] (≥95, <150) (n = 987) Mean ± SE	≥RNI, <UL [c] (≥150, 2400) (n = 3869) Mean ± SE	≥UL (≥2400) (n = 389) Mean ± SE		
Total						
Age	44.3 ± 0.8	44.4 ± 0.6	46.8 ± 0.3	50.7 ± 0.9	<.0001(+)	<.0001(+)
TSH (mIU/L)	2.5 ± 0.1	2.5 ± 0.1	2.8 ± 0.1	3.7 ± 0.4	0.008(+)	0.009(+)
UIC (μg/L)	111.1 ± 2.6	168.5 ± 3.4	632.6 ± 13.6	6903.2 ± 1202.3	<.0001(+)	<.0001(+)
FT4 (ng/dL)	1.3 ± 0.01	1.3 ± 0.01	1.2 ± 0.005	1.2 ± 0.01	<.0001(−)	<.0001(−)
Male						
Age	41.7 ± 1.1	42.8 ± 0.8	45.6 ± 0.3	50.1 ± 1.1	<.0001(+)	<.0001(+)
TSH (mIU/L)	2.1 ± 0.1	2.3 ± 0.1	2.6 ± 0.1	4.0 ± 0.7	0.024(+)	0.024(+)
UIC (μg/L)	109.8 ± 3.5	154.8 ± 3.9	580.0 ± 15.4	7404.0 ± 2222.9	0.002(+)	0.002(+)
FT4 (ng/dL)	1.3 ± 0.01	1.3 ± 0.0	1.3 ± 0.01	1.2 ± 0.02	<.0001(−)	0.002(−)
Female						
Age	46.0 ± 0.9	45.9 ± 0.8	48.3 ± 0.4	51.3 ± 1.3	0.002(+)	0.003(+)
TSH (mIU/L)	2.8 ± 0.1	2.8 ± 0.1	3.1 ± 0.1	3.4 ± 0.2	0.062(+)	0.079(+)
UIC (μg/L)	112.0 ± 3.3	181.6 ± 5.2	694.9 ± 21.6	6350.5 ± 597.7	<.0001(+)	<.0001(+)
FT4 (ng/dL)	1.2 ± 0.01	1.2 ± 0.01	1.2 ± 0.01	1.1 ± 0.01	0.0001(−)	0.001(−)

[a] EAR: Estimated average requirement; [b] RNI: Recommended nutrient intake; [c] UL: Tolerable upper intake; [d] All p for trend were calculated by surveyreg procedure of SAS; [e] Adjusted for age and energy intake (age was adjusted for energy intake).

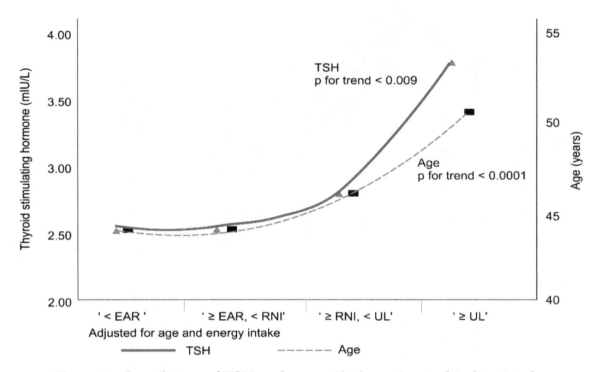

Figure 3. Correlation of TSH and age with the estimated iodine intake.

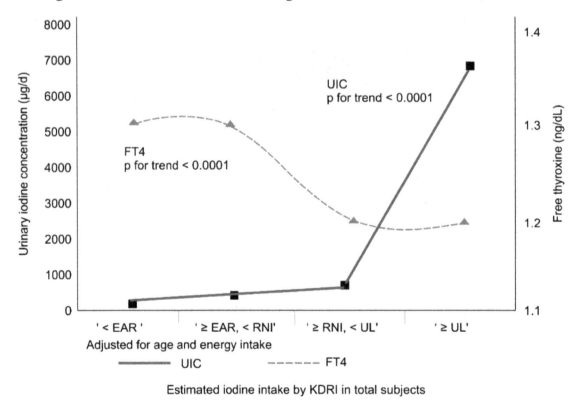

Figure 4. Correlation of UIC and free thyroxine (FT4) with the estimated iodine intake.

3.4. Prevalence of Thyroid Disease and Distribution of Iodine Intake According to the Estimated Iodine Intake by KDRI

The intake range, median, and mean of the estimated iodine intake classified by KDRI groups are shown in Table 3.

Table 3. Prevalence of thyroid disease, intake range, median, and mean according to the KDRI of the estimated iodine intake by sex.

Estimated Iodine Intake (μg/day)	Korean Dietary Reference Intake (KDRI) [a]				
	<EAR [c] (<95)	≥EAR, <RNI [d] (≥95, <150)	≥RNI, <UL [e] (≥150, 2400)	≥UL (≥2400)	Total
Total	n = 850	n = 987	n = 3869	n = 389	n = 6095
Intake Range	1.29–94.99	95.01–149.95	150.02–2399.36	2409.77–80672.0	1.29–80672.0
Median ± SE [b]	72.0 ± 1.2	122.5 ± 1.1	362.5 ± 7.1	4102.9 ± 152.3	256.4 ± 5.5
Mean ± SE	69.4 ± 0.8	122.2 ± 0.6	558.0 ± 9.7	6301.4 ± 672.7	790.1 ± 54.7
Prevalence of Thyroid Disease (n, weighted %)					
Non-Thyroid Disease	830 97.2	964 97.6	3744 96.9	370 94.4	5908
Thyroid Disease	20 2.8	23 2.4	125 3.1	19 5.6	187
Male	n = 296	n = 453	n = 1910	n = 193	n = 2852
Intake Range	2.79–94.99	95.03–149.76	150.02–2391.91	2414.16–80672.0	2.79–80672.0
Median ± SE	74.6 ± 1.7	122.0 ± 1.4	355.7 ± 8.3	3823.3 ± 227.3	270.9 ± 6.5
Mean ± SE	71.7 ± 1.2	122.1 ± 0.9	543.5 ± 12.8	6772.6 ± 1228.9	836.9 ± 96.9
Prevalence of Thyroid Disease (n, weighted %)					
Non-Thyroid Disease	293 98.2	449 99.1	1894 99.2	191 99.3	2827
Thyroid Disease	3 1.8	4 0.9	16 0.8	2 0.7	25
Female	n = 554	n = 534	n = 1959	n = 196	n = 3243
Intake Range	1.29–94.97	95.01–149.95	150.29–2399.36	2409.77–36494.0	1.29–36494.0
Median ± SE	70.3 ± 1.6	122.7 ± 1.8	372.8 ± 12.7	4285.4 ± 189.5	235.4 ± 8.1
Mean ± SE	67.9 ± 1.0	122.3 ± 0.9	575.3 ± 13.7	5781.4 ± 399.6	740.7 ± 38.7
Prevalence of thyroid disease (n, weighted %)					
Non-Thyroid Disease	537 96.4	515 96.1	1850 94.2	179 89.0	3081
Thyroid Disease	17 3.6	19 3.9	109 5.8	17 11.0	162

[a] KDRI group was classified based on the estimated iodine intake; [b] Standard error; [c] EAR: estimated average requirement; [d] RNI: Recommend nutrient intake; [e] UL: Tolerable upper intake.

The population distribution with respect to the dietary iodine intake and estimated iodine intake of all the subjects was divided into KDRI groups. The "≥RNI, <UL" group had the largest population—65.1% with respect to dietary iodine intake and 63.5% with respect to estimated iodine intake, while the "UL" group had the smallest population (Figure 5).

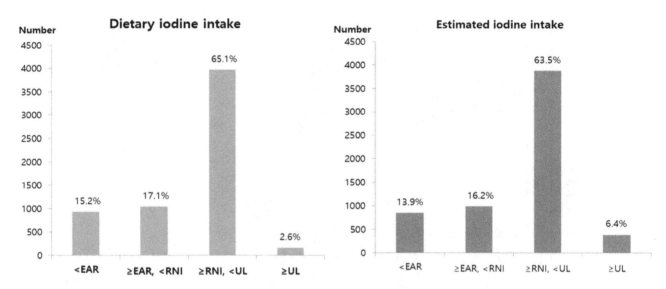

Figure 5. Population distribution of iodine intake by KDRI in the total subjects.

3.5. Relation between Thyroid Disease and the Estimated Iodine Intake by KDRI

The results of the relationship between the estimated iodine intake and the risk of thyroid disease incidence according to KDRI groups using logistic regression analysis are presented in Table 4.

In relation to the thyroid disease according to the estimated iodine intake, as the estimated iodine intake increased in Model 1, which was the unadjusted model in the female group, the odds ratio of the "≥UL" group was 2.940 (95% CI: 1.267–6.823), which showed a tendency to increase the risk of thyroid disease incidence (p for trend = 0.014). Additionally, as the iodine intake increased in Model 2 adjusted for age and energy intake, the odds ratio of Model 2 was 2.773 (95% CI: 1.198–6.420) in the "≥UL" group compared with the "<EAR" group, and the risk of thyroid disease tended to be increased (p for trend = 0.023). In Model 3, adjusted for age, energy intake, weight status, exercise status, smoking status, and alcohol consumption, the odds ratio was 2.686 (95% CI: 1.161–6.215) in the "≥UL" group compared with the "<EAR" group, and the risk of thyroid disease tended to be increased (p for trend = 0.026). Also, in Model 4 adjusted for age, energy intake, weight status, exercise status, smoking status, alcohol consumption, breakfast, and frequency of eating out, the odds ratio was 2.554 (95% CI: 1.113–5.861) in the "≥UL" group compared with the "<EAR" group, and the risk of thyroid disease tended to be increased (p for trend = 0.34). Lastly, in Model 5, adjusted for age, energy intake, weight status, exercise status, smoking status, alcohol consumption, breakfast, frequency of eating out, education level, region of residence, household income level, and occupation, the odds ratio was 2.418 (95% CI: 1.010–5.787) in the "≥UL" group compared with the "<EAR" group, and the risk of thyroid disease tended to be increased (p for trend = 0.038). However, there was no risk of iodine intake incidence and thyroid disease in the male group and in the total subjects.

This might support the idea that iodine intake by >UL (≥2400 µg/day) can increase the risk of thyroid disease in females (Figure 6). However, the same results were not observed in the male group. Also, dietary iodine intake did not indicate any risk of thyroid disease incidence.

Table 4. Logistic regression analysis of thyroid disease across KDRI of the estimated iodine intake by sex.

Estimated Iodine Intake (μg/day)	Korean Dietary Reference Intake (KDRI)				*p* for Trend [d]
	<EAR [a] (<95)	≥EAR, <RNI [b] (≥95, <150)	≥RNI, <UL [c] (≥150, 2400)	≥UL (≥2400)	
Total					
Model 1	1 [e]	0.832(0.409–1.692) [f]	1.084(0.634–1.854)	1.788(0.820–3.898)	0.059(+)
Model 2	1	0.854(0.416–1.750)	1.092(0.631–1.891)	1.692(0.773–3.704)	0.096(+)
Model 3	1	0.887(0.428–1.838)	1.144(0.657–1.992)	1.796(0.815–3.960)	0.076(+)
Model 4	1	0.891(0.422–1.882)	1.166(0.662–2.056)	1.846(0.840–4.058)	0.066(+)
Model 5	1	0.847(0.390–1.836)	1.095(0.612–1.957)	1.726(0.760–3.923)	0.085(+)
Male					
Model 1	1	0.499(0.095–2.620)	0.440(0.108–1.792)	0.414(0.051–3.359)	0.720(−)
Model 2	1	0.474(0.089–2.528)	0.390(0.095–1.609)	0.325(0.041–2.568)	0.607(−)
Model 3	1	0.397(0.075–2.098)	0.317(0.073–1.378)	0.251(0.034–1.839)	0.549(−)
Model 4	1	0.405(0.080–2.054)	0.353(0.079–1.566)	0.278(0.036–2.161)	0.582(−)
Model 5	1	0.419(0.084–2.084)	0.311(0.070–1.378)	0.240(0.029–1.954)	0.5573(−)
Female					
Model 1	1	1.056(0.492–2.263)	1.667(0.908–3.061)	2.940(1.267–6.823)	0.014(+)
Model 2	1	1.054(0.490–2.267)	1.629(0.887–2.989)	2.773(1.198–6.420)	0.023(+)
Model 3	1	1.063(0.488–2.315)	1.608(0.873–2.961)	2.686(1.161–6.215)	0.026(+)
Model 4	1	1.048(0.479–2.292)	1.561(0.846–2.881)	2.554(1.113–5.861)	0.034(+)
Model 5	1	0.979(0.438–2.192)	1.426(0.766–2.654)	2.418(1.010–5.787)	0.038(+)

[a] KDRI group was classified based on the estimated iodine intake; [b] Standard error; [c] EAR: Estimated average requirement; [d] *p* for trend was calculated by surveylogistic procedure of SAS; [e] Reference; [f] Odds ratio (95% CI, confidence interval); Model 1: Unadjusted model; Model 2: Adjusted for age and energy intake; Model 3: Adjusted for age, energy intake, weight status, exercise status, smoking status, and alcohol consumption; Model 4: Adjusted for age, energy intake, weight status, exercise status, smoking status, alcohol consumption, breakfast, and frequency of eating out; Model 5: Adjusted for age, energy intake, weight status, exercise status, smoking status, alcohol consumption, breakfast, frequency of eating out, education level, region of residence, household income level, and occupation.

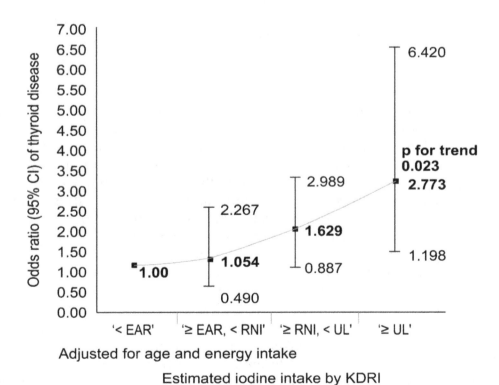

Figure 6. The odds ratio for thyroid disease by the estimated iodine intake in female.

4. Discussion

In this study, we investigated the relationship between iodine intake status and thyroid disease-related functions, and we found that as the estimated iodine intake increased, TSH increased and the risk of thyroid disease also increased. In Korea, iodine-replete areas generally have a high risk of thyroid disease and autoimmune thyroid disease tends to develop into hypothyroidism. Excessive iodine intake is considered to be an important factor in thyroid disease; however, the mechanism or cause is uncertain at present.

Currently, the iodine nutrition status is measured by dietary iodine intake or UIC. The dietary iodine intake is calculated by the iodine content of the food ingredient composition and measured using the 24 h dietary recall method, food record, and food frequency questionnaire. However, the 24 h dietary recall and food record methods do not accurately reflect the amount of iodine in soup stocks such as salt and kelp. In addition, the iodine content of the food composition varies greatly depending on the production area and production period. Also, the amount of iodine in the food is so low [3], and the dietary intake of iodine-rich foods also varies widely among individuals. Hence, it is very difficult to measure the amount of iodine in food and to obtain individual iodine intakes for meals [29,30].

Furthermore, iodine is mainly supplied by meals or drugs. The intake level is highly influenced by the environment, and iodine—which is a micronutrient—is present in a small amount in most foods and is concentrated in specific foods. It is difficult to accurately measure the iodine status [31,32]. Despite these limitations, the 24 h recall method is still valid for measuring dietary iodine intake in individuals. Hence, the UIC method is used more than the dietary iodine intake [8].

One of the most commonly used methods for measuring iodine nutrition status is the UIC as an epidemiologic criteria for the status of the population in the WHO [33]. Since, after metabolization in the body, more than 90% of iodine is excreted in the urine, UIC can estimate the recent intake of iodine by urinary iodine excretion amount and is used as a biomarker to determine the iodine status at the population level, which is a valuable and useful index [34,35]. However, UIC is inappropriate for evaluating the prevalence of iodine deficiency or excessive intake [16]. Therefore, in this study, we calculated and used the estimated iodine intake based on UIC.

Kim et al. [36] showed that 27 patients with Grave's disease showed higher urinary iodine excretion than the normal group, and in a similar article [37], urinary iodine excretion was higher in patients with simple goiter ($n = 17$; 2.88 mg/L), hyperthyroidism ($n = 42$; 4.90 mg/L), hypothyroidism ($n = 15$; 4.57 mg/L), and thyroid cancer ($n = 11$; 6.18 mg/L) than in the normal group (2.11 mg/L). Additionally, in our study, the mean UIC based on prevalence was higher in the thyroid disease group than in the non-thyroid disease group, and the estimated iodine intake showed the same result, although the difference was not significant. These results indicate that UIC concentration is higher in the thyroid disease (such as goiter, hypothyroidism, and hyperthyroidism) group than in the disease-free group.

In this study, the correlation between UIC and dietary iodine intake showed a significant correlation with the total subject ($r = 0.014$, $p < 0.001$) and also in the female group ($r = 0.089$, $p < 0.001$), but, as mentioned, the male group showed the opposite result ($r = -0.005$, $p < 0.001$). Also, in another study [38], UIC was associated with dietary iodine intake ($r = 0.60$, $p < 0.01$), and as iodine intake increased, the UIC gradually increased, which indicates a positive correlation between iodine intake and UIC. Additionally, the correlation between the estimated iodine intake and dietary iodine intake also showed a significant correlation with the total subjects ($r = 0.021$, $p < 0.001$) and also in the female group ($r = 0.095$, $p < 0.001$), but the male group showed the opposite result ($r = -0.001$, $p < 0.001$). Comparing the dietary iodine intake and UIC between these groups and understanding the differences will enable us to determine the iodine nutrition status of the population more accurately.

In this study, the estimated iodine intake, which was calculated from UIC and dietary iodine intake, was divided into KDRI intervals to determine the risk of thyroid disease. These results show that the intake of iodine in Korea is higher than that in other countries, but there were more subjects who consume <95 ug (<EAR) and ≥2400 ug (UL) (Figure 2). Most subjects consumed >150 µg and

<2400 μg, and 2.6% of them consume >2400 μg (dietary iodine intake) and 6.2% (estimated iodine intake) of iodine.

Furthermore, many other studies have shown that the median and upper limit of TSH increases with age [39–41]. In NHANES III, a higher TSH concentration was found to be associated with a higher UI/Cr excretion [42]. Additionally, TSH and FT4 levels were compared based on the presence of the disease. Moreover, similar results were found in the reference population: TSH levels were lower than that of the disease-free population. Therefore, a more in-depth study is required to clarify the link between TSH and iodine status; however, it has been confirmed that the excessive intake of iodine may be correlated with TSH.

In this study, the relationship between the estimated iodine intake, which was divided into KDRI intervals, and thyroid disease incidence was evaluated using the logistic regression analysis. It was found that the incidence of thyroid disease increased with increasing iodine intake. The correlation between the risk of thyroid disease according to the estimated iodine intake and the correlation between UIC and dietary iodine intake were significant only in the female group, but not in males.

These results support that the degree of response to iodine intake is higher due to the role of estrogen in women than in men, but more research is required on the concentration of estradiol and other cofactors [43–47].

One advantage of the study is that KNHANES VI (2013–2015) introduced TSH, FT4, TPOAb, and thyroid disease-related items, making it possible to observe the correlation of the iodine nutrition status with TSH and FT4 levels and to evaluate the effects of excessive iodine intake on thyroid disease. Additionally, the study cohort provided the most recently released nationally representative data of the Korean population.

However, there are some limitations to this study. First, KNHANES is a cross-sectional database; therefore, it cannot demonstrate the relationship between iodine intake and TSH or FT4 levels and thyroid disease, and it does not prove causality. Second, even though we have constructed a new iodine database for commercial foods in Korea, there is a limitation in the accurate determination of iodine intake by the food intake method. Finally, we did not consider various thyroid diseases.

The present study had limitations and further research is necessary to identify the factors contributing to the findings and to build accurate dietary sources. Despite these limitations and despite the need for further studies to identify the mechanisms involved in these findings and to build accurate dietary sources, this study provided important information. The study demonstrated the relationship between dietary iodine intake, UIC, and TSH along with a higher risk of thyroid disease-related hormone levels in groups with estimated iodine intake by over the UL (≥2400 μg/day).

Author Contributions: Conceptualization, Y.K.P., and J.Y.K.; Study design Y.K.P., and S.K. methodology, Y.S.K., and S.K.; formal analysis, Y.S.K., K.H.H., and S.K.; investigation, Y.S.K., and S.K.; writing –original draft preparation, S.K.; writing –review and editing, S.K., and Y.K.P.; validation, J.Y.K., and K.H.H.; visualization, S.K.; supervision, Y.K.P.

References

1.   Korean Food & Drug Administration. *Report on the Intake of Sugar, Sodium, and the Rest of Korean*; Korean Food & Drug Administration: Cheongju, Korea, 2007.

2.   Han, M.R.; Ju, D.L.; Park, Y.J.; Paik, H.Y.; Song, Y. An iodine database for common Korean foods and the association between iodine intake and thyroid disease in Korean adults. *Int. J. Thyroidol.* **2015**, *8*, 170–182. [CrossRef]

3.   Ko, Y.M.; Kwon, Y.S.; Park, Y.K. An iodine database establishment and iodine intake in Korean adults: Based on the 1998~2014 Korea National Health and Nutrition Examination Survey. *J. Nutr. Health* **2017**, *50*, 624–644. [CrossRef]

4. The Korean Nutrition Society. *Dietary Reference Intakes for Koreans*; The Korean Nutrition Society: Seoul, Korea, 2010.

5. Choi, J.; Kim, H.S.; Hong, D.J.; Lim, H.; Kim, J.H. Urinary iodine and sodium status of urban Korean subjects: A pilot study. *Clin. Biochem.* **2012**, *45*, 596–598. [CrossRef] [PubMed]

6. Institute of Medicine. *Dietary Reference Intakes for Vitamin A, Vitamin K, Arsenic, Boron, Chromium, Copper, Iodine, Iron, Molybdenum, Nickel, Silicon, Vanadium and Zinc. Food and Nutrition Board*; National Academy Press: Washington, DC, USA, 2001.

7. Hwang, S.; Lee, E.Y.; Lee, W.K.; Shin, D.Y.; Lee, E.J. Correlation between iodine intake and thyroid function in subjects with normal thyroid function. *Biol. Trace Elem. Res.* **2011**, *143*, 1393–1397. [CrossRef]

8. Lee, H.S.; Min, H. Iodine intake and tolerable upper intake level of iodine for Koreans. *Korean J. Nutr.* **2011**, *44*, 82–91. [CrossRef]

9. Laurberg, P.; Cerqueira, C.; Ovesen, L.; Rasmussen, L.B.; Perrild, H.; Andersen, S.; Pedersen, I.B.; Carlé, A. Iodine intake as a determinant of thyroid disorders in populations. *Best Pract. Res. Clin. Endocrinol. Metab.* **2010**, *24*, 13–27. [CrossRef]

10. Braverman, L.E. Iodine and the thyroid: 33 years of study. *Thyroid* **1994**, *4*, 351–356. [CrossRef]

11. Roti, E.; Uberti, E.D. Iodine excess and hyperthyroidism. *Thyroid* **2001**, *11*, 493–500. [CrossRef]

12. Laurberg, P.; Bulow Pedersen, I.; Knudsen, N.; Ovesen, L.; Andersen, S. Environmental iodine intake affects the type of nonmalignant thyroid disease. *Thyroid* **2001**, *11*, 457–469. [CrossRef]

13. Burgi, H. Iodine excess. *Best Pract. Res. Clin. Endocrinol. Metab.* **2010**, *24*, 107–115. [CrossRef]

14. Clark, O.H. Excess iodine intake and thyroid function and growth. *Thyroid* **1990**, *1*, 69–72. [CrossRef] [PubMed]

15. Sun, X.; Shan, Z.; Teng, W. Effects of increased iodine intake on thyroid disorders. *Endocrinol. Metab.* **2014**, *29*, 240–247. [CrossRef] [PubMed]

16. Zimmermann, M.B.; Andersson, M. Assessment of iodine nutrition in populations: Past, present, and future. *Nutr. Rev.* **2012**, *70*, 553–570. [CrossRef] [PubMed]

17. Zimmermann, M. Iodine deficiency and excess in children: Worldwide status in 2013. *Endocr. Pract.* **2013**, *19*, 839–846. [CrossRef] [PubMed]

18. Ross, D.S.; Burch, H.B.; Cooper, D.S.; Greenlee, M.C.; Laurberg, P.; Maia, A.L.; Rivkees, S.A.; Samuels, M.; Sosa, J.A.; Stan, M.N.; et al. 2016 American Thyroid Association Guidelines for Diagnosis and Management of Hyperthyroidism and Other Causes of Thyrotoxicosis. *Thyroid* **2016**, *26*, 1343–1421. [CrossRef] [PubMed]

19. Sheehan, M.T. Biochemical testing of the thyroid: TSH is the best and, oftentimes, only test needed—A review for primary care. *Clin. Med. Res.* **2016**, *14*, 83–92. [CrossRef] [PubMed]

20. Chaker, L.; Korevaar, T.I.; Medici, M.; Uiterlinden, A.G.; Hofman, A.; Dehghan, A.; Franco, O.H.; Peeters, R.P. Thyroid function characteristics and determinants: The Rotterdam study. *Thyroid* **2016**, *26*, 1195–1204. [CrossRef]

21. Ministry of Health and Welfare, Korea Centers for Disease Control and Prevention. Korea National Health and Nutrition Examination Survey (KNHANES VI). 2016. Available online: https://knhanes.cdc.go.kr/knhanes/main.do2016.

22. Kim, W.G.; Kim, W.B.; Woo, G.; Kim, H.; Cho, Y.; Kim, T.Y.; Kim, S.W.; Shin, M.-H.; Park, J.W.; Park, H.-L.; et al. Thyroid stimulating hormone reference range and prevalence of thyroid dysfunction in the Korean population: Korea National Health and Nutrition Examination Survey 2013 to 2015. *Endocrinol. Metab.* **2017**, *32*, 106–114. [CrossRef]

23. Leung, A.M.; Braverman, L.E. Consequences of excess iodine. *Nat. Rev. Endocrinol.* **2014**, *10*, 136. [CrossRef]

24. Kim, H.I.; Oh, H.K.; Park, S.Y.; Jang, H.W.; Shin, M.H.; Kim, S.W.; Kim, T.H.; Chung, J.H. Urinary iodine concentration and thyroid hormones: Korea National Health and Nutrition Examination Survey 2013–2015. *Eur. J. Nutr.* **2019**, *58*, 233–240. [CrossRef]

25. The Korean Nutrition Society. *Food Values*; The Korean Nutrition Society: Seoul, Korea, 2009.

26. National Rural Resources Development Institute. *Administration RD 9th Revision*; Rural Development Administration: Jeonju, Korea, 2018.

27. Ministry of Education, Culture, Sports, Science and Technology. *Japan Standard Tables of Food Composition in Japan*; Seventh Revised Version; Ministry of Education, Culture, Sports, Science and Technology: Tokyo, Japan, 2015.

28. Kweon, S.; Kim, Y.; Jang, M.J.; Kim, Y.; Kim, K.; Choi, S.; Chun, C.; Khang, Y.H.; Oh, K. Data resource profile: The Korea National Health and Nutrition Examination Survey (KNHANES). *Int. J. Epidemiol.* **2014**, *43*, 69–77. [CrossRef] [PubMed]

29. Freedman, L.S.; Commins, J.M.; Moler, J.E.; Willett, W.; Tinker, L.F.; Subar, A.F.; Spiegelman, D.; Rhodes, D.; Potischman, N.; Neuhouser, M.L. Pooled results from 5 validation studies of dietary self-report instruments using recovery biomarkers for potassium and sodium intake. *Am. J. Epidemiol.* **2015**, *181*, 473–487. [CrossRef] [PubMed]

30. McLean, R.M. Measuring population sodium intake: A review of methods. *Nutrients* **2014**, *6*, 4651–4662. [CrossRef] [PubMed]

31. Woeber, K.A. Iodine and thyroid disease. *Med. Clin. N. Am.* **1991**, *75*, 169–178. [CrossRef]

32. Winichagoon, P.; Svasti, S.; Munkongdee, T.; Chaiya, W.; Boonmongkol, P.; Chantrakul, N.; Fucharoen, S. Rapid diagnosis of thalassemias and other hemoglobinopathies by capillary electrophoresis system. *Transl. Res.* **2008**, *152*, 178–184. [CrossRef]

33. World Health Organization. *Urinary Iodine Concentrations for Determining Iodine Status in Populations*; World Health Organization: Geneva, Switzerland, 2013.

34. Nath, S.; Moinier, B.; Thuillier, F.; Rongier, M.; Desjeux, J. Urinary excretion of iodide and fluoride from supplemented food grade salt. *Int. J. Vitam. Nutr. Res.* **1992**, *62*, 66–72.

35. Jolin, T.; Escobar, D.R. Evaluation of iodine/creatinine ratios of casual samples as indices of daily urinary iodine output during field studies. *J. Clin. Endocrinol. Metab.* **1965**, *25*, 540–542. [CrossRef]

36. Kim, H.; Lee, H.; Park, K.; Joo, H.; Kim, K.; Hong, C.; Huh, K.; Lee, S.; Ryu, K. A study on the urinary iodide excretion in normal subjects and patients with thyroid disease. *Korean J. Intern. Med.* **1985**, *29*, 625–631.

37. Kim, J.Y.; Kim, K.R. Dietary iodine intake and urinary iodine excretion in patients with thyroid diseases. *Yonsei Med. J.* **2000**, *41*, 22–28. [CrossRef]

38. Kim, J.Y.; Moon, S.J.; Kim, K.R.; Sohn, C.Y.; Oh, J.J. Dietary iodine intake and urinary iodine excretion in normal Korean adults. *Yonsei Med. J.* **1998**, *39*, 355–362. [CrossRef]

39. Haymart, M.R.; Glinberg, S.L.; Liu, J.; Sippel, R.S.; Jaume, J.C.; Chen, H. Higher serum TSH in thyroid cancer patients occurs independent of age and correlates with extrathyroidal extension. *Clin. Endocrinol.* **2009**, *71*, 434–439. [CrossRef]

40. Hadlow, N.C.; Rothacker, K.M.; Wardrop, R.; Brown, S.J.; Lim, E.M.; Walsh, J.P. The relationship between TSH and free T4 in a large population is complex and monlinear and differs by age and sex. *J. Clin. Endocrinol. Metab.* **2013**, *98*, 2936–2943. [CrossRef] [PubMed]

41. Lee, Y.K.; Kim, J.E.; Oh, H.J.; Park, K.S.; Kim, S.K.; Park, S.W.; Kim, M.J.; Cho, Y.W. Serum TSH level in healthy Koreans and the association of TSH with serum lipid concentration and metabolic syndrome. *Korean J. Intern. Med.* **2011**, *26*, 432–439. [CrossRef] [PubMed]

42. Hollowell, J.G.; Staehling, N.W.; Flanders, W.D.; Hannon, W.H.; Gunter, E.W.; Spencer, C.A.; Braverman, L.E. Serum TSH, T4, and thyroid antibodies in the United States population (1988 to 1994): National Health and Nutrition Examination Survey (NHANES III). *J. Clin. Endocrinol. Metab.* **2002**, *87*, 489–499. [CrossRef]

43. Ishii, K.; Hayashi, A.; Tamaoka, A.; Mizusawa, H.; Shoji, S. A case of Hashimoto's encephalopathy with a relapsing course related to menstrual cycle. *Clin. Neurol.* **1993**, *33*, 995–997.

44. Leo, V.D.; D'Antona, D.; Lanzetta, D. Thyrotropin secretion before and after ovariectomy in premenopausal women. *Gynecol. Endocrinol.* **1993**, *7*, 279–283. [CrossRef]

45. Fujimoto, N.; Watanabe, H.; Ito, A. Blockade of the estrogen induced increase in progesterone receptor caused by propylthiouracil, an anti-thyroid drug, in a transplantable pituitary tumor in rats. *Endocr. J.* **1996**, *43*, 329–334. [CrossRef]

46. Ogard, C.G.; Ogard, C.; Almdal, T.P. Thyroid-associated orbitopathy developed during hormone replacement therapy. *Acta Ophthalmol. Scand.* **2001**, *79*, 426–427. [CrossRef]

47. Abalovich, M.; Gutierrez, S.; Alcaraz, G.; Maccallini, G.; Garcia, A.; Levalle, O. Overt and subclinical hypothyroidism complicating pregnancy. *Thyroid* **2002**, *12*, 63–68. [CrossRef]

Protective Effects of Myo-Inositol and Selenium on Cadmium-Induced Thyroid Toxicity in Mice

Salvatore Benvenga [1,†], Herbert R. Marini [1,†], Antonio Micali [2,*], Jose Freni [2], Giovanni Pallio [1], Natasha Irrera [1], Francesco Squadrito [1], Domenica Altavilla [2], Alessandro Antonelli [3], Silvia Martina Ferrari [3], Poupak Fallahi [3], Domenico Puzzolo [2] and Letteria Minutoli [1]

[1] Department of Clinical and Experimental Medicine, University of Messina, 98125 Messina, Italy; s.benvenga@live.it (S.B.); hrmarini@unime.it (H.R.M.); gpallio@unime.it (G.P.); nirrera@unime.it (N.I.); fsquadrito@unime.it (F.S.); lminutoli@unime.it (L.M.)

[2] Department of Biomedical and Dental Sciences and Morphofunctional Imaging, University of Messina, 98125 Messina, Italy; freni.jose@gmail.com (J.F.); daltavilla@unime.it (D.A.); puzzolo@unime.it (D.P.)

[3] Department of Clinical and Experimental Medicine, University of Pisa, 56126 Pisa, Italy; alessandro.antonelli@med.unipi.it (A.A.); sm.ferrari@int.med.unipi.it (S.M.F.); poupak.fallahi@unipi.it (P.F.)

* Correspondence: amicali@unime.it

† Both authors equally contributed.

Abstract: Cadmium (Cd) damages the thyroid gland. We evaluated the effects of myo-inositol (MI), seleno-L-methionine (Se) or their combination on the thyroids of mice simultaneously administered with Cd chloride ($CdCl_2$). Eighty-four male mice were divided into 12 groups (seven mice each). Six groups (controls) were treated with 0.9% NaCl (vehicle), Se (0.2 mg/kg/day), Se (0.4 mg/kg/day), MI (360 mg/kg/day), MI+Se (0.2 mg/kg) and MI+Se (0.4 mg/kg). The other six groups were treated with $CdCl_2$ (2 mg/kg), $CdCl_2$+MI, $CdCl_2$+Se (0.2 mg/kg), $CdCl_2$+Se (0.4 mg/kg), $CdCl_2$+MI+Se (0.2 mg/kg) and $CdCl_2$+MI+Se (0.4 mg/kg). An additional group of $CdCl_2$-challenged animals (n = 7) was treated with resveratrol (20 mg/kg), an effective and potent antioxidant. All treatments lasted 14 days. After sacrifice, the thyroids were evaluated histologically and immunohistochemically. $CdCl_2$ reduced the follicular area, increased the epithelial height, stroma, and cells expressing monocyte chemoattractant protein-1 (MCP-1) and C-X-C motif chemokine 10 (CXCL10). $CdCl_2$+Se at 0.2/0.4 mg/kg insignificantly reversed the follicular and stromal structure, and significantly decreased the number of MCP-1 and CXCL10-positive cells. $CdCl_2$+MI significantly reversed the thyroid structure and further decreased the number of MCP-1 and CXCL10-positive cells. $CdCl_2$+MI+Se, at both doses, brought all indices to those of $CdCl_2$-untreated mice. MI, particularly in association with Se, defends mice from Cd-induced damage. The efficacy of this combination was greater than that of resveratrol, at least when using the follicular structure as a read-out for a comparison. We suggest that the use of these nutraceuticals, more specifically the combination of MI plus SE, can protect the thyroid of Cd-exposed subjects.

Keywords: cadmium; nutraceuticals; myo-inositol; seleno-L-methionine; thyroid; MCP-1; CXCL10

1. Introduction

Thyroid disorders, including hypothyroidism, with its leading etiology (Hashimoto's thyroiditis) and cancer arising from the follicular epithelium, are very common diseases [1,2]. Indeed, with a prevalence of 10%–12% in the general population, Hashimoto's thyroiditis is the most common autoimmune disease [1]. The prevalence of thyroid cancer has increased considerably in recent decades.

Thyroid cancer incidence was relatively stable until the 1990s, when it began to increase dramatically. Overall, thyroid cancer incidence increased from 4.9 per 100,000 population to 14.7 per

100,000 population in 2011 [2]. Dysfunction, autoimmunity and cancer of the thyroid are triggered by environmental factors, including pollutants such as organochlorine compounds, polychlorinated biphenyls, polybrominated diphenylethers, bisphenol A, triclosan, perchlorates, thiocyanates, nitrates and heavy metals [3–8].

One such heavy metal is cadmium (Cd). Cd is found in food, cigarette smoke, mines, phosphate fertilizers and nickel–cadmium batteries [9]. Cd enters the body through the gastrointestinal tract and the alveolar epithelium [9] and passes through the systemic circulation, bound to albumin. Cd is then transported to the liver, where it is released and induces the synthesis of metallothionein (MT), a stress protein first discovered in 1957 in horse kidneys [10], which protects against Cd toxicity and oxidative stress [11]. The complex MT–Cd accumulates in the liver, kidneys, skeletal muscles and thyroid. With a biological half-life of 5 to 30 years, exposure over time to even environmentally low levels of Cd is associated with several toxic effects on the liver, kidneys, bones, testes and the cardiovascular system [12–15]. Persons living in Cd-polluted areas have an intrathyroid concentration of Cd that is threefold greater than control persons [16]. Finally, Cd has been classified as a group 1 human carcinogen, with evidence existing of its association with lung, prostate and kidney cancers [17], and a possible association with other malignancies, such as breast [18], pancreas [19], and urinary bladder cancer [20]. Concerning thyroid cancer, a recent study on 66 patients with papillary thyroid cancer (PTC) showed that the content of selenium (Se) was significantly decreased (66 vs. 132 ng/g), while the content of Cd (58 vs. 33 ng/g) and the resulting Cd/Se ratio (0.055 vs. 0.018) were significantly higher in the cancerous tissue compared to the healthy, noncancerous thyroid tissue [21]. Furthermore, Cd and the Cd/Se ratio were associated with the retrosternal thyroid growth of PTC [21].

Cd increases serum thyrotropin (TSH) concentration in rats [22,23] and humans [24]. After chronic exposure to Cd, the presence of desquamated cells in the follicles, mononuclear cell infiltration in the connective tissue and follicles lined by higher cells with light cytoplasm were observed [25]. In a similar manner to mercury (Hg), the interaction of Cd with Se, which is relatively abundant in the thyroid [26], as the inorganic component of the deiodinases [27–29], results in formation of insoluble complexes [27,28,30]. The consequence of such sequestration of Se is the impairment of selenoprotein synthesis and activities [28]. In over 5000 Chinese adults, blood levels of both Cd and lead (Pb) were directly correlated with both thyroid hypofunction and serum thyroid autoantibody levels [31], even if the risk of hypothyroidism increased incrementally with blood cadmium in men, but not in women [32]. In the study on 5628 Chinese adults, women showed a positive correlation between log (ln)-transformed blood concentrations of Cd and log (ln)-transformed blood concentrations of thyroglobulin autoantibodies (TgAb) [31]. In the adjusted logistic regression models, the log (ln)-transformed blood concentrations of Cd of women were positively related to their TgAb tertiles and hypothyroid status [31]. Cd exposure also causes increased susceptibility to testicular autoimmunity [33]. Indeed, the role of Cd in autoimmunity is supported by studies on 24 individuals, in whom the authors measured the blood levels of three heavy metals (Cd, Hg and Pb) and blood mRNA expression of 98 genes that are implicated in stress, toxicity, inflammation, and autoimmunity [34].

Among the different mechanisms involved in Cd-induced thyroid damage (genome influence, apoptosis, mitochondrial dysfunction, oxidative stress), the the last mechanism seems to play a relevant role [24]. Indeed, the said depletion of Se stores leads to its decreased availability to form glutathione (GSH) peroxidase, which is one of the main natural antioxidants [35]. Se supplementation exerts some beneficial effects on the thyroid of Cd-exposed rats. Histopathological analysis of the thyroid of young rats whose mothers received Cd during pregnancy demonstrated the presence of microfollicles lined by a single layer of columnar epithelium; Cd administration resulted in a sharp decrease in the height of epithelial cells [36]. Furthermore, treatment of Cd-exposed rats with Se partially attenuated the Cd-induced decrease in serum T4 levels [22].

Beneficial effects against Cd-induced damage of the thyroid or other organs were also described for other naturally occurring molecules that, like Se, are used as nutraceuticals. These molecules are quercetin [37] and myo-inositol (MI) [38–40]. Quercetin significantly increased serum thyroid hormones in rats treated with CdCl2, even if levels were significantly lower compared to unchallenged rats [37]. In mice, a 14-day treatment with $CdCl_2$ (2 mg/kg/day) plus MI (360 mg/kg/day) protected the testis [39] and the kidney [40] from the damage induced by $CdCl_2$. The Cd-induced testicular damage consisted of smaller tubules, the discontinuity of the seminiferous epithelium, the detachment of spermatogonia from the basal membrane, and reduced claudin-11 immunoreactivity [39]. The Cd-induced renal damage consisted of alterations in glomerular and tubular morphology [40]. Concerning the testis, experiments were also conducted with Se alone and with a combination MI plus Se-L-methionine [39], with such a combination having the greatest protective effects on the seminiferous tubules, and in particular on the blood–testis barrier.

Aside from the Cd setting, the beneficial effects of MI have been shown in human sperm [41,42] and oocytes [43]. The antioxidant properties of MI are demonstrated by the MI-induced increase in the intracellular levels of GSH, superoxide dismutase (SOD) and catalase (CAT) [44]. Starting from the knowledge that chemokines are mechanistically involved in the initiation and maintenance of Hashimoto's thyroiditis [45,46], it was shown that MI and, to a greater extent, the combination of MI plus Se-L-methionine, decreased serum levels and lymphocyte secretion of the investigated chemokines [47,48]. These chemokines were chemokine (C-C motif) ligand 2 (CCL2; also known as monocyte chemoattractant protein-1 (MCP-1)), C-X-C motif chemokine 9 (CXCL9; also known as monokine induced by gamma interferon (MIG)), and C-X-C motif chemokine 10 (CXCL10). Such effects on chemokines explain the benefits of the combination of MI plus Se-L-methionine in patients with Hashimoto's thyroiditis, in terms of decreased oxidative stress [38], decreased serum levels of thyroid autoantibodies and an improved hormone profile [47–49].

Based on this background, considering (i) that no morphometric analysis has been conducted in previous studies on protection from Cd-induced thyroid damage [24,36,50], (ii) the lack of data regarding the effects of MI alone and the association of MI plus Se with Cd-induced thyroid damage, and (iii) that MI, Se and other natural compounds are being increasingly used as nutraceuticals in clinical practice [38], we aimed to demonstrate their protective role in the structure of thyroid glands in mice exposed to Cd. We also wished to test whether Cd induced the expression of two aforementioned chemokines (MCP-1/CCL2 and CXCL10) and, if so, to test whether this expression could be counteracted by MI, Se or their combination.

2. Materials and Methods

2.1. Experimental Protocol

All procedures adhered to the standards for care and use of animals as per guidelines issued by Animal Research Reporting in Vivo Experiments (ARRIVE); the procedures were evaluated and approved by the Italian Health Ministry (project identification code: 112/2017-PR). Eighty-four male C57 BL/6J mice (25–30 g) were obtained from Charles River Laboratories Italia Srl (Calco, LC, Italy) and stored at the animal house faculty of our university hospital. A standard diet was provided ad libitum and the animals had free access to water; they were kept on a 12-h light/dark cycle. The animals were randomly distributed into twelve groups of seven mice each. Six groups (viz. 42 mice) were considered as controls (0.9% NaCl (vehicle, 1 mL/kg), seleno-L-methionine (Se) (0.2 mg/kg), Se (0.4 mg/kg), MI (360 mg/kg), MI (360 mg/kg) plus Se (0.2 mg/kg), MI (360 mg/kg) plus Se (0.4 mg/kg)). The other six groups were challenged with $CdCl_2$ (2 mg/kg) plus a vehicle, $CdCl_2$ (2 mg/kg) plus MI (360 mg/kg), $CdCl_2$ (2 mg/kg) plus Se (0.2 mg/kg), $CdCl_2$ (2 mg/kg) plus Se (0.4 mg/kg), $CdCl_2$ (2 mg/kg) plus MI (360 mg/kg) plus Se (0.2 mg/kg) and $CdCl_2$ (2 mg/kg) plus MI (360 mg/kg) plus Se (0.4 mg/kg). An additional group of $CdCl_2$-challenged animals ($n = 7$) were given 20 mg/kg of resveratrol [51,52], a biologically active compound with potent antioxidant properties [53]. $CdCl_2$ and NaCl were administered intraperitoneally (i.p.), while MI, Se and resveratrol per os. MI was ready for use, while $CdCl_2$ and Se were diluted in 0.9% NaCl before use. After 14 days of treatment, mice were sacrificed with an overdose of ketamine and xylazine, and their thyroids were collected and processed for histological and immunohistochemical procedures.

2.2. Histological Evaluation

The thyroid glands were fixed in 4% paraformaldehyde in 0.2 M phosphate buffer saline (PBS), dehydrated in ethanol, cleared in xylene and embedded in Paraplast (SPI Supplies, West Chester, PA, USA). Blocks were cut in a microtome (RM2125 RT, Leica Instruments, Nussloch, Germany), and 5 μm sections were cleared with xylene, rehydrated in ethanol and stained with hematoxylin and eosin (HE) and Sirius red (SR). All samples were observed with a Nikon Ci-L (Nikon Instruments, Tokyo, Japan) light microscope and the micrographs were obtained using a digital camera (Nikon Ds-Ri2) and saved as Tagged Image Format Files (TIFF) with the Adobe Photoshop CS5 12.1 software.

2.3. Immunohistochemistry for Monocyte Chemoattractant Protein-1 (MCP-1) and C-X-C Motif Chemokine 10 (CXCL10)

The same specimens used for histological evaluation were cut at 5 μm and the sections were placed on polysine slides (Thermo Fisher Scientific, Waltham, MA, USA), cleared with xylene and rehydrated in ethanol. Antigen retrieval was obtained in buffer citrate pH 6.0; endogenous peroxidase was blocked with 0.3% H_2O_2 in PBS. Incubation with primary antibodies (MCP-1, 1:150, Santa Cruz, Dallas, TX, USA; CXCL10, 1:100, Biorbyt, Cambridge, UK) was performed overnight at 4 °C in a moisturized chamber; then, secondary antibodies (anti-mouse and anti-rabbit, Vectastain, Vector, Burlingame, CA, USA) were added, and the reaction was evidenced with 3,3'-diaminobenzidine (DAB) (Sigma-Aldrich, Milan, Italy). Slides were counterstained in Mayer's hematoxylin. For each test, specific positive and negative controls were prepared. Micrographs were taken with a Nikon Ci-L (Nikon Instruments, Tokyo, Japan) light microscope using a digital camera (Nikon Ds-Ri2).

2.4. Morphometric and Immunohistochemical Evaluation

All micrographs were printed at the same final magnification (800×) and were blindly assessed by two trained observers, without knowledge of the previous treatment. Five microscopic fields (MFs), all including two entire thyroid follicles from ten non-serial sections stained with the HE of each group were considered.

As for the follicular compartment, a Peak Scale Loupe 7× (GWJ Company, Hacienda Heights, CA, USA) micrometer was used as a scale calibration standard to estimate the follicular diameters. The area (A) of each follicle was calculated by measuring the smaller inner diameter (d) and the larger inner diameter (D) of the follicle, both expressed in micrometers (μm). The estimated area of the follicular lumen was obtained by the following formula:

$$A = \pi . (d/2. D/2). \tag{1}$$

In each thyroid gland, we measured the area of 20 follicles. To calculate the epithelial height, a straight line perpendicular to the epithelium was traced and measured, and the results were expressed in micrometers.

For the evaluation of the stroma, a quantitative study of micrographs from 20 microscopic fields of Sirius Red (SR)-stained not-serial sections for each group was performed with the Adobe Photoshop CS5 12.1 software, acquiring the pink/red color of collagen fibers. Positive areas were automatically calculated based on their pixel number. Values were indicated as the pixel number of the positively stained area/unit area (UA). The area of the entire micrograph was evaluated as the UA.

For an assessment of the immunoreactivity of MCP-1/CCL2 and CXCL10, positive cells were counted from 10 non-serial sections of the thyroid, selecting two unit areas (UA) of 0.1 mm^2 (316 × 316 μm). Cells overlapping the right and top borders of the areas were not counted, while the cells overlapping the left and the bottom borders were considered.

2.5. Drugs and Chemicals

CdCl$_2$, Se and resveratrol were bought from Sigma-Aldrich Srl (Milan, Italy). LO.LI. Pharma Srl (Rome, Italy) kindly provided MI. All chemicals not otherwise mentioned were commercially available reagent grade quality.

2.6. Statistical Analysis

Values are expressed as the mean ± standard error (SE). The statistical significance of differences between group mean values was established using Student's t-test. The statistical evaluation of differences among groups was obtained with ANOVA. The statistical analysis of histological scores was done using the Mann–Whitney U test with Bonferroni correction. A p value of ≤ 0.05 was considered statistically significant.

3. Results

3.1. Histopathological Data

3.1.1. Follicular Epithelium

Images are presented in Figure 1A–G, with the quantification of the follicular area and the height of the follicular epithelium (thyrocytes) summarized in Figure 1H–I.

All control animals had thyroids with normal morphologies (results not shown). Therefore, for sake of simplicity, we present a single micrograph as representative of controls (Figure 1A). In the thyroid of mice challenged with CdCl$_2$, compared to controls, the follicular area was smaller and thyrocytes were taller but poorly stained (Figure 1B). In the thyroid of mice treated with CdCl$_2$ plus either dose of Se, compared to controls, the follicular area was also dose-dependently significantly smaller and the follicular epithelium was also dose-dependently significantly taller (Figure 1C,D), though the area and height changed to a lesser degree compared to mice treated with CdCl$_2$ alone (compare Figure 1C,D with Figure 1B, and corresponding points in Figure 1H,I). In the thyroid of mice treated with CdCl$_2$ plus MI, compared to controls, the follicular area was also significantly smaller, and the follicular epithelium was significantly taller (Figure 1E), while both the area and height changed to an even lesser degree compared to mice treated with CdCl$_2$ plus either dose of Se (compare Figure 1E with Figure 1B, and corresponding points in Figure 1H,I). In mice treated with CdCl$_2$ plus both MI and Se at either 0.2 or 0.4 mg/kg, the follicular area and epithelial height were no longer statistically different from the controls (Figure 1F,G), but both indices were statistically different from their counterparts in the other treated mice (compare Figure 1F,G with Figure 1B,G, and corresponding points in Figure 1H,I). Furthermore, the effect of the combination of MI plus Se on the follicular area and epithelial height was greater than that brought about by resveratrol, used for its potent antioxidant properties (see Supplemental materials Figure S1).

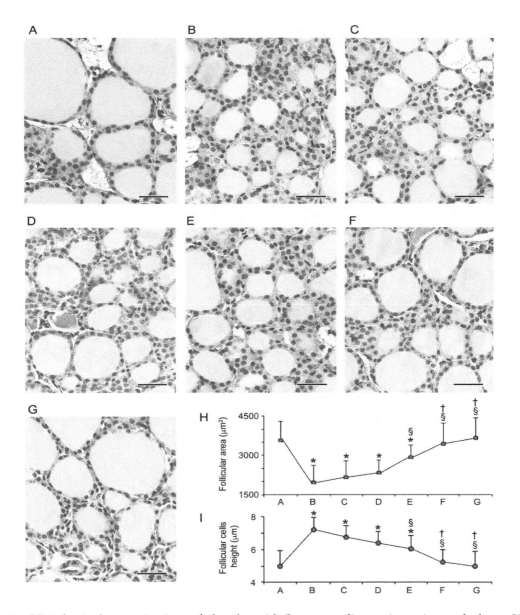

Figure 1. Histological organization of the thyroid (hematoxylin–eosin stain; scale bar: 25 μm). Mice groups (seven mice/group) are: controls (**A**), cadmium chloride ($CdCl_2$) plus vehicle (**B**), $CdCl_2$ plus seleno-L-methionine (Se) 0.2 mg/kg (**C**), $CdCl_2$ plus Se 0.4 mg/kg (**D**), $CdCl_2$ plus myo-inositol (MI) (**E**), $CdCl_2$ plus MI plus Se 0.2 mg/kg (**F**), $CdCl_2$ plus MI plus Se 0.4 mg/kg (**G**). A: Control mice have a normal thyroid structure, as demonstrated also by bar A in H and I. B: $CdCl_2$-treated mice show small follicles and less stainable follicular epithelium (thyrocytes), the height of which is increased, as shown by bar B in (**H,I**). C-D: In mice treated with $CdCl_2$ plus 0.2 mg/Kg Se or $CdCl_2$ plus 0.4 mg/kg Se, small follicles are present with thyrocytes of smaller height, as indicated by bars C and D in H and I. E: In mice treated with $CdCl_2$ plus MI, the follicles and thyrocytes show a tendency to acquire a normal size and height, even though both indices are significantly different from the controls; see also bar E in H and I. F-G: In mice treated with $CdCl_2$ plus MI and 0.2 mg/Kg Se or $CdCl_2$ plus MI and 0.4 mg/kg Se, follicles and epithelial cells were close to normal, as demonstrated by bars F and G in H and I. H: Mean ± standard error values of follicular area in the different groups of mice. I: Mean ± standard error values of epithelial cells height in the different groups of mice. * $p < 0.05$ versus control; § $p < 0.05$ versus $CdCl_2$ plus vehicle and $CdCl_2$ plus 0.2 or 0.4 mg/kg Se; † $p < 0.05$ versus $CdCl_2$ plus MI alone.

3.1.2. Stroma

As indicated in the Materials and Methods, Sirius Red staining allowed us to quantify the thyroid stroma, since stromal areas are positive to such staining. Positive areas were quantified by a software based on their pixel number. Data were expressed as the pixel number of the positively stained area/unit area (UA), considered to be the entire micrograph area. Matching the illustration of data for the epithelium (see above), images are presented in Figure 2A–G, with quantification also summarized in Figure 2H.

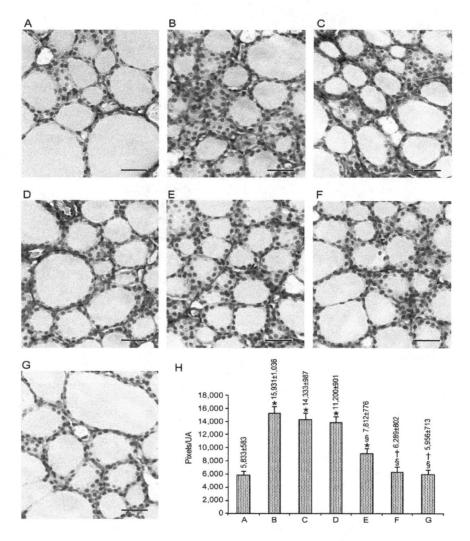

Figure 2. Structural organization of the thyroid stroma based on staining with Sirius Red (scale bar: 25 μm). Mice groups are as in Figure 1. (**A**): Control mice have a normal architecture of interstitial collagen, with well-stained fibrillary elements, as indicated by bar A in H. (**B**): In CdCl$_2$-treated mice, an increased amount of perifollicular connective tissue is present around the follicles, as indicated by bar B in H. (**C,D**): In mice challenged with CdCl$_2$ and 0.2 mg/kg Se or CdCl$_2$ and 0.4 mg/kg Se, stained areas are similar to mice challenged with CdCl$_2$, as shown by bars C and D in H. (**E**): CdCl$_2$ plus MI-treated mice have stained areas with a statistically significant decrease in the pink/red colored collagen fibers, as evident in H, bar E. (**F,G**): In mice treated with CdCl$_2$ plus MI and 0.2 mg/kg Se or CdCl$_2$ plus MI and 0.4 mg/kg Se, a significant reduction in the stained areas can be seen, as also demonstrated by bars F and G in H. (**H**): Mean ± standard error values of pixel numbers of Sirius Red (SR)-stained areas/unit areas (UA) in the different groups of challenged mice. * $p < 0.05$ versus control; § $p < 0.05$ versus CdCl$_2$ plus vehicle and CdCl$_2$ plus 0.2 or 0.4 mg/kg Se; † $p < 0.05$ versus CdCl$_2$ plus MI.

When comparing Figure 2H with Figure 1H,I, it is evident that changes in the stroma were parallel to changes in epithelial height and opposite to changes in follicular area. Compared to the amount of stroma in the seven untreated mice (5912 ± 556 pixels/UA (data not shown)), in the other 42 control mice, the variation was between −5.0% (mice treated with only 0.2 mg/kg Se) AND +2.1% (mice treated with vehicle) (data not shown). Accordingly, the value of 5833 ± 583 (mean ± SE of the 49 control mice; Figure 2A and bar A in Figure 2H) was taken as the reference to evaluate the effects of $CdCl_2$ alone or $CdCl_2$ co-administered with Se, MI, or their association. Exposure to $CdCl_2$ alone increased the amount of perifollicular connective tissue by almost threefold (compare Figure 2A,B, and bars A and B in Figure 2H). The co-administration of $CdCl_2$ and Se decreased—even though the $CdCl_2$-induced an insignificant increase in—thyroid connective tissue (compare Figure 2C,D with Figure 2B, and bars C and D with bar B in Figure 2H). MI co-administration was more effective compared to either dose of Se, since the increase in the amount of stroma was of a smaller magnitude (compare Figure 2E with Figure 2C,D, and bar E with bars C-D in Figure 2H) or approximately 1.5-fold higher when compared to controls (compare Figure 2E with Figure 2A, and bar E with bar A in Figure 2H). The association of MI with either dose of Se in mice that were simultaneously treated with $CdCl_2$ was even more effective, resulting in an amount of stroma superimposable to that of the control mice (compare Figure 2F,G with Figure 2A, and bars F-G with bar A in Figure 2H).

In summary, both the follicular epithelium and the connective tissue respond in a similar fashion to the administration of Se, MI or their combination in $CdCl_2$ co-treated mice. This response consists of a benefit that is modest in the case of Se, moderate in the case of MI, and high (full protection) in the case of MI combined with either dose of Se.

3.2. Immunohistochemical Expression of MCP-1/CCL2

To maintain the modality of illustrating results, images are presented in Figure 3A–G, with quantification also summarized in Figure 3H for MCP-1/CCL2, and in Figure 4A–G, with quantification also summarized in Figure 4H for CXCL10.

In the baseline condition represented by untreated mice, there were no cells at all that expressed MCP-1/CCL2 (data not shown), a pattern that was also true for the vehicle-treated mice and the other groups of control mice, except three groups. These three groups, in which only one cell was stained, were those treated with either concentrations of Se alone and the group treated with 0.4 mg/kg Se plus MI (data not shown). Overall, in the 49 mice from the seven control groups, the number of cells immunostained by the MCP-1/CCL2 averaged 0.35 ± 0.34/UA (Figure 3A, and bar A in Figure 3H). In contrast, $CdCl_2$ plus the vehicle induced a marked expression of MCP-1/CCL2, with a 60-fold increase in the number of thyrocytes immunostained (compare Figure 3B with Figure 3A, and bar B with bar A in Figure 3H). In the mice from the remaining groups, the over-expression induced by $CdCl_2$ was counteracted significantly by all of the tested compounds (Figure 3C–G, and bars C-G in Figure 3H). This antagonism was small with either the dose of Se alone (Figure 3C,D, and bars C-D in Figure 3H), moderate with MI alone (Figure 3E, and bar E in Figure 3H), and great with the dose of Se and MI (Figure 3F–G, and bars F-G in Figure 3H). Indeed, 0.4 mg/kg Se plus MI decreased the number of cells to 0.44 ± 0.39, which is statistically similar to the above 0.35 ± 0.34 for the 49 control mice.

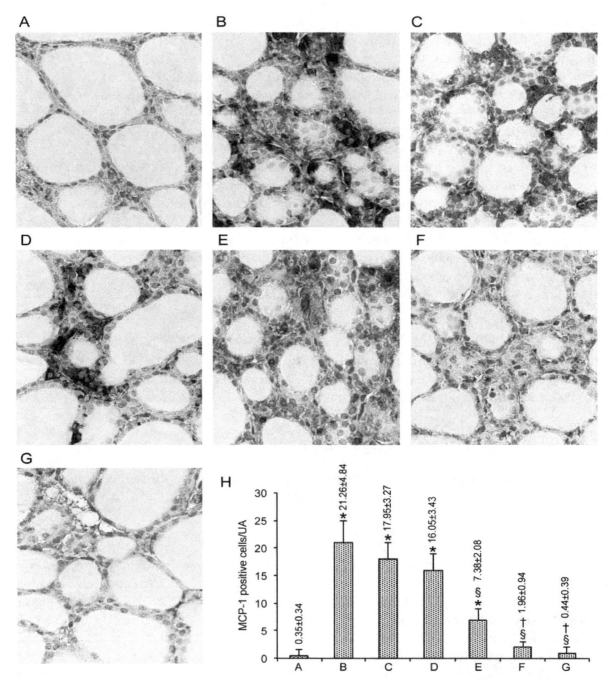

Figure 3. Immunohistochemical expression of monocyte chemoattractant protein-1 (MCP-1) in the thyroid (scale bar: 25 μm). Mice groups are as in Figure 1. (**A**): In controls, no MCP-1-positive cells are present, as shown by bar A in H. (**B**): CdCl$_2$-treated mice show a marked increase in MCP-1 immunoreactivity, as indicated by bar B in H; positive cells line the follicle wall with strong stains on their cytoplasm. (**C,D**): In mice treated with CdCl$_2$ plus 0.2 mg/kg Se or CdCl$_2$ plus 0.4 mg/kg Se, the number of MCP-1-positive cells is decreased, but still higher than controls, as evidenced by bars C and D in H. (**E**): CdCl$_2$ plus MI-treated mice, MCP-1-positive cells are fewer, as shown by bar E in H, and show reduced cytoplasmic staining. (**F,G**): In the thyroid of mice treated with CdCl$_2$ plus MI and 0.2 mg/Kg Se or CdCl$_2$ plus MI and 0.4 mg/kg Se, MCP-1 immunoreactivity is significantly decreased, as indicated by bars F-G in H. (**H**): The number of MCP-1-positive cells per microscopic field in the different groups of mice (mean ± standard error). * $p < 0.05$ versus control; § $p < 0.05$ versus CdCl$_2$ plus vehicle and CdCl$_2$ plus 0.2 or 0.4 mg/kg Se; † $p < 0.05$ versus CdCl$_2$ plus MI.

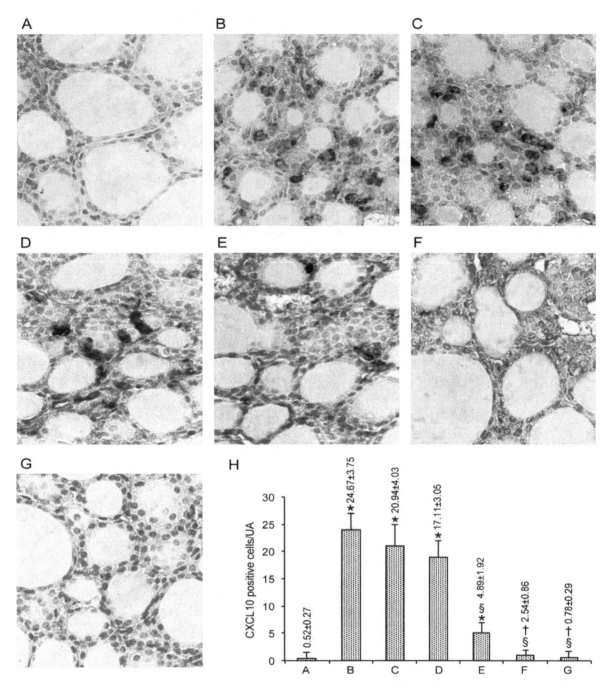

Figure 4. Immunohistochemical expression of C-X-C motif chemokine 10 (CXCL10) in the thyroid (scale bar: 25 μm). Mice groups are as in Figure 1. (**A**): In controls, no CXCL10-positive cells are evident, as shown by bar A in H. (**B**): In $CdCl_2$-treated mice, a large number of CXCL10-positive cells is present among the follicle walls, as indicated by bar B in H. (**C,D**): In mice treated with $CdCl_2$ plus 0.2 mg/kg Se or $CdCl_2$ plus 0.4 mg/kg Se, the number of CXCL10-positive cells is decreased, but still high, as evidenced by bars C and D in H. (**E**): In $CdCl_2$ plus MI-treated mice, only a few CXCL10-positive cells are present, as shown by bar E in H. (**F,G**): In the thyroid of $CdCl_2$ plus MI and 0.2 mg/kg Se or $CdCl_2$ plus MI and 0.4 mg/kg Se, no CXCL10 immunoreactivity is detectable, as indicated by bars F-G in H. (**H**): The number of CXCL10-positive cells per microscopic field in the different groups of mice (mean ± standard error).* $p < 0.05$ versus control; § $p < 0.05$ versus $CdCl_2$ plus vehicle and $CdCl_2$ plus Se 0.2 or 0.4 mg/kg Se; † $p < 0.05$ versus $CdCl_2$ plus MI.

3.3. Immunohistochemical Expression of CXCL10

When CXCL10 immunoreactivity was considered, the results mimicked those described above for MCP-1/CCL2. Thus, in the 49 mice from the seven control groups, the number of cells immunostained by the CXCL10 averaged 0.52 ± 0.27/UA (Figure 4A, and bar A in Figure 4H). The overexpression of CXLC10 induced by $CdCl_2$ plus the vehicle was fully counteracted by the combination of MI with either dose of Se (Figure 4F,G, and bars F-G in Figure 4H).

4. Discussion

In the present work, we have confirmed that Cd exposure has negative consequences for the murine thyroid. These consist of histologically demonstrable alterations in the follicular epithelium and stroma, and in the induced expression of two chemoattractant chemokines, an expression that is absent prior to Cd exposure.

In fact, after chronic exposure to Cd, desquamated cells into the follicles, mononuclear cell infiltration in the stroma and follicles lined by higher cells with light cytoplasm were observed [25]. Therefore, these Cd-elicited thyroid changes have consequences in terms of both thyroid dysfunction and autoimmunity [31,32,54].

Se is considered to exert an overall protection against toxicity induced by heavy metals such as Cd, Pb, As and Hg [55], mainly through the sequestration of these elements into biologically inert complexes and/or through the action of Se-dependent antioxidant enzymes [55]. This protection from Cd toxicity occurs regardless of the Se form (as selenite, selenomethionine, nanoSe, or Se from lentils) [56]. Furthermore, it was recently demonstrated that Se alleviated oxidative stress in chicken ovari and rat kidneys, and counteracted the endoplasmic reticulum stress able to induce apoptosis [57,58]. However, in this paper, we found that the trace element Se was less potent than the carbocyclic sugar MI in protecting mice from $CdCl_2$ thyroid toxicity, though the co-administration of Se amplified the protection conferred by MI alone. The complementary activity of the two antioxidants can be related to their distinctive mechanism of action. While Se is a vital constituent of the enzyme glutathione peroxidase that catalyzes the reaction between GSH and hydrogen peroxide, thus protecting against oxidative stress, MI is a hydroxyl radical scavenger, preventing lipid peroxidation. The combined action of the two compounds may enhance the antioxidant effect [39]. Interestingly the efficacy of this combination was greater that that of resveratrol (used for its potent antioxidant properties), at least when using the follicular area and the epithelial height as read-outs for a comparison evaluation.

One limitation of our work is the lack of hormone measurements. However, considering (i) the aforementioned Chinese study on the direct relationship between blood Cd levels with thyroid hypofunction and serum thyroid autoantibody levels [31], (ii) the association of insulin resistance with either decreased thyroid hormone levels or increased serum TSH [59–61], with counteracting effects by insulin-sensitizing agents [62–64], and (iii) the insulin-mimetic action of MI [54,65,66], we expected that Cd-exposed mouse thyroids would display decreased thyroid hormone levels and increased TSH compared to Cd-unexposed mice. We also expected that at least the combination of MI+Se would have fully counteracted these hormone changes induced by Cd.

On the other hand, the strengths of this study are the findings that are consistent with the previous literature concerning the benefits for the thyroid [38] and other endocrine organs, such as the testes [39], including consistency in the hierarchy of benefits (MI+Se > MI >> Se). In particular, $CdCl_2$ determined significant increase in MCP-1 and CXCL10-positive cell numbers. Our data clearly agree with many in vitro and in vivo experiments by different groups, showing that the production of these chemokines by thyrocytes may play a central role in the recruitment of monocytes and T-lymphocytes at immune inflammatory sites in the thyroid gland from the blood in humans, thus providing a possible mechanism by which thyrocytes themselves may participate in the processes of thyroid autoimmune and inflammatory disease [45,46]. After treatment with Se, MCP-1 and CXCL10-positive cell numbers were reduced. These data about the effects of Se on the thyroid gland, from our point of view, are not particularly surprising. In fact, the recent literature indicates that, regarding thyroid pathology, selenium intake has been associated with autoimmune disorders [67]. Our experimental data indicate the relative inefficacy of Se when administered alone, probably due to extensive detrimental effects of Cd on thyroid structure and function, not adequately counterbalanced by micronutrient administration alone. MI treatment significantly lowered MCP-1 and CXCL10-positive cell numbers, particularly in association with Se, thus confirming that this nutraceutical compound could impact different molecular pathways related to oxidative stress and inflammation, involving chemokines such as MCP-1 and CXCL10 [46].

In view of the "prophylactic" benefit reported in the present paper, it will now be interesting to investigate whether Se, MI and their combination (Se+MI) have "therapeutic" benefits. The demonstration of the latter's benefits requires that animals would be first exposed to $CdCl_2$ for a time sufficient to induce thyroid toxicity (14 days, based on the present work), and then administered Se, MI and Se+MI at doses equal to or greater than those used in the present work and for the same or a longer time (≥ 14 days), in order to show the reversal of the alterations induced by prior Cd exposure. Another translational implication of the data presented in this paper is that, because several pollutants, such as organochlorine compounds, polychlorinated biphenyls, polybrominated diphenylethers, bisphenol A, triclosan, perchlorates, thiocyanates, nitrates and heavy metals different from Cd [3–8] disturb thyroid homeostasis and confer increased environmental susceptibility to thyroid autoimmunity, it would be worthwhile to test whether the said molecules (particularly MI+Se) may have prophylactic and/or therapeutic effects against the thyroid alterations caused by exposure to a number of thyroid-disrupting chemicals.

Author Contributions: Conceptualization, S.B., H.R.M., A.M., A.A., F.S., L.M.; methodology and software, A.M., J.F.; formal analysis, D.P., N.I., G.P., D.A., S.B., L.M.; data curation, D.P., A.M., L.M.; writing the first draft of the manuscript, D.P., L.M.; writing sections of the manuscript, S.B., S.M.F., P.F.; reviewing the manuscript, H.R.M., S.B., A.M. All authors have read and agreed to the published version of the manuscript.

Acknowledgments: The authors thank LO.LI. Pharma S.r.l. (Rome, Italy) for the kind gift of MI.

References

1.   Wiersinga, W.M. Hashimoto's Thyroiditis. In *Thyroid Diseases. Pathogenesis, Diagnosis, and Treatment*; Vitti, P., Hegedus, L., Eds.; Springer: New York, NY, USA, 2018; pp. 205–247.

2.   Davies, L.; Morris, L.G.; Haymart, M.; Chen, A.Y.; Goldenberg, D.; Morris, J.; Ogilvie, J.B.; Terris, D.J.; Netterville, J.; Wong, R.J.; et al. AACE Endocrine Surgery Scientific Committee. American Association of Clinical Endocrinologists and American College of Endocrinology disease state clinical review: The increasing incidence of thyroid cancer. *Endocr. Pract.* **2015**, *21*, 686–696. [CrossRef] [PubMed]

3.   Köhrle, J. Environment and endocrinology: The case of thyroidology. *Ann. Endocrinol.* **2008**, *69*, 116–122. [CrossRef] [PubMed]

4.   Bajaj, J.K.; Salwan, P.; Salwan, S. Various possible toxicants involved in thyroid dysfunction: A review. *J. Clin. Diagn. Res.* **2016**, *10*, FE01. [CrossRef] [PubMed]

5.   Zoeller, T.R. Environmental chemicals targeting thyroid. *Hormones* **2010**, *9*, 28–40. [CrossRef]

6.   Maqbool, F.; Mostafalou, S.; Bahadar, H.; Abdollahi, M. Review of endocrine disorders associated with environmental toxicants and possible involved mechanisms. *Life Sci.* **2016**, *145*, 265–273. [CrossRef]

7.   Buha, A.; Matovic, V.; Antonijevic, B.; Bulat, Z.; Curcic, M.; Renieri, E.A.; Tsatsakis, A.M.; Schweitzer, A.; Wallace, D. Overview of Cadmium Thyroid Disrupting Effects and Mechanisms. *Int. J. Mol. Sci.* **2018**, *19*, 1501. [CrossRef]

8.   Benvenga, S.; Antonelli, A.; Vita, R. Thyroid nodules and thyroid autoimmunity in the context of environmental pollution. *Rev. Endocr. Metab. Disord.* **2015**, *16*, 319–340. [CrossRef]

9.   Thévenod, F.; Lee, W.K. Toxicology of cadmium and its damage in mammalian organs. *Met. Ions Life Sci.* **2013** *11*, 415–490. [CrossRef]

10. Margoshes, M.; Vallee, B.L. A cadmium protein from equine kidney cortex. *J. Am. Chem. Soc.* **1957**, *79*, 4813–4814. [CrossRef]

11. Klaassen, C.D.; Liu, J.; Diwan, B. Metallothionein protection of cadmium toxicity. *Toxicol. Appl. Pharmacol.* **2009**, *238*, 215–220. [CrossRef]

12. Matović, V.; Buha, A.; Bulat, Z.; Đukić-Ćosić, D. Cadmium Toxicity Revisited: Focus on Oxidative Stress Induction and Interactions with Zinc and Magnesium. *Arch. Ind. Hyg. Toxicol.* **2011**, *62*, 65–76. [CrossRef]

13. Matović, V.; Buha, A.; Dukić-Ćosić, D.; Bulat, Z. Insight into the oxidative stress induced by lead and/or cadmium in blood, liver and kidneys. *Food Chem. Toxicol.* **2015**, *78*, 130–140. [CrossRef] [PubMed]

14. Rinaldi, M.; Micali, A.; Marini, H.; Adamo, E.B.; Puzzolo, D.; Pisani, A.; Trichilo, V.; Altavilla, D.; Squadrito, F.; Minutoli, L. Cadmium, organ toxicity and therapeutic approaches: A review on brain, kidney and testis damage. *Curr. Med. Chem.* **2017**, *24*, 3879–3893. [CrossRef] [PubMed]

15. Mezynska, M.; Brzóska, M.M. Environmental exposure to cadmium—A risk for health of the general population in industrialized countries and preventive strategies. *Environ. Sci. Pollut. Res.* **2018**, *25*, 3211–3232. [CrossRef] [PubMed]

16. Uetani, M.; Kobayashi, E.; Suwazono, Y.; Honda, R.; Nishijo, M.; Nakagawa, H.; Kido, T.; Nogawa, K. Tissue cadmium (Cd) concentrations of people living in a Cd polluted area, Japan. *BioMetals* **2006**, *19*, 521–525. [CrossRef]

17. IARC. Personal Habits and Indoor Combustions. In *IARC Monographs on the Evaluation of Carcinogenic Risks to Humans*; International Agency for Research on Cancer: Lyon, France, 2012; Volume 100.

18. Larsson, S.C.; Orsini, N.; Wolk, A. Urinary cadmium concentration and risk of breast cancer: A systematic review and dose-response meta-analysis. *Am. J. Epidemiol.* **2015**, *182*, 375–380. [CrossRef]

19. Buha, A.; Wallace, D.; Matovic, V.; Schweitzer, A.; Oluic, B.; Micic, D.; Djordjevic, V. Cadmium Exposure as a Putative Risk Factor for the Development of Pancreatic Cancer: Three Different Lines of Evidence. *Biomed. Res. Int.* **2017**, *2017*, 1–8. [CrossRef]

20. Feki-Tounsi, M.; Hamza-Chaffai, A. Cadmium as a possible cause of bladder cancer: A review of accumulated evidence. *Environ. Sci. Pollut. Res.* **2014**, *21*, 10561–10573. [CrossRef]

21. Stojsavljević, A.; Rovčanin, B.; Krstić, Đ.; Jagodić, J.; Borković-Mitić, S.; Paunović, I.; Živaljević, V.; Mitić, B.; Gavrović-Jankulović, M.; Manojlović, D. Cadmium as main endocrine disruptor in papillary thyroid carcinoma and the significance of Cd/Se ratio for thyroid tissue pathophysiology. *J. Trace Elem. Med. Biol.* **2019**, *55*, 190–195. [CrossRef]

22. Hammouda, F.; Messaoudi, I.; El Hani, J.; Baati, T.; Saïd, K.; Kerkeni, A. Reversal of cadmium-induced thyroid dysfunction by selenium, zinc, or their combination in rat. *Biol. Trace Elem. Res.* **2008**, *126*, 194–203. [CrossRef]

23. Buha, A.; Antonijević, B.; Bulat, Z.; Jaćević, V.; Milovanović, V.; Matović, V. The impact of prolonged cadmium exposure and co-exposure with polychlorinated biphenyls on thyroid function in rats. *Toxicol. Lett.* **2013**, *221*, 83–90. [CrossRef] [PubMed]

24. Jancic, S.A.; Stosic, B.Z. Cadmium effects on the thyroid gland. *Vitam. Horm.* **2014**, *94*, 391–425. [CrossRef] [PubMed]

25. Piłat-Marcinkiewicz, B.; Brzóska, M.M.; Sawicki, B.; Moniuszko-Jakoniuk, J. Structure and function of thyroid follicular cells in female rats chronically exposed to cadmium. *Bull. Vet. Inst. Pulawy* **2003**, *47*, 157–163.

26. Aaseth, J.; Frey, H.; Glattre, E.; Norheim, G.; Ringstad, J.; Thomassen, Y. Selenium concentrations in the human thyroid gland. *Biol. Trace Elem. Res.* **1990**, *24*, 147–152. [CrossRef]

27. Köhrle, J.; Jakob, F.; Contempré, B.; Dumont, J.E. Selenium, the thyroid, and the endocrine system. *Endocr. Rev.* **2005**, *26*, 944–984. [CrossRef]

28. Köhrle, J. Selenium and the thyroid. *Curr. Opin. Endocrinol. Diabetes Obes.* **2015**, *22*, 392–401. [CrossRef]

29. Duntas, L.H.; Benvenga, S. Selenium: An element for life. *Endocrine* **2015**, *48*, 756–775. [CrossRef]

30. Ralston, N.V.; Raymond, L.J. Dietary selenium's protective effects against methylmercury toxicity. *Toxicology* **2010**, *278*, 112–123. [CrossRef]

31. Nie, X.; Chen, Y.; Chen, Y.; Chen, C.; Han, B.; Li, Q.; Zhu, C.; Xia, F.; Zhai, H.; Wang, N.; et al. Lead and cadmium exposure, higher thyroid antibodies and thyroid dysfunction in Chinese women. *Environ. Pollut.* **2017**, *230*, 320–328. [CrossRef]

32. Chung, S.M.; Moon, J.S.; Yoon, J.S.; Won, K.C.; Lee, H.W. Sex-specific effects of blood cadmium on thyroid hormones and thyroid function status: Korean nationwide cross-sectional study. *J. Trace Elem. Med. Biol.* **2019**, *53*, 55–61. [CrossRef]

33. Ogawa, Y.; Itoh, M.; Hirai, S.; Suna, S.; Naito, M.; Qu, N.; Terayama, H.; Ikeda, A.; Miyaso, H.; Matsuno, Y.; et al. Cadmium exposure increases susceptibility to testicular autoimmunity in mice. *J. Appl. Toxicol.* **2013**, *33*, 652–660. [CrossRef] [PubMed]

34. Monastero, R.N.; Vacchi-Suzzi, C.; Marsit, C.; Demple, B.; Meliker, J.R. Expression of Genes Involved in Stress, Toxicity, Inflammation, and Autoimmunity in Relation to Cadmium, Mercury, and Lead in Human Blood: A Pilot Study. *Toxics* **2018**, *6*, 35. [CrossRef] [PubMed]

35. Rani, A.; Kumar, A.; Lal, A.; Pant, M. Cellular mechanisms of cadmium-induced toxicity: A review. *Int. J. Environ. Health Res.* **2014**, *24*, 378–399. [CrossRef] [PubMed]

36. Bekheet, S.H. Comparative effects of repeated administration of cadmium chloride during pregnancy and lactation and selenium protection against cadmium toxicity on some organs in immature rats' offsprings. *Biol. Trace Elem. Res.* **2011**, *144*, 1008–1023. [CrossRef] [PubMed]

37. Badr, G.M.; Elsawy, H.; Sedky, A.; Eid, R.; Ali, A.; Abdallah, B.M.; Alzahrani, A.M.; Abdel-Moneim, A.M. Protective effects of quercetin supplementation against short-term toxicity of cadmium-induced hematological impairment, hypothyroidism, and testicular disturbances in albino rats. *Environ. Sci. Pollut. Res. Int.* **2019**, *26*, 8202–8211. [CrossRef] [PubMed]

38. Benvenga, S.; Feldt-Rasmussen, U.; Bonofiglio, D.; Asamoah, E. Nutraceutical Supplements in the Thyroid Setting: Health Benefits beyond Basic Nutrition. *Nutrients* **2019**, *11*, 2214. [CrossRef]

39. Benvenga, S.; Micali, A.; Pallio, G.; Vita, R.; Malta, C.; Puzzolo, D.; Irrera, N.; Squadrito, F.; Altavilla, D.; Minutoli, L. Effects of Myo-inositol Alone and in Combination with Seleno-L-methionine on Cadmium-Induced Testicular Damage in Mice. *Curr. Mol. Pharmacol.* **2019**, *12*, 311–323. [CrossRef]

40. Pallio, G.; Micali, A.; Benvenga, S.; Antonelli, A.; Marini, H.R.; Puzzolo, D.; Macaione, V.; Trichilo, V.; Santoro, G.; Irrera, N.; et al. Myo-inositol in the protection from cadmium-induced toxicity in mice kidney: An emerging nutraceutical challenge. *Food Chem. Toxicol.* **2019**, *132*, 110675. [CrossRef]

41. Condorelli, R.A.; La Vignera, S.; Di Bari, F.; Unfer, V.; Calogero, A.E. Effects of myoinositol on sperm mitochondrial function in-vitro. *Eur. Rev. Med. Pharmacol. Sci.* **2011**, *15*, 129–134.

42. Condorelli, R.A.; La Vignera, S.; Bellanca, S.; Vicari, E.; Calogero, A.E. Myoinositol: Does it improve sperm mitochondrial function and sperm motility? *Urology* **2012**, *79*, 1290–1295. [CrossRef]

43. Caprio, F.; D'Eufemia, M.D.; Trotta, C.; Campitiello, M.R.; Ianniello, R.; Mele, D.; Colacurci, N. Myo-inositol therapy for poor-responders during IVF: A prospective controlled observational trial. *J. Ovarian Res.* **2015**, *8*, 37. [CrossRef]

44. Jiang, W.D.; Wu, P.; Kuang, S.Y.; Liu, Y.; Jiang, J.; Hu, K.; Li, S.H.; Tang, L.; Feng, L.; Zhou, X.Q. Myo-inositol prevents copper-induced oxidative damage and changes in antioxidant capacity in various organs and the enterocytes of juvenile Jian carp (Cyprinus carpio var. Jian). *Aquat. Toxicol.* **2011**, *105*, 543–551. [CrossRef] [PubMed]

45. Kasai, K.; Banba, N.; Motohashi, S.; Hattori, Y.; Manaka, K.; Shimoda, S.I. Expression of monocyte chemoattractant protein-1 mRNA and protein in cultured human thyrocytes. *FEBS Lett.* **1996**, *394*, 137–140. [CrossRef]

46. Fallahi, P.; Ferrari, S.M.; Elia, G.; Ragusa, F.; Paparo, S.R.; Caruso, C.; Guglielmi, G.; Antonelli, A. Myo-inositol in autoimmune thyroiditis, and hypothyroidism. *Rev. Endocr. Metab. Disord.* **2018**, *19*, 349–354. [CrossRef]

47. Ferrari, S.M.; Fallahi, P.; Di Bari, F.; Vita, R.; Benvenga, S.; Antonelli, A. Myo-inositol and selenium reduce the risk of developing overt hypothyroidism in patients with autoimmune thyroiditis. *Eur. Rev. Med. Pharmacol. Sci.* **2017**, *21*, 36–42. [PubMed]

48. Benvenga, S.; Vicchio, T.; Di Bari, F.; Vita, R.; Fallahi, P.; Ferrari, S.M.; Catania, S.; Costa, C.; Antonelli, A. Favorable effects of myo-inositol, selenomethionine or their combination on the hydrogen peroxide-induced oxidative stress of peripheral mononuclear cells from patients with Hashimoto's thyroiditis: Preliminary in vitro studies. *Eur. Rev. Med. Pharmacol. Sci.* **2017**, *21*, 89–101. [PubMed]

49. Nordio, M.; Basciani, S. Treatment with Myo-Inositol and Selenium Ensures Euthyroidism in Patients with Autoimmune Thyroiditis. *Int. J. Endocrinol.* **2017**, *2017*, 2549491. [CrossRef]

50. Gupta, P.; Kar, A. Role of ascorbic acid in cadmium-induced thyroid dysfunction and lipid peroxidation. *J. Appl. Toxicol.* **1998**, *18*, 317–320. [CrossRef]

51. Eleawa, S.M.; Alkhateeb, M.A.; Alhashem, F.H.; Bin-Jaliah, I.; Sakr, H.F.; Elrefaey, H.M.; Elkarib, A.O.; Alessa, R.M.; Haidara, M.A.; Shatoor, A.S.; et al. Resveratrol reverses cadmium chloride-induced testicular damage and subfertility by downregulating p53 and Bax and upregulating gonadotropins and Bcl-2 gene expression. *J. Reprod. Dev.* **2014**, *60*, 115–127. [CrossRef]

52. Rafati, A.; Hoseini, L.; Babai, A.; Noorafshan, A.; Haghbin, H.; Karbalay-Doust, S. Mitigating Effect of Resveratrol on the Structural Changes of Mice Liver and Kidney Induced by Cadmium; A Stereological Study. *Prev. Nutr. Food Sci.* **2015**, *20*, 266–275. [CrossRef]

53. Salehi, B.; Mishra, A.P.; Nigam, M.; Sener, B.; Kilic, M.; Sharifi-Rad, M.; Fokou, P.; Martins, N.; Sharifi-Rad, J. Resveratrol: A Double-Edged Sword in Health Benefits. *Biomedicines* **2018**, *6*, 91. [CrossRef] [PubMed]

54. Giammanco, M.; Leto, G. Selenium and autoimmune thyroiditis. *EC Nutr.* **2019**, *14*, 449–450.

55. Rahman, M.M.; Hossain, K.F.B.; Banik, S.; Sikder, M.T.; Akter, M.; Bondad, S.E.C.; Rahaman, M.S.; Hosokawa, T.; Saito, T.; Kurasaki, M. Selenium and zinc protections against metal-(loids)-induced toxicity and disease manifestations: A review. *Ecotoxicol. Environ. Saf.* **2019**, *168*, 146–163. [CrossRef] [PubMed]

56. Zwolak, I. The Role of Selenium in Arsenic and Cadmium Toxicity: An Updated Review of Scientific Literature. *Biol. Trace Elem. Res.* **2020**, *193*, 44–63. [CrossRef] [PubMed]

57. Wan, N.; Xu, Z.; Liu, T.; Min, Y.; Li, S. Ameliorative Effects of Selenium on Cadmium-Induced Injury in the Chicken Ovary: Mechanisms of Oxidative Stress and Endoplasmic Reticulum Stress in Cadmium-Induced Apoptosis. *Biol. Trace Elem. Res.* **2018**, *184*, 463–473. [CrossRef]

58. Chen, Z.J.; Chen, J.X.; Wu, L.K.; Li, B.Y.; Tian, Y.F.; Xian, M.; Huang, Z.P.; Yu, R.A. Induction of Endoplasmic Reticulum Stress by Cadmium and Its Regulation on Nrf2 Signaling Pathway in Kidneys of Rats. *Biomed. Environ. Sci.* **2019**, *32*, 1–10. [CrossRef]

59. Benvenga, S.; Antonelli, A. Inositol(s) in thyroid function, growth and autoimmunity. *Rev. Endocr. Metab. Disord.* **2016**, *17*, 471–484. [CrossRef]

60. Brenta, G.; Caballero, A.S.; Nunes, M.T. Case finding for hypothyroidism should include type 2 diabetes and metabolic syndrome patients: A Latin American Thyroid Society (LATS) position statement. *Endocr. Pract.* **2019**, *25*, 101–105. [CrossRef]

61. Chang, Y.C.; Hua, S.C.; Chang, C.H.; Kao, W.Y.; Lee, H.L.; Chuang, L.M.; Huang, Y.T.; Lai, M.S. High TSH Level within Normal Range Is Associated with Obesity, Dyslipidemia, Hypertension, Inflammation, Hypercoagulability, and the Metabolic Syndrome: A Novel Cardiometabolic Marker. *J. Clin. Med.* **2019**, *8*, 817. [CrossRef]

62. Lupoli, R.; Di Minno, A.; Tortora, A.; Ambrosino, P.; Lupoli, G.A.; Di Minno, M.N. Effects of treatment with metformin on TSH levels: A meta-analysis of literature studies. *J. Clin. Endocrinol. Metab.* **2014**, *99*, E143–E148. [CrossRef]

63. Dimic, D.; Golubovic, M.V.; Radenkovic, S.; Radojkovic, D.; Pesic, M. The effect of metformin on TSH levels in euthyroid and hypothyroid newly diagnosed diabetes mellitus type 2 patients. *Bratisl. Med. J.* **2016**, *117*, 433–435. [CrossRef] [PubMed]

64. Wang, J.; Gao, J.; Fan, Q.; Li, H.; Di, Y. The Effect of Metformin on Thyroid-Associated Serum Hormone Levels and Physiological Indexes: A Meta-Analysis. *Curr. Pharm. Des.* **2019**, *25*, 3257–3265. [CrossRef] [PubMed]

65. D'Anna, R.; Di Benedetto, A.; Scilipoti, A.; Santamaria, A.; Interdonato, M.L.; Petrella, E.; Neri, I.; Pintaudi, B.; Corrado, F.; Facchinetti, F. Myo-inositol Supplementation for Prevention of Gestational Diabetes in Obese Pregnant Women: A Randomized Controlled Trial. *Obstet. Gynecol.* **2015**, *126*, 310–315. [CrossRef] [PubMed]

66. D'Anna, R.; Santamaria, A.; Alibrandi, A.; Corrado, F.; Di Benedetto, A.; Facchinetti, F. Myo-Inositol for the Prevention of Gestational Diabetes Mellitus. A Brief Review. *J. Nutr. Sci. Vitaminol.* **2019**, *65*, S59–S61. [CrossRef]

67. Ventura, M.; Melo, M.; Carrilho, F. Selenium and Thyroid Disease: From Pathophysiology to Treatment. *Int. J. Endocrinol.* **2017**, *2017*, 1297658. [CrossRef]

Breast Milk Iodine Concentration is Associated with Infant Growth, Independent of Maternal Weight

Lindsay Ellsworth [1], Harlan McCaffery [2], Emma Harman [3], Jillian Abbott [4] and Brigid Gregg [5,*]

[1] Division of Neonatal-Perinatal Medicine, Department of Pediatrics, University of Michigan, Ann Arbor, MI 48109, USA; ellsworl@med.umich.edu

[2] Center for Human Growth and Development, University of Michigan, Ann Arbor, MI 48109, USA; hmccaff@umich.edu

[3] School of Public Health, University of Michigan, Ann Arbor, MI 48109, USA; erharman@umich.edu

[4] Metals Laboratory, Division of Clinical Biochemistry and Immunology, Mayo Clinic, Rochester, MN 55905, USA; abbott.jillian@mayo.edu

[5] Division of Pediatric Endocrinology, Department of Pediatrics, University of Michigan, Ann Arbor, MI 48109, USA

* Correspondence: greggb@med.umich.edu

Abstract: In breastfed infants, human milk provides the primary source of iodine to meet demands during this vulnerable period of growth and development. Iodine is a key micronutrient that plays an essential role in hormone synthesis. Despite the importance of iodine, there is limited understanding of the maternal factors that influence milk iodine content and how milk iodine intake during infancy is related to postnatal growth. We examined breast milk samples from near 2 weeks and 2 months post-partum in a mother-infant dyad cohort of mothers with pre-pregnancy weight status defined by body mass index (BMI). Normal (NW, BMI < 25.0 kg/m^2) is compared to overweight/obesity (OW/OB, BMI $\geq$ 25.0 kg/m^2). The milk iodine concentration was determined by inductively coupled plasma mass spectrometry. We evaluated the associations between iodine content at 2 weeks and infant anthropometrics over the first year of life using multivariable linear mixed modeling. Iodine concentrations generally decreased from 2 weeks to 2 months. We observed no significant difference in iodine based on maternal weight. A higher iodine concentration at 2 weeks was associated with a larger increase in infant weight-for-age and weight-for-length Z-score change per month from 2 weeks to 1 year. This pilot study shows that early iodine intake may influence infant growth trajectory independent of maternal pre-pregnancy weight status.

Keywords: iodine status; human milk; lactation; infant growth

1. Introduction

Iodine is a key micronutrient required for adequate growth and development through its critical role in thyroid hormone synthesis [1]. Deficiency in iodine during the neonatal and infant periods may result in impairments in brain development, cognitive outcomes, motor function, and growth stunting. Exposure to excess iodine can lead to iodine-induced hyperthyroidism or hypothyroidism [2–5]. Newborns are a particularly vulnerable population for iodine related disorders given their low storage of iodine in the thyroid at birth and their relatively high requirements for iodine relative to their body size [2,3,6–9].

Exclusively breast-fed infants depend primarily on breast milk iodine to meet their daily iodine needs [7,10]. The United States Institute of Medicine recommends 110 μg/day iodine intake for infants from birth to 6 months of age, while the World Health Organization (WHO) recommends 90 μg/day to achieve adequate intake [11,12]. In order to support fetal and neonatal development, the American

Thyroid Association recommends all pregnant and lactating women supplement their iodine intake with 150 µg/day iodine [3,13]. Iodine supplementation for mothers is intended to achieve the United States Institute of Medicine recommendation of 290 µg/day iodine intake and WHO recommendation of 250 µg/day. Through this degree of supplementation during lactation, the goal is to reach a sufficient breast milk iodine concentration (BMIC) to support a breast-fed infant's daily requirements [5,13]. However, the exact BMIC needed to meet infant needs is not universally defined [3,14].

BMIC is impacted by the maternal degree of iodine sufficiency from dietary iodine sources or supplementation. BMIC also varies based on the time point during lactation, maternal smoking, maternal health conditions, and with day to day fluctuation [3,15–19]. In establishing maternal iodine insufficiency, iodine is thought to be secreted into breast milk rather than excreted into the urine, to promote adequate levels of intake for offspring. The concentrating ability of mammary epithelial cells has been modeled with in vivo rat studies showing that the sodium/iodine symporter (NIS) mediates transport; however, published studies on the activity of the NIS in human mammary epithelial cells remain limited [20]. BMIC is a stronger marker of maternal iodine status than urine concentration [7,10,14,21–25]. BMIC is the greatest in the colostrum and then decreases in early lactation, with an over 40% reduction over the first 6 months of lactation [2,3,6,7,10,15,16]. To date, the impact of maternal health factors on BMIC has not been well described.

In pregnant and non-pregnant women, body mass index (BMI) has been negatively associated with urinary iodine concentration, which is measured as an indicator of iodine status [26–28]. Iodine deficiency has also been reported to be higher in those with morbid obesity [29]. The evaluation of BMIC in the establishment of obesity during pregnancy and lactation has not been well studied. Given the documented relationship with BMI, BMIC may have an important connection with rising levels of obesity in adulthood, as well as a potential contributing factor to childhood obesity. Iodine studies in mother-infant cohorts have shown mixed results regarding birth anthropometric outcomes, with some studies associated with an increased mean birth weight with improved maternal iodine status [30–34]. Postnatal studies of iodine levels have shown an impact on growth factors but have not shown a consistent association with infant growth [1,31,35–38].

With this study, we aimed to determine maternal BMIC over the first 2 months of lactation in mothers with normal weight compared to mothers with elevated pre-pregnancy BMI to characterize the impact of maternal metabolic factors on BMIC. We also assessed the impact of BMIC on infant growth trajectory over the first year of life while taking into account maternal pre-pregnancy weight status to gain a greater understanding of the impact of iodine on post-natal growth.

2. Materials and Methods

2.1. Subjects and Methods

This pilot study included a subset of 57 mother-infant dyads recruited in 2016 to 2018 at the University of Michigan and St. Joseph Mercy Ann Arbor Hospital during hospital admission at the time of infant delivery as part of the prospective Infant Metabolism and Gestational Endocrinopathies (IMAGE) cohort. This study was developed to detect differences in breast milk insulin concentration. This is a secondary analysis of the collected breast milk samples. The mothers included in this study were enrolled if they (1) planned to breastfeed their infant, (2) were > 18 years of age, and (3) had a healthy singleton infant delivered at ≥ 35 weeks gestation. Maternal health conditions, including obesity, gestational diabetes, and polycystic ovary syndrome were included. Maternal demographics and health history were obtained through an electronic medical record review and paper surveys. The maternal pre-pregnancy weight status was determined through a calculation of BMI using obstetrics recorded pre-pregnancy or the early first trimester weight and height as documented in the medical record. Mother-infant dyads were categorized by maternal pre-pregnancy weight status as normal weight (NW, BMI < 25.0 kg/m^2) or overweight/obese (OW/OB, BMI ≥ 25.0 kg/m^2).

The study was approved by the institutional review boards at the University of Michigan (HUM00107801, approved 01/05/2016) and St. Joseph Mercy Ann Arbor Hospital (HSR-17–1686, approved 03/07/17). Mothers gave written informed consent for themselves and assent for their infants prior to participation in the study. The study was conducted in accordance with the protocol approved by the institutional review boards. Participants received reimbursement for their involvement in this study.

2.2. Milk Collection

A written milk collection protocol was provided to the mothers, and in person verbal instruction was given by the study team. Mothers were instructed to collect a 25 mL milk sample on the morning of their infant's 2 week (transitional milk) and 2 month (mature milk) routine well-child visit. The milk collection protocol was based on the published methods by Fields and Demerath, with modifications as described [39]. Mothers collected milk samples between 8:00 and 10:00 am and at least 2 h after feeding their infant by hand expression or pumping of an entire breast based on the maternal preference of expression type. Mothers expressed milk into a large container and then mixed the milk by inversion before the milk was transferred to five glass vials (5 mL each). Samples were immediately placed in the mother's home freezer and then transported on ice to the clinic for storage at −20 °C prior to transport on ice to the final storage location at −80 °C within one week. The milk was thawed on ice for subsequent analyses, at which time 250 μL was aliquoted for further iodine assessment after refreezing at −80 °C and shipment on dry ice.

2.3. Laboratory Analysis

Frozen whole milk 250 μL aliquots were shipped on dry ice to the Mayo Clinic Metals Laboratory (Rochester, MN) for iodine analysis. PerkinElmer Sciex ELAN Dynamic Reaction Cell (DRC) II Inductively Coupled Plasma Mass Spectrometer (ICP-MS), manufactured in Waltham, Massachusetts, USA was used for testing. The gold standard of ICP-MS was used [3]. All samples had one freeze-thaw cycle additional before dilution and were tested within an International Standards Organization (ISO) class 7 cleanroom. The analysis performed followed the standard operating procedure of a test that was developed and consistent with Clinical Laboratory Improvement Amendments (CLIA) requirements. The method used commercially prepared calibrators (Inorganic Ventures, Christiansburg, VA, USA) in 1% TMAH, 7.5 g/L NaCl and 0.5 g/L CaCl$_2$ matrix with iodine concentrations at 0, 10, 100, 500, 1000, 5000 μg/L, having an analytical measurement range (AMR) from 10 to 40,000 μg/L, with the use of 10,000 μg/L and 40,000 μg/L linearity standards. Results above linearity were diluted with SRW (≥18 MΩ cm Special Reagent Water using a NANOpure system, Thermo Scientific, Waltham, MA, USA).

To assess the degree of error for the test method, a recovery study was performed on 3 breast milk samples by spiking them with iodine calibration standards (0, 100 and 500 μg/L) and two levels of Quality Control UTAK Serum Trace Element (UTAK Laboratories, Inc. Valencia, CA, USA), as shown in Table 1. Initial dilutions were repeated five times in duplicate for an intra-assay coefficient of variation (CV). Samples were then run with subsequent loads over a period of five days for an inter-assay CV. The average percentages of recovery were all within 10% of the expected values and <10% for the intra and inter-assay CV.

Table 1. Performance characteristics of the iodine assay.

Target	0 Standard	100 µg/L	500 µg/L	NR UTAK QC	HR UTAK QC
		Breast Milk Precision and Recovery			
Mean	42.89	145.56 µg/L	551.52 µg/L	49 ng/mL	186 ng/mL
CV%	9.32%	6.65%	0.43%	9.6%	2.5%
Recovery		97.40 µg/L	450.9 µg/L	46 µg/L	179 µg/L
% Recovery		97.40%	90.18%	93.88%	96.24%

The same levels of UTAK Serum Trace Elements were used for the Quality Control Analysis; levels were analyzed identically to those of the patient samples in duplicate. QC was run after every 20 samples and at the end of each load. During the sample preparation step each specimen was thoroughly vortexed immediately before performing a two-step dilution using a Hamilton MicorLab diluter (Hamilton Company, Reno, NV, USA) to aspirate 60 µg/L of the sample and 60 µg/L of the Iodine 0 Solution, combined with Iodine Diluent (50 µg/L Te (30% HCl *v/v*) and 10 µg/L Rh (21% HCl *v/v*) in 1% TMAH) for a total of 3 mL. The iodine concentration was measured in ng/mL. Samples were analyzed in duplicate, and the results were averaged for reporting.

One milk sample at 2 weeks had a significantly elevated iodine concentration upon initial analysis, which was consistent on repeat analysis at a separate run time point; given this outlier concentration of >7000 ng/mL without biological plausibility, this value was truncated to the next highest iodine concentration value in our cohort (649.1 ng/mL). A potential etiology may include iodine exposure peri-partum through antiseptics; however, this was unable to be verified.

2.4. Infant Anthropometric Measurements

Infant health history was reviewed from the electronic medical record, including documentation of birth history during hospital admission and follow-up routine outpatient well-child pediatric visits. The type of nutritional intake, such as human milk, formula, or combinations, was determined from the pediatrician notes at the well-child visits. Infant growth anthropometric measures were extracted from the medical record measurements for weight and length obtained in the hospital at birth and during outpatient well-child visits at 2 weeks, 2 months, 6 months, and 1 year. Age and sex specific WHO Z-scores for weight-for-age (WFA), length-for-age (LFA), and weight-for-length (WFL) were extracted from the medical record [40].

2.5. Statistical Analysis

The statistical analysis was completed using R version 3.6.1 (R Foundation for Statistical Computing, Vienna, Austria) and the package nlme version 3.1–140 for this pilot study. Descriptive statistics, comparisons of overweight and obese mothers, and unadjusted comparisons of log(BMIC) were done using Fisher's exact tests or *t*-tests, as appropriate, on all dyads with complete data for each test ($n = 49$ for comparisons involving 2 week BMIC; $n = 50$–57 for all other covariates).

Linear mixed models with random intercepts at the subject level were fit using the 35 dyads that had exclusively breast milk feedings at 2 weeks and 2 months, with BMIC measured at 2 weeks. WFA Z-score (WFAZ), LFA Z-score (LFAZ), and WFL Z-score (WFLZ) were considered dependent variables. Estimates were obtained for the fixed effects for the following independent variables: 2 weeks BMIC, time (in months, 0.5, 2, 6, 12), birth anthropometric Z-score, maternal BMI, gender, interaction of maternal BMI and time, and interaction of 2 week BMIC and time. The interaction of BMIC and time was used to test the association between BMIC and infant growth, and the interaction of maternal BMI and time was included to control for the effects of maternal BMI on infant growth. An initial time point of 2 weeks was used due to the anticipated fluid shift in the first 2 weeks of life in newborns. Parameter estimates were considered statistically significant at $p < 0.05$.

3. Results

This mother-infant cohort included 57 dyads with infant growth measures from birth to 1 year of age, with the descriptive analysis shown in Table 2. Of the 57 dyads, 25 mothers provided milk samples only at 2 weeks, 8 mothers provided milk samples only at 2 months, and 24 mothers provided milk samples at both 2 weeks and 2 months. Mothers in our Midwestern population were primarily Caucasian in the OW/OB maternal group compared to the NW maternal group. Infants were delivered at term gestational age, with 47% male infants. At the 2 week time point of milk collection (mean 16.5 days, SD 3.0 days), 49 milk samples were available for analysis. At the 2 month time point of time collection (mean 63.0 days, SD 5.6 days), 32 milk samples were available for analysis. At the 2 week time point with milk samples collected, 86% of the infants were reported to be exclusively breastfed, 10% received breast milk and formula, 4% did not have their nutrition intake reported, and no infants were exclusively formula fed. By the 2 month time point after the milk samples were collected, 81% of infants received exclusively breast milk, 12% of infants received breast milk and formula, 6% of infants did not have their nutritional intake documented, and no infants were exclusively formula fed. Higher rates of formula supplementation were seen among mothers with OW/OB at 2 weeks (17%) and 2 months (20%). The exact amount of formula supplementation was not quantified.

Table 2. Participant demographics.

Participant Characteristics	NW (n = 24)	OW/OB (n = 33)	p
Maternal Age: years, mean (SD)	31.00 (3.66)	31.61 (3.06)	0.5
* Maternal Pre-Pregnancy BMI: kg/m^2, mean (SD)	21.25 (1.99)	30.95 (4.69)	<0.001
* Maternal Race/Ethnicity			
Caucasian, no. (%)	11 (46)	28 (85) *	
African American, no. (%)	2 (8)	1 (3)	
Hispanic/Latino, no. (%)	4 (17)	1 (3)	0.002
Asian/Pacific Islander, no. (%)	6 (25)	1 (3)	
Indian, no. (%)	1 (4)	0 (0)	
N/A, no. (%)	0 (0)	2 (6)	
Gestational Age: weeks, mean (SD)	39.5 (1.0)	39.1 (1.3)	0.16
Mode of Delivery			
Vaginal, no. (%)	18 (75)	20 (60)	0.39
C-section, no. (%)	6 (25)	13 (40)	
Country			
Washtenaw, no. (%)	18 (75)	17 (52)	0.1
Other, no. (%)	6 (25)	16 (49)	
Maternal income: dollars, mean (SD)			
<60,000, no. (%)	21 (88)	19 (68)	
>60,000, no. (%)	3 (12)	9 (32)	0.04
Unknown, no. (%)	0 (0)	5 (15)	
Smoker			
Yes, no. (%)	1 (4)	1 (3)	
No, no. (%)	19 (80)	27 (82)	>0.99
N/A, no. (%)	4 (17)	5 (15)	
Infant birth weight: kg mean (SD)	3.42 (0.36)	3.52 (0.42)	0.35
Infant birth weight: Z-score mean (SD)	0.33 (0.78)	0.42 (0.81)	0.68
Infant sex			
Male, no. (%)	11 (54)	16 (49)	>0.99
Female, no. (%)	13 (54)	17 (51)	
Infant age at 2 week time point: days, mean (SD)	15.9 (3)	16.9 (3)	0.27
Infant age at 2 month time point: days, mean (SD)	62.0 (7.2)	62.5 (6.7)	0.8

Descriptive statistics on maternal and infant demographics from the cohort of 57 mother-infant dyads presented as the mean (standard deviation) or number (percentage). The sample size is slightly smaller than the totals presented for infants aged at 2 weeks (missing data for 9 infants). Statistical analysis using a t-test or Fischer's exact test. * represents statistical significance, with a p-value < 0.05. Abbreviations: normal weight (NW), overweight and obesity (OW/OB), not available (N/A) number (no.). BMI p < 0.001, Maternal race/ethnicity p = 0.002.

BMIC ranged from 16.0 to 649.1 ng/mL in samples collected near 2 weeks and 2 months. The median BMIC at 2 weeks was 160.7 ng/mL, and, by 2 months, it was 86.0 ng/mL. For comparisons of the mean BMIC, we used a log-transformation BMIC to satisfy the normality assumptions ($p = 0.73$ and 0.56 for the 2 week and 2 month BMIC, respectively, with a Shapiro-Wilk test). There was no significant difference in the log-BMIC between NW and OW/OB mothers at 2 weeks ($p = 0.54$) or at 2 months ($p = 0.57$). The log-BMIC decreased from 2 weeks to 2 months by 0.59 (39%, $p = 0.007$) in the 24 mothers who had iodine measurements at both time points. There was no impact of infant sex, maternal county of residence, or maternal income on BMIC. Untransformed BMIC is shown by the weight status and time of measurement in Figure 1.

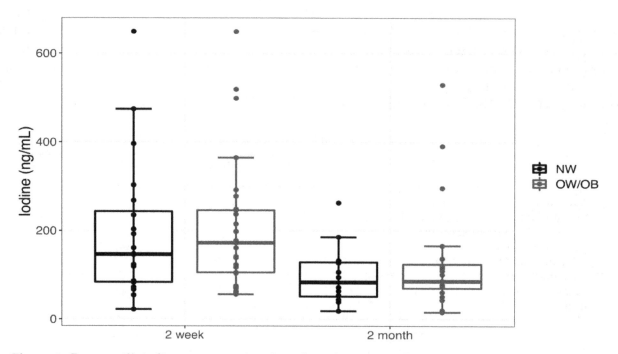

Figure 1. Breast milk iodine concentration (based on the maternal pre-pregnancy weight status for normal weight (NW) compared to overweight and obese (OW/OB) mothers) in transitional milk at 2 weeks (NW $n = 20$, OW/OB $n = 29$) and mature milk at 2 months (NW $n = 12$, OW/OB $n = 20$). Data are represented as a box plot, with the box showing median (IQR) and the whiskers equal to the farthest observation less than 1.5 times IQR from the box edge.

We then explored the impact of maternal weight and BMIC on infant growth from 2 weeks to 1 year using linear mixed models, with a subset of dyads who had complete data for all variables included in the model, and who were exclusively breastfed at 2 weeks and 2 months ($n = 35$). We evaluated infant growth by testing the interactions of maternal BMI with time, and BMIC at 2 weeks with time, using an anthropometric Z-score through the first year of life, with the WFA, LFA, and WFL Z-scores as dependent variables. We found no significant interactions between maternal pre-pregnancy BMI and time for WFA ($\beta = -0.00126$, $p = 0.534$), LFA ($\beta = 0.00359$, $p = 0.118$), or WFL ($\beta = -0.00452$, $p = 0.089$) Z-score changes per month from 2 weeks to 1 year. A higher milk iodine concentration at 2 weeks was associated with a larger increase in infant WFA ($\beta = 0.00033$, $p = 0.0007$) and WFL Z-score ($\beta = 0.00029$, $p = 0.0212$) change per month from 2 weeks to 1 year, with no significant association with LFA ($\beta = 0.00015$, $p = 0.154$), as shown in Table 3. Figure 2 represents the model interaction terms of BMIC and time, showing the predicted WFAZ, LFAZ, and WFLZ for a male infant with a mean birth Z-score, breastfed by a mother with mean BMI based on a 2 week BMIC mean, mean +1 standard deviation (SD), and −1 SD.

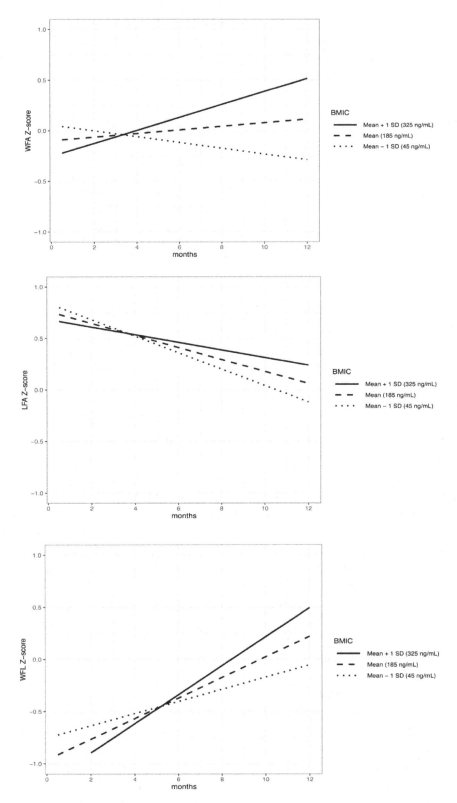

Figure 2. Infant growth anthropometric Z-score from 2 weeks to 1 year, with BMIC predicted by linear mixed models (model *n* = 35). Graphs depict the difference in the predicted growth lines for the mean ± 1 standard deviation BMIC as measured at 2 weeks for dyads with a male infant, the mean birth anthropometric Z-score, and the mean maternal BMI. Interaction effect of BMIC and time (months) on infant WFA (β = 0.00033, *p* < 0.001), infant LFA (β = 0.00015, *p* = 0.154), and infant WFL (β = 0.00029, *p* = 0.021). Abbreviations: weight-for-age Z-score (WFA), length-for-age Z-score (LFA), and weight-for-length Z-score (WFL); breast milk iodine concentration (BMIC).

Table 3. Association of maternal weight status and 2 week breast milk iodine concentration with change in weight-for-age, length-for-age, and weight-for-length Z-score across the first year of life.

Variables	Model n	WFAZ	LFAZ	WFLZ
		Difference (β (p-value)) in change in infant anthropometry Z-score		
BMIC at 2 weeks (ng/mL)	35	−0.1883 (0.706)	1.23581 (0.028) *	−1.1945 (0.053)
Time (months)	35	−0.0011 (0.170)	−0.00056 (0.527)	−0.0015 (0.136)
Birth WFAZ	35	0.53027 (0.0006) *	−0.18117 (0.002) *	0.16434 (0.016) *
Maternal BMI (kg/m^2)	35	−0.00532 (0.769)	0.42163 (0.0004) *	0.24395 (0.022) *
Infant sex	35	0.23087 (0.247)	−0.03543 (0.080)	0.01866 (0.411)
Maternal BMI interaction with time	35	−0.00126 (0.536)	0.00359 (0.118)	−0.00452 (0.089)
BMIC at 2 weeks interaction with time	35	0.00033 (0.0007) *	0.00015 (0.154)	0.00029 (0.021) *

* Statistical significance based on an estimation of the fixed effects in linear mixed models, with a significance threshold at $p < 0.05$. Abbreviations: weight-for-age Z-score (WFAZ), length-for-age Z-score (LFAZ), weight-for-length Z-score (WFLZ), body mass index (BMI), and breastmilk iodine concentration (BMIC).

4. Discussion

In the maternal-infant dyads in this study, transitional milk BMIC was positively associated with infant WFA and WFL Z-score changes over the first year of life, and these iodine-related growth differences were not related to maternal pre-pregnancy weight status based on this pilot study. The importance of early milk iodine may point to a critical period of offspring development during high vulnerability and a time during which formula fed infants may consume less iodine than breastfed infants.

Milk iodine concentrations were not associated with maternal pre-pregnancy weight status in our cohort. While literature on adult obesity has described iodine deficiency as associated with elevated BMI, we did not find similar findings related to BMI as a marker of iodine status [26–29]. Limited literature on BMIC during lactation has focused on the maternal health influences on milk iodine concentration [26,27,29]. A study by Dumrongwongsiri, in Thailand, showed an association of BMIC with maternal weight; however, there was no association with maternal age or lactation stage [41]. This study did not define the time point of maternal weight measurement and may not reflect the weight prior to pregnancy, as assessed in our study. It is important for future studies on BMIC to include an analysis of maternal pre-pregnancy weight status in order to understand the role of maternal health on milk micronutrient composition.

The milk iodine concentrations in our cohort showed considerable variability. The BMIC to achieve adequate iodine delivery to infants is debated, with the lower most BMIC proposed to range from 60 to 150 ng/mL [3,13,14,22]. While exact values of the ideal BMIC for sufficient infant intake ranges are not well described, a goal of 150 ng/mL in breast milk has been reported [3]. The levels in our study showed a high degree of values below 150 ng/mL at 2 weeks (47%) and even more below 150 ng/mL at 2 months (81%). These results are higher than those of a study from the Netherlands, showing that 33% of infants were anticipated to be iodine deficient based on BMIC <1.1 µmol/L (139 ng/mL) [42]. Mothers with low BMIC may signify a population with iodine insufficiency, as BMIC has been shown to be positively correlated with maternal urinary iodine concentration, the standard measure of iodine sufficiency [43]. Currently, the United States has salt iodization programs, with a reported use near 90% due to a decline in iodized salt into the 1990s, based on National Health and Nutrition Examination Survey (NHANES) data [44]. Additionally, the NHANES reports on iodine status during pregnancy showed a concerning degree of iodine insufficiency (56.9%) in 2005–2008 [45]. Previous cohorts from Boston have shown a similar degree of iodine insufficiency (47%) based on estimated infant milk intake; however, this group had higher milk iodine concentrations (median 155 ng/mL) at a median of 48 days collection compared to BMIC at our 2 month time point (median 86 ng/mL) [43]. A meta-analysis by Nazeri described overall lower mature milk iodine level in iodine sufficient countries (mean 71.5 ng/mL) [46]. This difference may represent population, geographic, or nutritional intake differences.

While our cohort may be a population at risk for infant iodine insufficiency based on BMIC, we also noted some elevated BMIC levels in both NW and OW/OB throughout the first 2 months of lactation. The level of BMIC that may lead to iodine excess has not been defined in the same manner that urinary iodine concentration >300 ng/mL in children and >500 ng/mL in pregnancy is defined as iodine excess [47]. Prior studies of high iodine exposure through elevated water iodine levels by Liu identified a BMIC >200 ng/mL in mothers with high iodine intake [48]. A further evaluation of excessive iodine exposure through breast milk is necessary to determine the safe levels of exposure, particularly in mothers at risk for iodine excess, including those with high dietary, oral, or topical iodine exposure [49].

Our data on BMIC overall, independent of maternal pre-pregnancy weight status, suggests a relationship between infant iodine exposure and growth, with a higher BMIC at 2 weeks associated with an increased change in Z-score for WFA and WFL over the first year of life. However, the clinical implications of these small growth changes are unclear, and future long-term studies into childhood growth and adiposity are needed. Prior literature has focused on the impact of iodine status and supplementation on prenatal growth, with a systematic review showing low quality evidence for increased birth weight in infants of mothers with severe iodine deficiency who are receiving iodine supplementation [31]. Postnatal growth studies are limited in both observational and iodine supplementation intervention studies during lactation [31]. In a study performed in China by Yang, a maternal iodine deficiency based on urinary iodine levels <50 μg/L during lactation was linked to a decreased infant WFA and LFA for infants <6 months of age, with positive effects of maternal iodine status on infant weight; however, BMIC was not measured to determine infant intake [1]. A review of survey data by Mason showed a positive relationship with iodine salt use and increased infant WFA and mid-upper-arm-circumference at 2 years. This study also assessed maternal BMI, showing that the positive relationship between iodinated salt use and WFA was increasingly greater with a lower maternal BMI [50]. However, there have been opposing trials and systematic reviews showing no impact of iodine intake on infant growth. In a multicenter randomized control trial of iodine supplementation during infancy in breastfeeding infants compared to placebo or formula fed infants, there was no difference found for 12 month WFA Z-score or WFL Z-score in infants receiving high or low iodine supplementation; however, infants receiving no intervention had higher LFA Z-scores and formula fed infants had higher WFA, WFL, and LFA Z-scores [51]. In a systematic review by Farebrother, on the impact of iodine supplementation on postnatal growth outcomes based on limited supplementation studies during pregnancy and one randomized clinical trial of preterm infant formula supplementation, there was no difference at 12 and 24 months in infant weight, length, or head circumference with maternal iodine supplementation [31].

Our prospective observational cohort study without specific iodine supplementation evaluated the association of BMIC with infant anthropometrics and found positive associations between growth over the first year and early BMIC near 2 weeks. The potential mechanisms for iodine related infant growth may be related to the role of iodine in the endocrine pathways of the thyroid hormone (TH) and growth hormone-insulin-like growth factor (GH-IGF) axis [31,32]. Zimmerman showed in a prospective intervention of iodine repletion in school age children that there was improved somatic growth in the WFA and head circumference-for-age Z-score associated with increased IGF-I and IGF binding protein-3 (IGFBP-3) concentrations in children [38]. Future work evaluating the link between BMIC, infant somatic growth, and growth related hormone levels (TSH, free thyroxine, IGF-1, and IGFBP-3) may provide further insight into mediators and identify areas for intervention for the promotion of iodine sufficient status during lactation.

This study provides insight into longitudinal BMIC in a United States Midwestern population, with corresponding assessments of infant growth through the first year of life in this pilot study. The strength of this study is that the population was selected for their initial plans to breastfeed without selection for predetermined maternal iodine status. This pilot study is limited by the small sample size used for its secondary analysis, which the initial study was not powered for; the mixed modeling involved a large number of parameters for the sample size, which could raise questions about the generalizability of these models among the larger population. However, the significant associations with BMIC and infant growth seen with these small numbers highlights the importance of consideration for BMIC analysis in more expansive mother-infant lactation focused cohorts to further understand this potential early programming influence. Additional limitations, including the assessment of infant growth outcomes, were measured by medical staff at pediatrician well-child visits, possibly resulting in inaccurate anthropometrics. Infant growth is complex, and this study is not able to address the numerous factors contributing to infant growth, which are not limited to genetic, environmental, later formula supplementation quantity, complimentary feedings, milk volume intake, and the complex composition of human milk, including macronutrients, micronutrients, bioactive factors, growth hormones, and immune factors [52,53]. Our cohort did not assess iodine status during pregnancy, which could impact fetal growth and development. Maternal iodine intake was also not quantified in this study. This will be important in future studies to provide a further explanation for the high BMIC among the population of lactating mothers. An assessment of infant iodine status will also be an important addition to future work to determine the relationship with BMIC based on detailed 24 h infant breast milk volume intake.

5. Conclusions

While the importance of maternal health during pregnancy and lactation in promoting infant growth and development cannot be understated, this study did not show the impact of maternal pre-pregnancy BMI on BMIC. We have identified a positive association between transitional BMIC and infant weight and weight-for-length growth over the first year of life based on a Z-score irrespective of maternal pre-pregnancy weight status. These findings highlight the critical need for knowledge of breast milk composition, particularly in micronutrients (such as iodine), which play a key role in infant growth. A further evaluation of the complex components in breast milk and the impact of these components during ongoing organ development in infancy is necessary to promote targeted interventions to support optimal childhood health.

Author Contributions: Conceptualization, L.E. and B.G.; formal analysis, L.E. and H.M.; methodology, L.E., E.H., J.A., and B.G.; supervision, B.G.; validation, J.A.; Writing-original draft, L.E., E.H., J.A., and B.G.; writing-review and editing, L.E., H.M., E.H., J.A., and B.G. All authors have read and agreed to the published version of the manuscript.

Acknowledgments: Thanks to all of the participating families for allowing this research to be possible. We appreciate the assistance from Judith Ivacko for help in coordinating our research sites. This project was made possible by biostatistics support from the University of Michigan Center for Human Growth and Development with guidance by Niko Kaciroti.

References

1.   Yang, J.; Zhu, L.; Li, X.; Zheng, H.; Wang, Z.; Hao, Z.; Liu, Y. Maternal iodine status during lactation and infant weight and length in Henan Province, China. *BMC Pregnancy Childbirth* **2017**, *17*. [CrossRef] [PubMed]
2.   Azizi, F.; Smyth, P. Breastfeeding and maternal and infant iodine nutrition. *Clin. Endocrinol. (Oxf)* **2009**, *70*, 803–809. [CrossRef] [PubMed]
3.   Dror, D.K.; Allen, L.H. Iodine in Human Milk: A Systematic Review. *Adv. Nutr. (Bethesda, Md.)* **2018**, *9*, 347S–357S. [CrossRef]

4. Michaelsen, K.F.; Larsen, P.S.; Thomsen, B.L.; Samuelson, G. The Copenhagen Cohort Study on Infant Nutrition and Growth: Breast-milk intake, human milk macronutrient content, and influencing factors. *Am. J. Clin. Nutr.* **1994**, *59*, 600–611. [CrossRef] [PubMed]
5. Zimmermann, M.B. The role of iodine in human growth and development. *Semin. Cell Dev. Biol.* **2011**, *22*, 645–652. [CrossRef] [PubMed]
6. Etling, N.; Padovani, E.; Fouque, F.; Tato, L. First-month variations in total iodine content of human breast milks. *Early Hum. Dev.* **1986**, *13*, 81–85. [CrossRef]
7. Semba, R.D.; Delange, F. Iodine in human milk: Perspectives for infant health. *Nutr. Rev.* **2001**, *59*, 269–278. [CrossRef]
8. van den Hove, M.F.; Beckers, C.; Devlieger, H.; de Zegher, F.; De Nayer, P. Hormone synthesis and storage in the thyroid of human preterm and term newborns: Effect of thyroxine treatment. *Biochimie* **1999**, *81*, 563–570. [CrossRef]
9. Zimmermann, M.B. Are weaning infants at risk of iodine deficiency even in countries with established iodized salt programs? *Nestle Nutr. Inst. Workshop Ser.* **2012**, *70*, 137–146. [CrossRef]
10. Mulrine, H.M.; Skeaff, S.A.; Ferguson, E.L.; Gray, A.R.; Valeix, P. Breast-milk iodine concentration declines over the first 6 mo postpartum in iodine-deficient women. *Am. J. Clin. Nutr.* **2010**, *92*, 849–856. [CrossRef]
11. WHO. *Reaching Optimal Iodine Nutrition in Pregnant and Lactating Women and Young Children*; World Health Organization: Geneva, Switzerland, 2007.
12. Institute of Medicine (US). Panel on Micronutrients. Dietary Reference Intakes for Vitamin A, Vitamin K, Arsenic, Boron, Chromium, Copper, Iodine, Iron, Manganese, Molybdenum, Nickel, Silicon, Vanadium, and Zinc. 2001. Available online: https://www.ncbi.nlm.nih.gov/books/NBK222310/ (accessed on 10 November 2019).
13. ACOG Committee opinion No. 549: Obesity in pregnancy. *Obstet. Gynecol.* **2013**, *121*, 213–217.
14. Dold, S.; Zimmermann, M.B.; Baumgartner, J.; Davaz, T.; Galetti, V.; Braegger, C.; Andersson, M. A dose-response crossover iodine balance study to determine iodine requirements in early infancy. *Am. J. Clin. Nutr.* **2016**, *104*, 620–628. [CrossRef]
15. Chierici, R.; Saccomandi, D.; Vigi, V. Dietary supplements for the lactating mother: Influence on the trace element content of milk. *Acta Paediatr. (Oslo, Norway: 1992) Suppl.* **1999**, *88*, 7–13. [CrossRef]
16. Henjum, S.; Lilleengen, A.M.; Aakre, I.; Dudareva, A.; Gjengedal, E.L.F.; Meltzer, H.M.; Brantsaeter, A.L. Suboptimal Iodine Concentration in Breastmilk and Inadequate Iodine Intake among Lactating Women in Norway. *Nutrients* **2017**, *9*. [CrossRef]
17. Osei, J.; Andersson, M.; Reijden, O.V.; Dold, S.; Smuts, C.M.; Baumgartner, J. Breast-Milk Iodine Concentrations, Iodine Status, and Thyroid Function of Breastfed Infants Aged 2–4 Months and Their Mothers Residing in a South African Township. *J. Clin. Res. Pediatr. Endocrinol.* **2016**, *8*, 381–391. [CrossRef]
18. Sabatier, M.; Garcia-Rodenas, C.L.; Castro, C.A.; Kastenmayer, P.; Vigo, M.; Dubascoux, S.; Andrey, D.; Nicolas, M.; Payot, J.R.; Bordier, V.; et al. Longitudinal Changes of Mineral Concentrations in Preterm and Term Human Milk from Lactating Swiss Women. *Nutrients* **2019**, *11*. [CrossRef]
19. Chen, Y.; Gao, M.; Bai, Y.; Hao, Y.; Chen, W.; Cui, T.; Guo, W.; Pan, Z.; Lin, L.; Wang, C.; et al. Variation of iodine concentration in breast milk and urine in exclusively breastfeeding women and their infants during the first 24 wk after childbirth. *Nutrition (Burbank, Los Angeles County, Calif.)* **2019**, *71*, 110599. [CrossRef]
20. Tazebay, U.H.; Wapnir, I.L.; Levy, O.; Dohan, O.; Zuckier, L.S.; Zhao, Q.H.; Deng, H.F.; Amenta, P.S.; Fineberg, S.; Pestell, R.G.; et al. The mammary gland iodide transporter is expressed during lactation and in breast cancer. *Nat. Med.* **2000**, *6*, 871–878. [CrossRef]
21. Brown-Grant, K. The iodide concentrating mechanism of the mammary gland. *J. Physiol* **1957**, *135*, 644–654. [CrossRef]
22. Dold, S.; Zimmermann, M.B.; Aboussad, A.; Cherkaoui, M.; Jia, Q.; Jukic, T.; Kusic, Z.; Quirino, A.; Sang, Z.; San Luis, T.O.; et al. Breast Milk Iodine Concentration Is a More Accurate Biomarker of Iodine Status Than Urinary Iodine Concentration in Exclusively Breastfeeding Women. *J. Nutr.* **2017**, *147*, 528–537. [CrossRef]
23. Eskin, B.A.; Bartuska, D.G.; Dunn, M.R.; Jacob, G.; Dratman, M.B. Mammary gland dysplasia in iodine deficiency. Studies in rats. *JAMA* **1967**, *200*, 691–695. [CrossRef] [PubMed]
24. Nazeri, P.; Dalili, H.; Mehrabi, Y.; Hedayati, M.; Mirmiran, P.; Azizi, F. Breast Milk Iodine Concentration Rather than Maternal Urinary Iodine Is a Reliable Indicator for Monitoring Iodine Status of Breastfed Neonates. *Biol. Trace Elem. Res.* **2018**, *185*, 71–77. [CrossRef] [PubMed]

25. Strum, J.M. Effect of iodide-deficiency on rat mammary gland. *Virchows Arch. B Cell Pathol. Incl. Mol. Pathol.* **1979**, *30*, 209–220. [CrossRef] [PubMed]
26. Robinson, S.M.; Crozier, S.R.; Miles, E.A.; Gale, C.R.; Calder, P.C.; Cooper, C.; Inskip, H.M.; Godfrey, K.M. Preconception Maternal Iodine Status Is Positively Associated with IQ but Not with Measures of Executive Function in Childhood. *J. Nutr.* **2018**, *148*, 959–966. [CrossRef]
27. Soriguer, F.; Valdes, S.; Morcillo, S.; Esteva, I.; Almaraz, M.C.; de Adana, M.S.; Tapia, M.J.; Dominguez, M.; Gutierrez-Repiso, C.; Rubio-Martin, E.; et al. Thyroid hormone levels predict the change in body weight: A prospective study. *Eur. J. Clin. Invest.* **2011**, *41*, 1202–1209. [CrossRef]
28. Torlinska, B.; Bath, S.C.; Janjua, A.; Boelaert, K.; Chan, S.Y. Iodine Status during Pregnancy in a Region of Mild-to-Moderate Iodine Deficiency is not Associated with Adverse Obstetric Outcomes; Results from the Avon Longitudinal Study of Parents and Children (ALSPAC). *Nutrients* **2018**, *10*. [CrossRef]
29. Lecube, A.; Zafon, C.; Gromaz, A.; Fort, J.M.; Caubet, E.; Baena, J.A.; Tortosa, F. Iodine deficiency is higher in morbid obesity in comparison with late after bariatric surgery and non-obese women. *Obes. Surg.* **2015**, *25*, 85–89. [CrossRef]
30. Alvarez-Pedrerol, M.; Guxens, M.; Mendez, M.; Canet, Y.; Martorell, R.; Espada, M.; Plana, E.; Rebagliato, M.; Sunyer, J. Iodine levels and thyroid hormones in healthy pregnant women and birth weight of their offspring. *Eur. J. Endocrinol.* **2009**, *160*, 423–429. [CrossRef]
31. Farebrother, J.; Naude, C.E.; Nicol, L.; Sang, Z.; Yang, Z.; Jooste, P.L.; Andersson, M.; Zimmermann, M.B. Effects of Iodized Salt and Iodine Supplements on Prenatal and Postnatal Growth: A Systematic Review. *Adv. Nutr. (Bethesda, Md.)* **2018**, *9*, 219–237. [CrossRef]
32. Gunnarsdottir, I.; Dahl, L. Iodine intake in human nutrition: A systematic literature review. *Food Nutr. Res.* **2012**, *56*. [CrossRef]
33. Rydbeck, F.; Rahman, A.; Grander, M.; Ekstrom, E.C.; Vahter, M.; Kippler, M. Maternal urinary iodine concentration up to 1.0 mg/L is positively associated with birth weight, length, and head circumference of male offspring. *J. Nutr.* **2014**, *144*, 1438–1444. [CrossRef] [PubMed]
34. Iodine supplementation for women during the preconception, pregnancy and postpartum period - Harding, KB - 2017. *Cochrane Libr.* **2019**. [CrossRef]
35. Aboud, F.E.; Bougma, K.; Lemma, T.; Marquis, G.S. Evaluation of the effects of iodized salt on the mental development of preschool-aged children: A cluster randomized trial in northern Ethiopia. *Matern. Child Nutr.* **2017**, *13*. [CrossRef]
36. Gowachirapant, S.; Jaiswal, N.; Melse-Boonstra, A.; Galetti, V.; Stinca, S.; Mackenzie, I.; Thomas, S.; Thomas, T.; Winichagoon, P.; Srinivasan, K.; et al. Effect of iodine supplementation in pregnant women on child neurodevelopment: A randomised, double-blind, placebo-controlled trial. *Lancet Diabetes Endocrinol.* **2017**, *5*, 853–863. [CrossRef]
37. Zimmermann, M.B.; Connolly, K.; Bozo, M.; Bridson, J.; Rohner, F.; Grimci, L. Iodine supplementation improves cognition in iodine-deficient schoolchildren in Albania: A randomized, controlled, double-blind study. *Am. J. Clin. Nutr.* **2006**, *83*, 108–114. [CrossRef]
38. Zimmermann, M.B.; Jooste, P.L.; Mabapa, N.S.; Schoeman, S.; Biebinger, R.; Mushaphi, L.F.; Mbhenyane, X. Vitamin A supplementation in iodine-deficient African children decreases thyrotropin stimulation of the thyroid and reduces the goiter rate. *Am. J. Clin. Nutr.* **2007**, *86*, 1040–1044. [CrossRef]
39. Fields, D.A.; Demerath, E.W. Relationship of insulin, glucose, leptin, IL-6 and TNF-alpha in human breast milk with infant growth and body composition. *Pediatr. Obes.* **2012**, *7*, 304–312. [CrossRef]
40. WHO Child Growth Standards based on length/height, weight and age. *Acta Paediatr. (Oslo, Norway: 1992) Suppl.* **2006**, *450*, 76–85.
41. Dumrongwongsiri, O.; Chatvutinun, S.; Phoonlabdacha, P.; Sangcakul, A.; Chailurkit, L.O.; Siripinyanond, A.; Suthutvoravut, U.; Chongviriyaphan, N. High Urinary Iodine Concentration Among Breastfed Infants and the Factors Associated with Iodine Content in Breast Milk. *Biol. Trace Elem. Res.* **2018**, *186*, 106–113. [CrossRef]
42. Stoutjesdijk, E.; Schaafsma, A.; Dijck-Brouwer, D.A.J.; Muskiet, F.A.J. Iodine status during pregnancy and lactation: A pilot study in the Netherlands. *Neth J. Med.* **2018**, *76*, 210–217.
43. Pearce, E.N.; Leung, A.M.; Blount, B.C.; Bazrafshan, H.R.; He, X.; Pino, S.; Valentin-Blasini, L.; Braverman, L.E. Breast milk iodine and perchlorate concentrations in lactating Boston-area women. *J. Clin. Endocrinol. Metab.* **2007**, *92*, 1673–1677. [CrossRef]

44. Hollowell, J.G.; Staehling, N.W.; Hannon, W.H.; Flanders, D.W.; Gunter, E.W.; Maberly, G.F.; Braverman, L.E.; Pino, S.; Miller, D.T.; Garbe, P.L.; et al. Iodine nutrition in the United States. Trends and public health implications: Iodine excretion data from National Health and Nutrition Examination Surveys I and III (1971–1974 and 1988–1994). *J. Clin. Endocrinol. Metab.* **1998**, *83*, 3401–3408. [CrossRef]

45. Caldwell, K.L.; Makhmudov, A.; Ely, E.; Jones, R.L.; Wang, R.Y. Iodine status of the U.S. population, National Health and Nutrition Examination Survey, 2005–2006 and 2007–2008. *Thyroid* **2011**, *21*, 419–427. [CrossRef]

46. Nazeri, P.; Kabir, A.; Dalili, H.; Mirmiran, P.; Azizi, F. Breast-Milk Iodine Concentrations and Iodine Levels of Infants According to the Iodine Status of the Country of Residence: A Systematic Review and Meta-Analysis. *Thyroid* **2018**, *28*, 124–138. [CrossRef]

47. WHO. Assessment of Iodine Deficiency Disorders and Monitoring Their Elimination. Available online: https://apps.who.int/iris/bitstream/handle/10665/43781/9789241595827_eng.pdf (accessed on 24 October 2019).

48. Liu, L.; Liu, J.; Wang, D.; Shen, H.; Jia, Q. Effect of Urinary Iodine Concentration in Pregnant and Lactating Women, and in Their Infants Residing in Areas with Excessive Iodine in Drinking Water in Shanxi Province, China. *Biol. Trace Elem. Res.* **2019**. [CrossRef]

49. Iodine. In *Drugs and Lactation Database (LactMed) [Internet]*, [Updated 2019 Feb 28] ed.; National Library of Medicine (US): Bethesda, MD, USA, 2006.

50. Mason, J.B.; Deitchler, M.; Gilman, A.; Gillenwater, K.; Shuaib, M.; Hotchkiss, D.; Mason, K.; Mock, N.; Sethuraman, K. Iodine fortification is related to increased weight-for-age and birthweight in children in Asia. *Food Nutr. Bull.* **2002**, *23*, 292–308. [CrossRef]

51. Nazeri, P.; Tahmasebinejad, Z.; Mehrabi, Y.; Hedayati, M.; Mirmiran, P.; Azizi, F. Lactating Mothers and Infants Residing in an Area with an Effective Salt Iodization Program Have No Need for Iodine Supplements: Results from a Double-Blind, Placebo-Controlled, Randomized Controlled Trial. *Thyroid* **2018**, *28*, 1547–1558. [CrossRef]

52. Ballard, O.; Morrow, A.L. Human milk composition: Nutrients and bioactive factors. *Pediatr. Clin. N. Am.* **2013**, *60*, 49–74. [CrossRef]

53. Eriksen, K.G.; Christensen, S.H.; Lind, M.V.; Michaelsen, K.F. Human milk composition and infant growth. *Curr. Opin. Clin. Nutr. Metab. Care* **2018**, *21*, 200–206. [CrossRef]

Permissions

List of Contributors

Elizabeth R. Eveleigh, Lisa J. Coneyworth, Amanda Avery and Simon J. M. Welham
Division of Food, Nutrition & Dietetics, School of Biosciences, The University of Nottingham, Sutton Bonington LE12 5RD, UK

Ahmed A Madar and Espen Heen
Department of Community Medicine and Global Health, Institute of Health and Society, University of Oslo, 0318 Oslo, Norway

Laila A Hopstock
Department of Community Medicine, Faculty of Health Sciences, UiT The Arctic University of Norway, 9037 Tromsø, Norway

Monica H Carlsen
Department of Nutrition, Institute of Basic Medical Sciences, University of Oslo, 0318 Oslo, Norway

Haakon E Meyer
Department of Community Medicine and Global Health, Institute of Health and Society, University of Oslo, 0318 Oslo, Norway
Division of Mental and Physical Health, Norwegian Institute of Public Health, 0213 Oslo, Norway

Natale Musso, Lucia Conte, Beatrice Carloni, Claudia Campana, Maria C. Chiusano and Massimo Giusti
Centre for Secondary Hypertension, Unit of Clinical Endocrinology, Department of Internal Medicine, University of Genoa Medical School, IRCCS Ospedale Policlinico San Martino, 16132 Genova, Italy

Karen E. Charlton
School of Medicine, University of Wollongong, Wollongong 2500, New South Wales, Australia
Illawarra Health and Medical Institute, University of Wollongong, Wollongong 2500, New South Wales, Australia

Lisa J. Ware
Hypertension in Africa Research Team (HART), North-West University, Potchefstroom 2531, North West Province, South Africa
MRC/Wits Developmental Pathways for Health Research Unit, University of the Witwatersrand, Johannesburg 2193, Gauteng, South Africa

Jeannine Baumgartner
Centre of Excellence for Nutrition (CEN), North-West University, Potchefstroom 2531, North West Province, South Africa

Marike Cockeran
Statistical Consultation Services, North-West University, 11 Hoffman Street, Potchefstroom; Private Bag X6001, Potchefstroom 2520, North West Province, South Africa

Aletta E. Schutte
Hypertension in Africa Research Team (HART), North-West University, Potchefstroom 2531, North West Province, South Africa
MRC Research Unit for Hypertension and Cardiovascular Disease, North-West University, Potchefstroom 2531, North West Province, South Africa

Nirmala Naidoo
World Health Organization (WHO), Avenue Appia 20, CH-1211 Geneva 27, Switzerland

Paul Kowal
World Health Organization (WHO), Avenue Appia 20, CH-1211 Geneva 27, Switzerland
Research Centre for Generational Health and Ageing, University of Newcastle, Newcastle 2308, New South Wales, Australia

Maria Bouga, Michael E. J. Lean and Emilie Combet
Human Nutrition, School of Medicine, College of Medical, Veterinary and Life Sciences, 10–16 Alexandra Parade, University of Glasgow, Glasgow G31 2ER, UK

Enke Baldini and Salvatore Ulisse
Department of Surgical Sciences, "Sapienza" University of Rome, 00161 Rome, Italy

Camilla Virili and Marco Centanni
Department of Medico-Surgical Sciences and Biotechnologies, "Sapienza" University of Rome, 04100 Latina, Italy

Eleonora D'Armiento
Department of Internal Medicine and Medical Specialties, "Sapienza" University of Rome, 00161 Rome, Italy

Giuseppe Lisco
ASL Brindisi, Unit of Endocrinology, Metabolism &
Clinical Nutrition, Hospital "A. Perrino", Strada per
Mesagne 7, 72100 Brindisi, Puglia, Italy

Anna De Tullio and Vincenzo Triggiani
Interdisciplinary Department of Medicine—Section of
Internal Medicine, Geriatrics, Endocrinology and Rare
Diseases, University of Bari "Aldo Moro", School of
Medicine, Policlinico, Piazza Giulio Cesare 11, 70124
Bari, Puglia, Italy

Vito Angelo Giagulli
Interdisciplinary Department of Medicine—Section of
Internal Medicine, Geriatrics, Endocrinology and Rare
Diseases, University of Bari "Aldo Moro", School of
Medicine, Policlinico, Piazza Giulio Cesare 11, 70124
Bari, Puglia, Italy
Clinic of Endocrinology and Metabolic Disease,
Conversano Hospital, Via Edmondo de Amicis 36,
70014 Conversano, Bari, Puglia, Italy

Giovanni De Pergola
Department of Biomedical Sciences and Human
Oncology, Section of Internal Medicine and Clinical
Oncology, University of Bari Aldo Moro, Piazza Giulio
Cesare 11, 70124 Bari, Puglia, Italy

Renuka Jayatissa
Department of Nutrition, Medical Research Institute,
Danister De Silva Mawatha, Colombo 8, Sri Lanka

Jonathan Gorstein
University of Washington, Department of Global
Health, Seattle, WA 98195, USA

**Onyebuchi E. Okosieme, John H. Lazarus and
Lakdasa D. Premawardhana**
Centre for Endocrine and Diabetes Sciences and
Thyroid Research Group, C2 Link Corridor,
University Hospital of Wales, Heath Park, Cardiff
CF14 4XN, UK

**Silvia Martina Ferrari, Giusy Elia, Francesca Ragusa,
Armando Patrizio, Sabrina Rosaria Paparo, Stefania
Camastra and Alessandro Antonelli**
Department of Clinical and Experimental Medicine,
University of Pisa, 56126 Pisa, Italy

Poupak Fallahi
Department of Translational Research and New
Technologies in Medicine and Surgery, University of
Pisa, 56126 Pisa, Italy

Demetre E. Gostas and D. Enette Larson-Meyer
Department of Family and Consumer Sciences,
University of Wyoming, Laramie, WY 82071, USA

Hillary A. Yoder
Division of Kinesiology, University of Alabama,
Tuscaloosa, AL 35487, USA

Ainsley E. Huffman
University of Utah School of Medicine, Salt Lake City,
UT 84108, USA

Evan C. Johnson
Division of Kinesiology & Health, University
of Wyoming, Laramie, WY 82070, USA

**Alexandra C. Purdue-Smithe, Sunni L. Mumford and
James L. Mills**
Epidemiology Branch, Division of Intramural
Population Health Research, Eunice Kennedy Shriver
National Institute of Child Health and Human
Development, National Institutes of Health, Bethesda,
MD 20892, USA

Eila Suvanto
Northern Finland Laboratory Centre NordLab, 90120
Oulu, Finlan

Tuija Männistö
Northern Finland Laboratory Centre NordLab, 90120
Oulu, Finlan
Department of Clinical Chemistry, University of Oulu,
90120 Oulu, Finland
Medical Research Center Oulu, Oulu University
Hospital and University of Oulu, 90120 Oulu, Finland
Finnish Institute for Health andWelfare, 00290
Helsinki, Finland

Griffith A. Bell
Ariadne Labs, Brigham and Women's Hospital,
Harvard T.H. Chan School of Public Health, Boston,
MA 02115, USA
Harvard T.H. Chan School of Public Health, Department
of Health Policy and Management, Boston, MA 02115,
USA

Aiyi Liu
Biostatistics and Bioinformatics Branch, Division
of Intramural Population Health Research, Eunice
Kennedy Shriver National Institute of Child Health
and Human Development, National Institutes of
Health, Bethesda, MD 20892, USA

Kurunthachalam Kannan and Un-Jung Kim
Wadsworth Center, New York State Department of
Health, Albany, NY 12201, USA

Mika Gissler
Finnish Institute for Health and Welfare, 00290
Helsinki, Finland
Karolinska Institute, 17177 Stockholm, Sweden

Heljä-Marja Surcel
Biobank Borealis of Northern Finland, Oulu University Hospital, 90120 Oulu, Finland
Faculty of Medicine, University of Oulu, 90120 Oulu, Finland

Salvatore Benvenga
Department of Clinical and Experimental Medicine-Endocrinology, University of Messina, via Consolare Valeria-Gazzi, 98125 Messina, Italy
Interdepartmental Program on Molecular and Clinical Endocrinology and Women's Endocrine Health, AOU Policlinico G. Martino, via Consolare Valeria-Gazzi, 98125 Messina, Italy
Master Program on Childhood, Adolescent and Women's Endocrine Health, Department of Clinical and Experimental Medicine, University of Messina, 98125 Messina

Ulla Feldt-Rasmussen
Medical Endocrinology and Metabolism PE 2132, Rigshospitalet, Copenhagen University Hospital, Blegdamsvej 9, DK-2100 Copenhagen, Denmark

Ernest Asamoah
Community Physicians Network, Diabetes & Endocrinology Care, 8435 Clearvista Place, Suite 101, Indianapolis, IN 46256, USA

Ines Barone
Department of Pharmacy, Health and Nutritional Sciences, University of Calabria, 87036 Rende (CS), Italy

Cinzia Giordano, Stefania Marsico, Rosalinda Bruno, Daniela Bonofiglio, Stefania Catalano and Sebastiano Andò
Department of Pharmacy, Health and Nutritional Sciences, University of Calabria, 87036 Rende (CS), Italy
Centro Sanitario, University of Calabria, 87036 Rende (CS), Italy

Lanfranco D'Elia
World Health Organization Collaborating Centre for Nutrition, University of Warwick, Coventry CV4 7AL, UK
Department of Clinical Medicine and Surgery, "Federico II" University of Naples, 80131 Naples, Italy

Galina Obreja
Department of Social Medicine and Health Management, State University of Medicine and Pharmacy Nicolae Testemitanu, 2004 Chi‚sinău, Moldova

Angela Ciobanu
World Health Organization Country Office, 2012 Chişinău, Moldova
World Health Organization European Office for Prevention and Control of Noncommunicable Diseases, 2100 Copenhagen, Denmark

Joao Breda
World Health Organization European Office for Prevention and Control of Noncommunicable Diseases, 229994 Moscow, Russia

Jo Jewell
World Health Organization European Office for Prevention and Control of Noncommunicable Diseases, 2100 Copenhagen, Denmark
United Nations Children's Fund, UNICEF, New York, NY 10017, USA

Francesco P. Cappuccio
World Health Organization Collaborating Centre for Nutrition, University of Warwick, Coventry CV4 7AL, UK
Division of Health Sciences, Warwick Medical School, University of Warwick, Coventry CV4 7AL, UK

Yoo Kyoung Park
Department of Medical Nutrition, Graduate School of East-West Medical Science, Kyung Hee University, Yongin 17104, Korea

Sohye Kim
Department of Medical Nutrition, Graduate School of East-West Medical Science, Kyung Hee University, Yongin 17104, Korea
Nutrition Care Services, Seoul National University of Bundang Hospital, Seongnam 13620, Korea

Yong Seok Kwon
F&D Communication, Gyeonggi 10433, Korea

Ju Young Kim
Department of Family Medicine, Seoul National University of Bundang Hospital, Seongnam 13620, Korea

Kyung Hee Hong
Department of Food Science and Nutrition, Dongseo University, Pusan 47011, Korea

Herbert R. Marini, Giovanni Pallio, Natasha Irrera, Francesco Squadrito and Letteria Minutoli
Department of Clinical and Experimental Medicine, University of Messina, 98125 Messina, Italy

Domenica Altavilla, Domenico Puzzolo, Antonio Micali and Jose Freni
Department of Biomedical and Dental Sciences and Morphofunctional Imaging, University of Messina, 98125 Messina, Italy

Alessandro Antonelli, Silvia Martina Ferrari and Poupak Fallahi
Department of Clinical and Experimental Medicine, University of Pisa, 56126 Pisa, Italy

Lindsay Ellsworth
Division of Neonatal-Perinatal Medicine, Department of Pediatrics, University of Michigan, Ann Arbor, MI 48109, USA

Harlan McCaffery
Center for Human Growth and Development, University of Michigan, Ann Arbor, MI 48109, USA

Emma Harman
School of Public Health, University of Michigan, Ann Arbor, MI 48109, USA

Jillian Abbott
Metals Laboratory, Division of Clinical Biochemistry and Immunology, Mayo Clinic, Rochester, MN 55905, USA

Brigid Gregg
Division of Pediatric Endocrinology, Department of Pediatrics, University of Michigan, Ann Arbor, MI 48109, USA

Index

A

Alanine Aminotransferase, 110

Aliquots, 45, 231

Ammonium Persulfate, 23, 45, 102, 189

Anemia, 114, 131, 157, 159

Antioxidant Enzymes, 110, 117, 166, 224

Apoptosis, 75, 88, 112, 115-116, 120, 122, 126, 128, 166, 174, 215, 224, 228

Atrial Fibrillation, 36, 162

Autoimmune Disorders, 131, 140, 225

B

Blood Pressure, 34-35, 39, 41, 44, 53-54, 187, 189, 196

Body Mass Index, 22, 24, 34, 47, 60, 87, 132, 135, 149, 151-152, 200, 229-230, 236

C

Cardiovascular Events, 34, 40, 187

Cell Damage, 82

Cell Lines, 111, 113, 115-116, 118, 126, 174

Clinical Thyroidology, 108-109, 122, 158

Cognitive Development, 56, 95

Creatinine Excretion, 38, 41, 45-46, 50, 188, 190, 195, 198

D

Diabetes, 36, 40, 54, 72, 88, 99, 107, 121-122, 129, 131, 144, 146, 151-152, 156, 158, 165, 174, 197, 226, 228, 230, 240

Dietary Assessment Method, 21, 30

Dietary Components, 108-109, 122, 158

Dietary Sodium, 15, 34, 40, 190, 197-198

Drug Consumption, 34, 36, 41

E

Endemic Cretinism, 35, 56, 106

Endemic Goiter, 31, 35, 40, 97, 130, 144, 177-181, 183, 185

Endocrine Disrupting Chemicals, 82, 91

Energy Intake, 24, 26-27, 29, 57, 201, 203-205, 208-209

Estimated Average Requirement, 22, 32, 42-43, 46, 48, 199, 204-205, 207, 209

F

Fetal Growth, 153, 155, 177, 238

Flavonoids, 108-109, 111-113, 122, 125, 166

Folic Acid, 61-63, 81

Food Frequency Questionnaire, 19, 21, 26, 31, 56, 58, 61, 71, 73, 130, 132, 136-137, 142, 210

G

Gestational Age, 147-149, 151-152, 233

Glutathione Peroxidase, 110, 117, 166, 224

H

Homeostasis, 82-83, 85-89, 92, 109, 112, 128, 175, 225

Hormone Synthesis, 82, 84, 88-89, 92, 177, 199, 229, 239

Hydration Status, 50, 131

Hypertension, 34, 36, 39-40, 42, 53, 144, 151-152, 189-190, 197-198, 228

Hyperthyroidism, 2, 50, 84, 110, 114, 119-120, 126, 128, 134, 138, 145, 163, 166, 168-169, 173, 175, 200, 210, 212, 229

Hypothyroidism, 2, 75-76, 80, 82-84, 86-88, 96, 111-118, 120-121, 124, 126-131, 134, 138, 140, 148, 153, 155-157, 163-164, 168-169, 173, 180, 200, 210, 213-215, 227-229

I

Inositol, 108-110, 121-122, 129, 158, 160-161, 163-165, 169, 172-174, 214-215, 219, 227-228

Iodine Deficiency, 1-3, 6, 8, 13, 16-23, 29, 31, 34-35, 39-40, 43-44, 46, 50-52, 54, 56, 71-80, 84, 86-87, 92, 96-97, 99-100, 104, 106-107, 112, 118, 125, 130-132, 138, 140-141, 143-146, 148, 153-157, 174, 176-187, 193-194, 197, 200, 210, 212, 230, 236-237, 239-241

Iodine Fortification, 13, 22, 40, 50-51, 68, 70, 73, 184, 241

Iodine Intake, 1-3, 6, 8, 11-24, 26-35, 38-44, 46-48, 50-51, 53-54, 56-61, 63, 66-68, 70, 72-75, 77-80, 84, 86, 88, 92, 105, 107, 130-132, 134-141, 145-146, 148, 153, 156, 177-178, 180-187, 193, 195, 198-202, 204-213, 229-230, 237-240

Iodine Metabolism, 17, 83, 91-92, 106

Iodine Prophylaxis, 41, 75-78, 97, 107, 177-183, 185, 198

Iodine Status, 1-4, 6, 8, 11, 13-14, 16-23, 29-32, 34, 40, 42-44, 46, 50-54, 57, 68-69, 71-73, 75-77, 88, 91-92, 94, 97, 99-100, 102, 104-105, 107, 130-132, 134-135, 137-141, 144-145, 147-148, 152-157, 177-179, 182-185, 187, 195-196, 200, 210-211, 213, 229-230, 236-241

Iodoprophylaxis, 76

L

Lactating Women, 2, 22, 29, 31, 54, 75, 84, 94, 200, 230, 239, 241

Lactation, 2, 50, 57-60, 62-63, 65, 71, 73, 79, 81, 84, 88, 118, 127, 155, 227, 229-230, 236-241

Lipid Metabolism, 115, 125-126, 164

M

Melatonin, 108-110, 113-115, 122, 126, 158, 160-161, 165, 169, 172-174

Midwives, 56, 62-64, 67-69, 73-74, 79, 81

Mineral Supplements, 27, 167

Mixed Diet, 3

Morning Sickness, 56, 64
Multivitamin Supplements, 56, 62, 67

N
Natrium-iodide Symporter, 82-83
Nutraceuticals, 79, 108-109, 122, 158-161, 168-169, 171-172, 214-216
Nutrient Intakes, 18, 32, 51

O
Odds Ratios, 147, 149, 151-152, 199, 202

P
Perinatal Period, 56, 61, 70
Pescatarians, 1, 12-13
Prediction Equations, 42-44, 46, 48, 50, 52
Pregnancy Nutrition, 56, 62-63, 70

R
Recommended Daily Intake, 22, 26, 31
Reproductive Age, 13, 43, 130
Resveratrol, 108-110, 116-117, 122, 127, 158, 160-161, 166, 169, 172, 174, 214, 216, 218, 224, 228

S
Salivary Glands, 83, 111
Salt Iodization, 21-22, 31, 34, 40, 43, 107, 177-178, 182, 187, 193-195, 236, 241
Selenium, 17, 20, 92, 108-110, 117-118, 122, 127, 129, 145, 158, 160-161, 163, 166-169, 172-176, 214-215, 225-228
Serum Iodine, 147, 151, 153-154, 156
Spot Urine, 29, 34-35, 42-45, 50-54, 76, 146, 156, 178, 195

T
Thyroid Autoimmunity, 83-84, 92, 176, 225
Thyroid Function, 2, 17-18, 50, 54, 72, 78-79, 82-84, 86-88, 91-92, 94-95, 97, 108-109, 112, 114, 119-122, 125, 127, 129-131, 134, 138, 140-141, 146-149, 155-156, 158-159, 162, 164-167, 169, 173-174, 176, 185, 200-201, 212, 226-228, 239
Thyroid Hormones, 2, 21, 35, 56, 63, 75, 83-85, 95, 114, 117, 121, 125-126, 129-130, 148, 151, 153, 155-156, 161-165, 167, 175, 195, 200, 212, 215, 227, 240
Thyroid Stimulating Hormone, 31, 84, 130-131, 148, 151-152, 162, 212
Thyroxine, 2, 21, 75, 86-87, 93, 95, 99, 110, 128-130, 146, 172, 199-200, 206, 237, 239
Triiodothyronine, 2, 21, 75, 83, 86, 99, 110, 129-130, 172, 200

U
Urinary Creatinine, 38, 41-42, 45-46, 50, 188, 190, 195
Urinary Iodine Concentration, 2-3, 6, 21-22, 31, 40, 42-43, 47, 50, 52-54, 56, 71, 75-76, 107, 131-132, 135, 137-138, 146, 152, 156, 177, 180-182, 199-200, 203, 212, 230, 236-237, 239-241
Urinary Iodine Excretion, 18, 21, 23, 29-32, 34-35, 40, 42, 44, 47-48, 50-53, 57, 72, 92, 145-146, 156, 180, 185, 187, 191, 194-195, 210, 213
Urine Iodine, 23, 34, 51, 99-101, 104, 148, 199
Urine Volume, 21-24, 45-46, 50-51

V
Vegetarian Diets, 1, 3, 6, 8, 11-14, 16-18
Vitamin D, 61, 63, 110, 119-120, 128, 132, 142-143, 145, 170-171

W
Water Iodine, 99, 105, 237

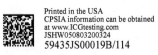